TRANSFUSION MEDICINE MADE EASY FOR STUDENTS OF ALLIED MEDICAL SCIENCES AND MEDICINE

Authored by **Osaro Erhabor** and **Teddy Charles Adias**

Transfusion Medicine Made Easy for Students of Allied Medical Sciences and Medicine
Authored by: **Dr Osaro Erhabor** (Ph.D, CSci, FIBMS) and **Dr Teddy Charles Adias** (Ph.D, FIBMS)

Edition 2014

Published by InTech
Janeza Trdine 9, 51000 Rijeka, Croatia

Publishing Process Manager Silvia Vlase
Typesetting Vladimir Sijan
Cover InTech Design Team

Additional hard copies can be obtained from orders@intechopen.com

Transfusion Medicine Made Easy for Students of Allied Medical Sciences and Medicine
Authored by: Dr Osaro Erhabor (Ph.D, CSci, FIBMS) and Dr Teddy Charles Adias (Ph.D, FIBMS)
p. cm.
ISBN 978-953-51-0523-7

For EU product safety concerns:
IN TECH d.o.o., Prolaz Marije Krucifikse Kozulić 3, 51000 Rijeka, Croatia,
info@intechopen.com or visit our website at intechopen.com.

Meet the authors

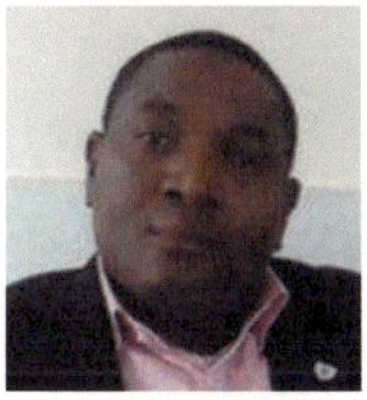

Dr Osaro Erhabor is an Immuno-Haematologist, a Chartered Scientist, Registration Portfolio Verifier and a Fellow of the Institute of Biomedical Medical Science, London. He is a seasoned Biomedical Scientist and Lecturer. He holds a Ph.D in Immuno-Haematology. He has taught best practices in Transfusion Medicine for several years to students in both the United Kingdom and Nigeria. A recipient of several scientific awards, member of the editorial boards, an article reviewer to several scientific journals, a well published author and speaker in several international scientific conferences. His current research interest includes transfusion safety and alternatives and haematology of infectious diseases.

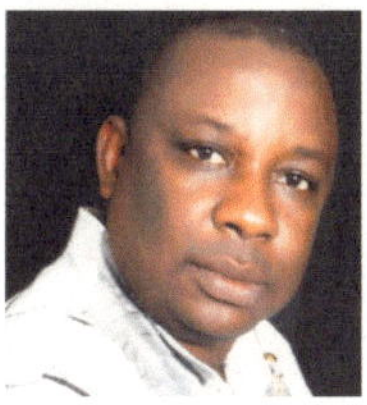

Dr Teddy Charles Adias is currently the Provost of the Bayelsa State College of Health Technology, Ogbia-Town, Nigeria. He holds a Ph.D in Immuno-Haematology, as well as a Fellow of the Institute of Biomedical Science (FIBMS), London. He had held several Adjunct academic appointments with various Nigerian universities and had taught at both post graduate and undergraduate levels for over nine years. His current research interest is focus on Transfusion immunology, safety and alternatives, and haematology of infectious diseases. Recent publications have included articles in Journals such as the Journal of Blood Medicine; Transfusion Clinque et Biologique, Pathology and Laboratory Medicine International amongst others.

Contents

Transfusion Medicine Made Easy for Students of Allied Medical Sciences and Medicine

Dr Erhabor Osaro (Ph.D, CSci, FIBMS)
Dr Adias Teddy Charles (Ph.D, FIBMS)

Blood Sciences Department
Royal Bolton Hospital
UK

Preface

Blood transfusion is a field where there has been, and continue to be, significant advances in science, technology and most particularly governance. The aim of this book is to provide students of allied medical sciences, medicine and transfusion practitioners with a comprehensive overview of both the scientific and managerial aspects of blood transfusion. The book is intended to equip biomedical, clinical and allied medical professionals with practical tools to allow for an informed practice in the field of blood transfusion management.

Dr Erhabor Osaro

Acknowledgements

The authors are indebted to Prof E.K Uko and Prof E.A Usanga both of the Haematology and blood transfusion Department of the University of Calabar in Nigeria for taking time out to review this book. We are also grateful to the publishers InTech. Our sincere thanks goes to members of our families and friend for the encouragement while we put this material that will improve the quality of transfusion medicine training and by extension transfusion service delivery particularly in Africa. We are eternally grateful to God for this opportunity to in our own little way improve the quality of transfusion medicine training offered to students of biomedical, medical and allied medical sciences. To God alone be all the glory.

1. History of blood transfusion

The first historical attempt at blood transfusion was described by the 17th century chronicler Stefano Infessura. Infessura relates that, in 1492, as Pope Innocent VIII sank into a coma, the blood of three boys was infused into the dying pontiff (through the mouth, as the concept of circulation and methods for intravenous access did not exist at that time) at the suggestion of a physician. The boys were ten years old, and had been promised a ducat each. However, not only did the pope die, but so did the three children. Some authors have discredited Infessura's account, accusing him of anti-papalism.

Beginning with Harvey's experiments with circulation of the blood, more sophisticated research into blood transfusion began in the 17th century, with successful experiments in transfusion between animals. However, successive attempts on humans continued to have fatal results.

The first fully documented human blood transfusion was administered by Dr. Jean-Baptiste Denys, eminent physician to King Louis XIV of France, on June 15, 1667. He transfused the blood of a sheep into a 15-year-old boy, who survived the transfusion. Denys performed another transfusion into a labourer, who also survived. Both instances were likely due to the small amount of blood that was actually transfused into these people. This allowed them to withstand the allergic reaction. Denys' third patient to undergo a blood transfusion was Swedish Baron Bonde. He received two transfusions. After the second transfusion Bonde died. In the winter of 1667, Denys performed several transfusions on Antoine Mauroy with calf's blood, who on the third account died. Much controversy surrounded his death. Mauroy's wife asserted Denys was responsible for her husband's death; she was accused as well. Though it was later determined that Mauroy actually died from arsenic poisoning, Denys' experiments with animal blood provoked a heated controversy in France. Finally, in 1670 the procedure was banned. In time, the British Parliament and even the pope followed suit. Blood transfusions fell into obscurity for the next 150 years.

Richard Lower examined the effects of changes in blood volume on circulatory function and developed methods for cross-circulatory study in animals, obviating clotting by closed arteriovenous connections. His newly devised instruments eventually led to actual transfusion of blood.

Towards the end of February 1665 he selected one dog of medium size, opened its jugular vein, and drew off blood, until its strength was nearly gone. Then, to make up for the great loss of this dog by the blood of a second, I introduced blood from the cervical artery of a fairly large mastiff, which had been fastened alongside the first, until this latter animal showed it was overfilled by the inflowing blood." After he "sewed up the jugular veins," the animal recovered "with no sign of discomfort or of displeasure."

Lower had performed the first blood transfusion between animals. He was then requested by the Honorable Robert Boyle to acquaint the Royal Society with the procedure for the whole experiment," which he did in December of 1665 in the Society's Philosophical Transactions. On 15 June 1667 Denys, then a professor in Paris carried out the first transfusion between humans and claimed credit for the technique, but Lower's priority cannot be challenged.

Six months later in London, Lower performed the first human transfusion in Britain, where he "superintended the introduction in a patient's arm at various times of some ounces of sheep's blood at a meeting of the Royal Society, and without any inconvenience to him." The recipient was Arthur Coga, "the subject of a harmless form of insanity." Sheep's blood was used because of speculation about the value of blood exchange between species; it had been suggested that blood from a gentle lamb might quiet the tempestuous spirit of an agitated person and that the shy might be made outgoing by blood from more sociable creatures. Lower wanted to treat Coga several times, but his patient refused. No more transfusions were performed. Shortly before, Lower had moved to London, where his growing practice soon led him to abandon research.

In 1667 - Jean-Baptiste Denis in France reported successful transfusions from sheep to humans. In 1678 transfusion from animals to humans, having been tried in many different ways, was confirmed to be unsuccessful, and was subsequently outlawed by the Paris Society of Physicians because of reactions and associated mortality. In 1795 in Philadelphia USA, an American physician Philip Syng Physick, performed the first known human Blood transfusion, although he did not publish the details of his findings. In 1818 James Blundell, a British obstetrician, performed the first successful transfusion of human blood to a patient for the treatment of post partum haemorrhage. Using the patient's husband as a donor, he extracted a small amount of Blood from the husband's arm and using a syringe, he successfully transfused the wife. Between 1825 and 1830 he performed ten documented transfusions, five of which proved beneficial to his patients, and published these results. He also devised various instruments for performing Blood transfusions. 1840 in London England, Samuel Armstrong Lane, aided by consultant Dr. Blundell, performed the first successful whole Blood transfusion to treat haemophilia. In 1867 English surgeon Joseph Lister utilized antiseptics to control infection during Blood transfusions. In 1901 - Karl Landsteiner, an Austrian physician, and the most important individual in the field of Blood transfusion, documented the first three human Blood groups (A, B and O). A year later in 1902 a fourth main blood type, AB was found by A. Decastrello and A. Sturli. In 1907 Hektoen suggested that the safety of transfusion might be improved by cross-matching blood between donors and patients to exclude incompatible mixtures. Reuben Ottenberg performed the first blood transfusion using blood typing and cross-matching. Ottenberg also observed the 'Mendelian inheritance' of blood groups and recognized the "universal" utility of group O donors. In 1908 - French surgeon Alexis Carrel devised a way to prevent blood from clotting. His method involved joining an artery in the donor, directly to a vein in the recipient with surgical sutures. He first used this technique to save the life of the son of a friend, using the father as donor. This procedure, not feasible for Blood transfusion, paved the way for successful organ transplantation, for which Carrel received the Nobel Prize in 1912. In 1908 - Carlo Moreschi documented the antiglobulin reaction. In 1914 long-term anticoagulants, among them sodium citrate, were developed, allowing longer preservation of Blood. In 1915 at Mt. Sinai Hospital in New York City, Richard Lewisohn was documented to have used sodium citrate as an anticoagulant which in the future transformed transfusion procedure from one that had to be performed with both the donor and the receiver of the transfusion in the same place at the same time, to basically the Blood banking system in use today. Further, in the same time period, R. Weil demonstrated the feasibility of refrigerated storage of such anticoagulated Blood. In 1916 Francis Rous and J. R. Turner introduced a citrate-glucose solution that permitted storage of Blood for several days after collection. Also, as in the 1915 Lewisohn discovery allowed for Blood to be stored in containers for later transfusion, and aided in the transition from the vein-to-vein method to direct transfusion. This discovery also directly led to the establishment of the first Blood depot by the British during World War I. Oswald Robertson was credited as the creator of the Blood depots. In 1925 - Karl Landsteiner, then working in New York City, in collaboration with Phillip Levine, discovered three more Blood groups: M, N and P. View Nobel Biography. In 1926 the British Red Cross instituted the first human Blood transfusion service in the world. In 1932, the first facility functioning as a Blood bank was established in a Leningrad Russia hospital. 1937, Bernard Fantus, director of therapeutics at the Cook County Hospital in Chicago, Illinois (U. S.), established the first hospital Blood bank in the United States. In creating a hospital laboratory that could preserve and store donor Blood, Fantus originated the term 'Blood bank. In 1939 and 1940 - The Rh Blood group system was discovered by Karl Landsteiner, Alex Wiener, Philip Levine and R. E. Stetson and was soon recognized as the cause of the then majority of transfusion reactions. Known as the Rhesus (Rh) system, once this reliable test for this grouping had been established, transfusion reactions became rare. Identification of the Rh factor has stood next to ABO as another important breakthrough in Blood banking.

2. Antigen

An antigen is a substance which in an appropriate biological circumstance can stimulate the production of an antibody. Such substances will react specifically with the antibody in an observable manner. Such observable ways includes;agglutination(the clumping of red blood cells in the presence of an antibody. The antibody or other molecule binds multiple particles and joins them, creating a large complex) and precipitation (the coalescing of small particles that are suspended in a solution; these larger masses are then (usually) precipitated. Blood group antigens are located within the red cell membrane. Antigens are made up of antigenic determinants (antigen binding sites). There are more antigenic determinants on a red cell of an individual who is homozygote for a particular antigen compared to a heterozygote. For example a homozygote (DD) individual has about 25-37,000 Rh (DD) antigenic determinants compared to 10,000-15,000 for a heterozygote (Dd). Similarly a homozygote show a stronger reaction with the corresponding group specific antibody compared to a heterozygote. This is the reason why red cells with homozygous antigen expression is preferred as a red cell reagent used for antibody detection and identification.

Characteristics of antigens. In order for a substance to be an antigen to you it must be foreign (not found in the host). The more foreign a substance the better it is an antigen. Antigens can either be autologous or homologous. Autologous antigens are your own antigens (not foreign to you). Homologous, or allogeneic, antigens are antigens from someone else (within the same species) that may be foreign to you.

Antigens must be chemically complex. Proteins and polysaccharides are antigenic due to their complexity. On the other hand, lipids are antigenic only if coupled to protein or sugar. Besides being chemically complex, antigens must also be large enough to stimulate antibody production. Their molecular weight needs to be at least 10,000. Due to the complexity of these molecules there are specific antigenic determinants (antigen sites) which are those portions of the antigen that reacts specifically with the antibody.

Antigen-antibody reaction occurs in 2 stages; sensitization and agglutination. The characteristics of an antigen and antibody reaction include; the antigen reacts with thegroup specific antibody and the reaction occurs in optimum proportion. Factors affecting antigen –antibody reaction includes:

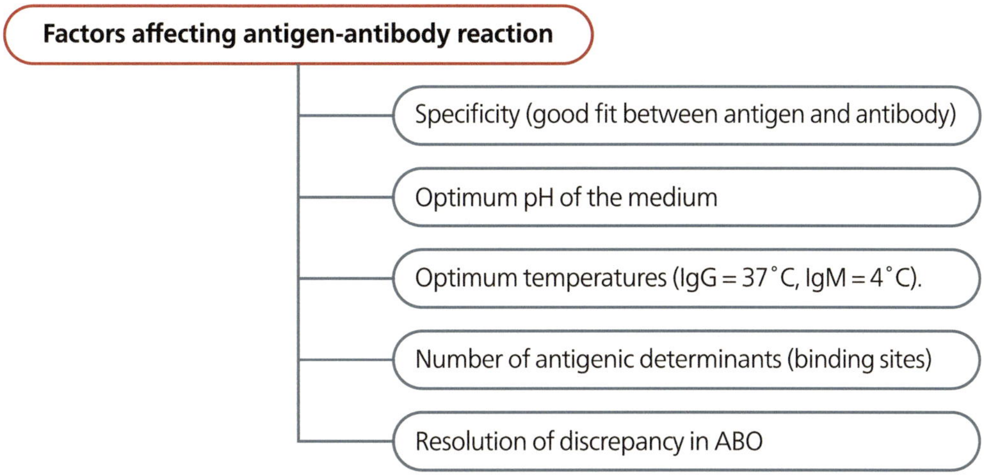

Factors that play a role in antigen antibody reactions

Techniques used in identification. ABO blood group antibodies bind red cells (containing the group specific antigen) suspended in saline. ABO blood group antibodies are IgM antibodies. They are high molecular weight antibodies that can span the distance that red cells keep apart (zeta potential) when suspended in saline whereas Rh antibodies are IgG antibodies and will require antihuman globulin (AHG) and or enzyme techniques for its detection.

Effect of enzymes. Enzymes like papain (from paw paw) and ficin (from figs) and bromelin (pineapple) can either enhance the reactivity of antigen-antibody reaction (Rhesus) or destroy (remove) antigen structures of some antigens (Duffy). Characteristics of an antigen includes; foreign (not found in the host) and react specifically with corresponding antibody.

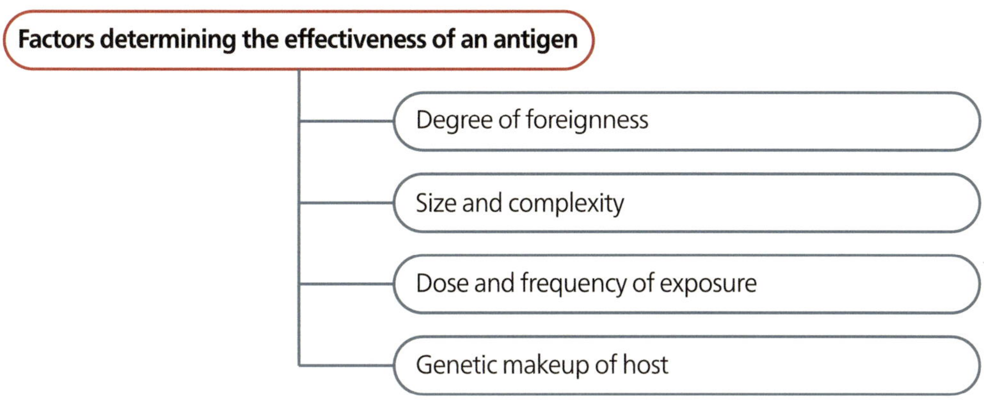

Factors determining the effectiveness or whether an antigen will stimulate an antibody response:

Red cell agglutination. Agglutination is the clumping of particles. The word agglutination comes from the Latin word agglutinare, meaning to glue. Red cell agglutination occurs when antigens on the red cell membrane of the red cells are cross-linked with their group specific antibody to form a three–dimensional lattice structure (clumps). Agglutination occur in 2 phases; primary (antibody sensitization) and the secondary phase (agglutination). Each of these phases are affected by certain factors.

Primary phase (Sensitization). Sensitization is a chemical reaction (interaction) between an antigen and the group specific antibody. It is the coating of the antigen by the group specific antibody. It is a reaction in which antigen and antibody associate and dissociate until equilibrium is reached. Sensitization is governed by the law of mass action and it is concentration dependent. The higher the concentration of the antigen and antibody the more the AG-AB complexes formed and the stronger the agglutination. These complexes are held together by ionic, hydrogen, hydrophobic bonds as well as covalent van der Waal's forces. Sensitization is affected by factors such as;

1. **Temperature**. The type of antigen-antibody bonding determines the optimum reactive temperation. Some antigens particularly carbonhydrate antigens (A, B, P1 H, Lea, Leb and I) form hydrogen bonds which dissipitate the heat generated during Ag-Ab reaction. These antigens reacts optimally at a cold (exothermic) temperation of 4-20°C. Non exothermic protein antigens (Rh, Duffy, Kell, Kidd and Lutheran) non-hydrogen bonding antigens react optimally at a warmer temperature of 37°C. Most IgM antibodies (ABO) reacts optimally at cold temperature while IgG antibody (Rh) react optimally at 37°C.

2. **Ionic strength of the medium**. Red cells when suspended in saline becomes negatively charged and repel each other. Antigens and antibody molecules are themselves charged molecules. Reduction of the charge (reduced Na+ and Cl- ions per unit volume) of the medium in which the red cells are suspended reduces the electrostatic barrier that exist between red cells suspended in saline (Zeta potential) facilitates faster antigen-antibody reaction. The surface of red cells carry a negative charge due to the ionization of the carboxyl group of NeuNac (N-acetyl neuraminic acid), also called NANA or sialic acid. In saline, red cells will attract positively charged Na+, and an ionic cloud will form around each cell. Thus the cells will be repelled and stay a certain distance apart. Zeta potential is a measure of this repulsion and is measured in microvolts at the boundary of sheer or slipping plane. Zeta potential is measured at the "slipping plane" and results from the difference in electrostatic potential at the surface of the RBCS and the boundary of shear (slipping plane). When zeta potential decreases, the RBCS can come closer together, allowing them to be agglutinated by the small IgG molecule. For IgG molecules to span the distance between red cells in saline, the ZP must be reduced so the cells can come closer. Reduc-

tion of the ionic strength reduces the interfering effect of the electrostatic barrier and facilitates better attraction between the antigen and antibody. Lower ionic strength saline (LISS) (0.003M saline plus glycine) produces an isotonic environment due to the reduced Na+ and Cl- ions concentration. LISS facilitate better agglutination and thus shorter incubation times compared to normal saline. LISS is not a potentiating medium (does not reduce the ionic cloud that exist between red cells suspended in saline and thus does not reduce the distance between red cells like Bovine Serum Albumin. It merely facilitates the non-specific interaction between red cells and antibody. This is why the the ionic strength and the optimum antigen and antibody ratio are most important factors in agglutination reaction.

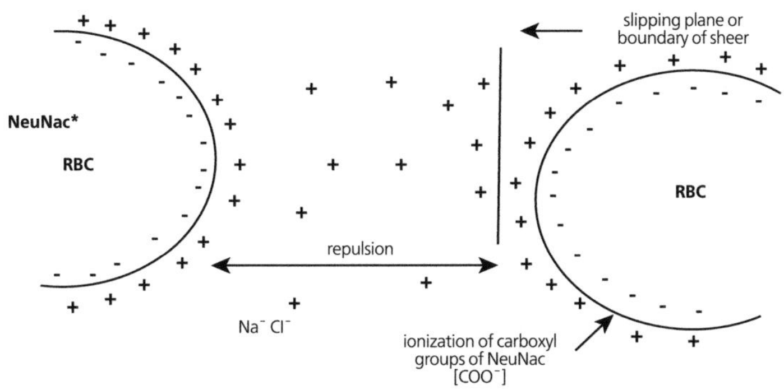

Figure 1: Demonstration of the effect of zeta potential on agglutination reaction

3. **pH of the medium in which the red cells are suspended.** Since the immunoglobulins and the red cell membranes both have an electrical charge, there is an optimum pH. pH differences cause differences in chemical structures of antigens/antibodies, affecting the "fit".
4. **Shape and structure of antigen and antibody (fit).** Specificity between antigens and antibodies depends on the spatial and chemical "fit" between antigen and antibody. The better the fit between the antigenic determinants (antigen site) and the antibody combining sites, the better the agglutination.

Effect of pH

Demonstration of the effect of pH of medium of cell suspension on agglutination reaction

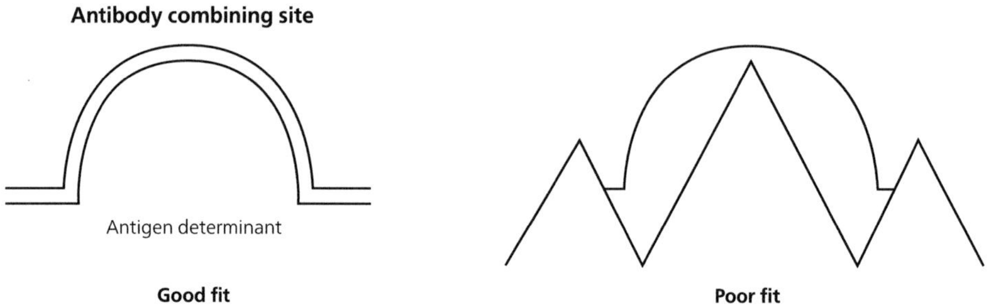

Demonstration of the effect of shape and structure on agglutination

1. **The antigen-antibody ratio.** The greater the antibody amount for a given antigen the more antibodies will be bound to the corresponding antigen and the greater the agglutination reaction. The more the antibody bound to a red cell (sensitization) and more the agglutination. Antigen and antibody reaction occur in optimum proportion. If the antibody concentration is high (excess) and the antigen concentration is low, the antigen sites (antigenic determinants) becomes saturated with more antibodies competing for the few antigen sites present resulting in few agglutination (Prozone effect). The optimum ratio is 80 parts antibody to 1 part antigen. There are specific terms for variations in this ratio. In order to get optimum antigen-antiboy concentration in Blood Banking we make washed 3% saline suspension of red cells to mix with our reagents.

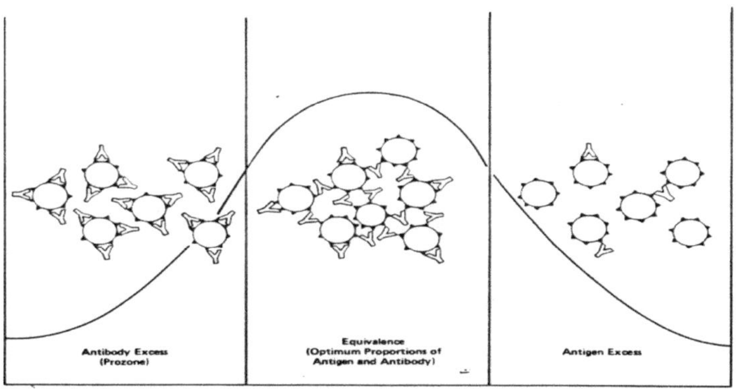

Demonstration of the effect of antigen-antibody ratio on agglutination reaction

2. **Prozone effect.** Excess antibodies saturates all the antigen sites leaving no room for the formation of cross-linkages between sensitized cells. Thus even though there are antibodies in the plasma that are specific against the corresponsing antigens on the red cells suspended in saline a false negative reaction with no agglutination observed may be evident. Zone of equivalence: Antibodies and antigens present in optimum proportion and significant agglutination is formed. Zone of antigen excess: Too many antigens are present to bind with fewer antibodies. Thus the agglutina-

tion formed is often super-imposed by the large masses of unagglutinated antigens. This can cause a false negative reaction.

Secondary stage of agglutination reaction

The second phase of the agglutination process involves the cell to cell cross linking by antibodies. The level of agglutination observed is affected by the rate at which red cells sensitized with antibody collide with each other. Red cell collision (attraction) is dependent on the following aggregating forces:

1. **Gravity**. Red cells are attracted together by gravity. This attraction can be facilitated by centrifugation. Centrifugation of the cells attempts to bring the red blood cells closer together, but even then the smaller IgG antibodies usually can not reach between two cells. The larger antibodies, IgM, can reach between cells that are further apart and cause agglutination. The second phase of agglutination involving an IgG antibody can only be enhanced either by altering the suspending environment by using an aggregating or potentiating mwdium (20% BSA) or by altering the red cell membrane of the red cells using enzyme treatment (papain, ficin or bromelin) or by using an additional cross linking reagent (anti- human globulin) to facilitate agglutination.

2. **Surface tension.** The concept Zeta potential is important to understand why the cells will maintain a certain distance from each other. Zeta potential refers to the repulsion between the red blood cells. It is due to an electric charge surrounding cells suspended in saline. It is caused by sialic acid groups on the red blood cell membrane which gives the cells a negative charge. The positive ions in saline are attracted to the negatively charged red blood cells. The net positive charge surrounding the cells in saline keeps them far apart due to repulsion from electric charges. Smaller antibodies (IgG) cannot cause agglutination when zeta potential exists. To overcome the effect of the zeta potential, there is the need to neutralize these charges. One of the commonest technique is to add a potentiating medium (Bovine Serum Albumin 22%) to the mixture. The hydroxyl group (OH-) neutralizes the net postitive charge and and draw the red cells closer to each other reducing the gap between the red cells. This facilitate the ability of low molecular weight IgG antibody to bridge the gap between red cells and cause agglutination. The effect of these aggregating forces are ofter resisted by the zeta potential (occurs when negatively charged red cells suspended in saline repel each other creating an ionic cloud between themselves). The minimum distance between red cells suspended in saline is > 14nm. Thus the closest the cells can approach each other is the edge of their individual ionic clouds (slipping plane). IgG antibodies are low molecular weight antibodies (150,000) and thus are unable to span the slipping plane that exist beween cells suspended in saline. IgM antiboies on the other hand are a high molecular weight (900,000) molecule

that is large enogh to bridge this slipping plane and cause agglutination. IgM can agglutinate cells suspended in saline while IgG antibodies cannot. IgG antibody will however require an alteration to the environment by a potentiating medium to be able to agglutinate cells containing the group specigen antigens suspended in saline.

3. **Antigen-antibody ratio:** Antigen- antibody reaction occurs in optimum proportion. The optimum ratio is 80 parts of antibody to 1 part of antigen. If the antigen –antibody ratio is optimum, agglutination occurs (zone of equivalence) but if the antibody ration is higher than the antigen a false negative reaction (prozone effect) results. But if the antigen ration exceeds the antibody ration the agglutinated red cells are masked by masses of the unagglutinated antigens (Post-zone effect).

Examples of such potentiating medium are:

1. **Bovine serum albumin:** Bovine albumin (20- 22%) or polybrene (hexadimethrine bromide) can potentially reduce the dielectric constant (charge density) of the red cell suspension medium thereby reducing the net repulsive force between cells suspended in saline. This potentially reduced the distance apart between red cells allowing low molecular weight IgG antibody to span the gap and cause a reversible aggregation. This aggregation cross linkages between antibody sensitized red cells to produce agglutination. Polyethylene glycol (PEG) can potential enhance the uptake of antibody onto the red cells and can be used in conjunction with the AHG technique.

2. **Enzyme (Papain, ficin and bromelin).** The negative charge on the red cells is carried on the glycoprotein molecule of the red cell membrane. Proteolytic enzymes at the correct concentration can potentially remove some of these protein molecules and thus reduce the negative charge on the red cells and thus reduces the gap allowing IgG antibody to be able to span the gap and produce agglutination. However removal of these glycoprotein molecules by enzyme treatment can potential expose some antigenic specificities by removing charge proteins physically close to the antigen (reduction of steric hindrance) and facilitate their reaction with antibody containg the corresponding group specific antibodies. Enzyme treatment facilitate the reaction by Rh and Kell antigens. Enzyme treat however destroy certain proteins present with the glycoproteins. Such antigens are therefore not detectable by enzyme technique (Fya, Fyb, Xga, S, s, M and N).

3. **Anti humanglobulin (AHG) reagent**. Anti-human globulin reagent are antibodies produced against human globulin (IgG) and will detect the presence of human globulin coating on red cells (sensitized red cells) by forming cross linksbetween the IgG antibody coating on sensitized red cells. The Fab

portion of the anti-human globulin cross link with the Fc portion of the IgG molecule and help overcome the challenge caused by the zeta potential allowing the reaction links between the antigens on the red cells and antibodies in the plasma to be visualized in the form of agglutination. Antiglobulin test is one of the most important serological tests done in a routine blood transfusion laboratory. It utilizes the anti-human globulin (AHG) reagent to bring about agglutination of red cells coated with immunoglobulin or complement component, which do not show any agglutination in saline. Red cells which are coated with incomplete (IgG) antibodies show agglutination on addition of anti-human globulin (AHG or Coombs; reagent). The coating can occur either in vivo or in vitro following incubation with serum containing the antibody. The majority of incomplete antibodies are IgG which attach to the red cell membrane by he Fab portion. The two arm of IgG molecule are unable to bridge the gap between red cells which are separated from each other because of the negative charge on their surface. While this results in sensitization of the cells, agglutination is not seen as the RBCs do not form lattice. Addition of AHG reagent results in the Fab portion of the AHG molecule combining with the Fc portion of two adjacent IgG molecules, thereby bridging the gap between the red cells and causing agglutination.

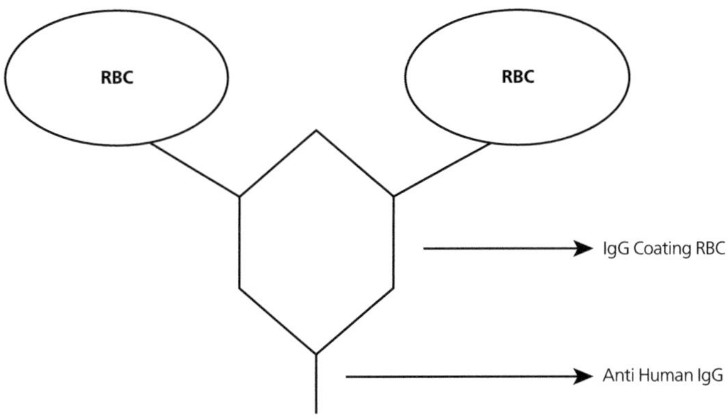

Demonstration of role of AHG reagent in causing agglutination of IgG sensitizes RBCS

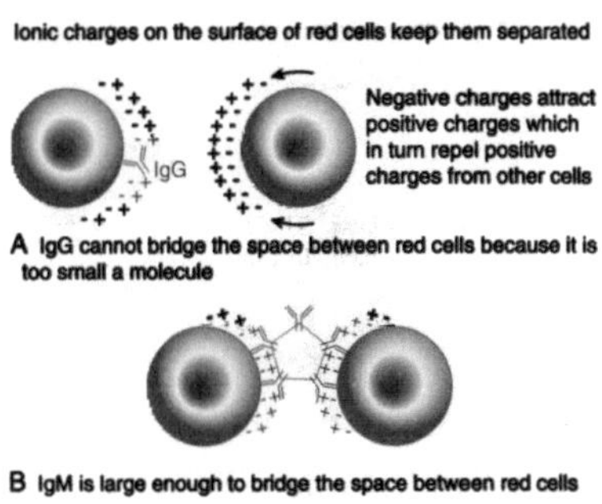

Figure 5: Effect of surface tension on agglutination reaction

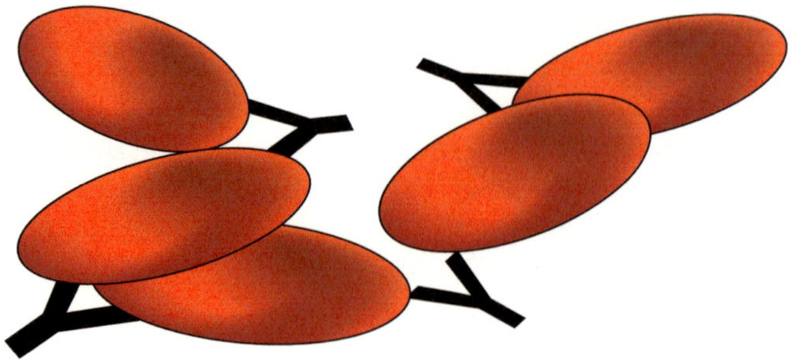

Demonstration of the first stage of agglutination (Sensitization).

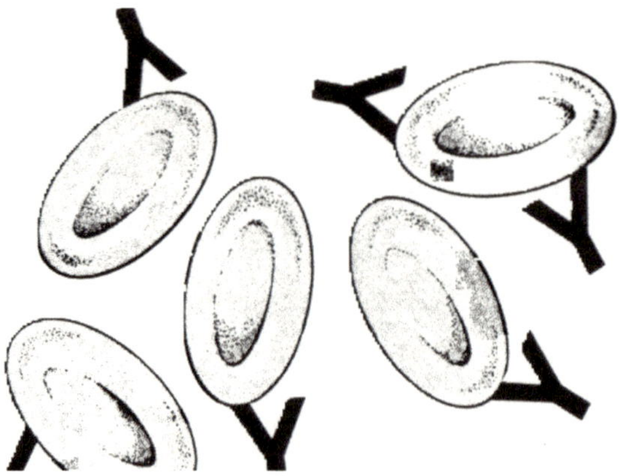

Demonstration of the second stage of the agglutination process (Clumping)

Red Cell Membrane. The red cell membrane is made up of lipids (40%), proteins (49%) and carbohydrate (7%). The membrane of the red blood cell plays many roles that aid in regulating their surface deformability, flexibility, adhesion to other cells and immune recognition. The red blood cell membrane is composed of 3 layers: the glycocalyx on the exterior, which is rich in carbohydrates; the lipid bilayer which contains many transmembrane proteins, besides its phoslipid main constituents; and the membrane skeleton, a structural network of proteins located on the inner surface of the lipid bilayer. The erythrocyte cell membrane comprises a typical lipid bilayer, similar to what can be found in virtually all human cells. Simply put, this lipid bilayer is composed of cholesterol and phospholipids in equal proportions by weight. The lipid composition is important as it defines many physical properties such as membrane permeability and fluidity.

Lipids. Phospholipids are the major lipid component of the red cells and constitute 75% of the lipid component. The lipid bilayer is made up of a hydrophilic water soluble head and two hydrophobic water insoluble tail groups. This bilayer confers the property of impemeability to ions and other metabolites as well as the deformability.

Proteins. The interaction of proteins and the lipid bilayer allow for selective transport across the membrane bi-layer as well as the maintenance of the skeletal function. Red cell protein appears either as free component or anchored to the ankrin and spectrin protein underneath the phospholipid bi-layer. Proteins of the membrane skeleton are responsible for the deformability, flexibility and durability of the red blood cell, enabling it to squeeze through tiny capillaries. There are currently more than 50 known membrane proteins. Approximately 25 of these membrane proteins carry the various blood group antigens, such as the A, B and Rh antigens. These membrane proteins can perform a wide diversity of functions, such as transporting ions and molecules across the red cell membrane, adhesion and interaction with other cells. Disorders of the proteins in these membranes are associated with many disorders, such as hereditary spherocytosis, hereditary elliptocytosis, hereditary stomatocytosis, and paroxysmal nocturnal hemoglobinuria. The red blood cell membrane proteins organized according to their function. Red Blood Cell membrane major proteins performs 3 major functions; selective transport across the membrane barrier, cell adhesion and structural role.

Carbonhydrate. The following blood group antigens (ABO, Lewis) are essentially carbohydrates. Majority of the carbonhydrate components of the red cell membrane occur either as glycoproteins (Rh, Kidd, Lutheran, Kell, Duddy) or glycolipids (P antigen). Glycolipid constitutes 5% of the total lipid component of the red cell membrane. The glycoproteins sialoglycoproteins) constitute a significant portion of the red cell membrane Sialic acid (N-acetylneuramic acid) component. Sialic acid is a major charged molecule of the red cell membrane that confers the red cell with a net negative charge. Examples of sialoglycoproteins include glycophorin A (MN antigens) and B (Ss antigens).

Red cell membrane function	Associated blood group antigens
Complement regulation	Cromer and Knops
Membrane transport	Rhesus, Kidd, Diego, Colton and Kx
Cell adhesion molecules	Lutheran, LW, XG and Indian
Membrane bound enzymes	Kell and Cartwright
Structural assembly	MNSs and Gerbich
Chemokine receptor	Duffy

Blood group antigen and associated red cell membrane functions

Functions of the red cell membrane. The red cell membrane plays an active role in selective transport. Band 3 is an anion transporter that defines the Diego blood group. It is also an important structural component of the erythrocyte cell membrane (makes up to 25% of the cell membrane surface and each red cell contains approximately one million copies). Aquaporin 1 is a water transport protein and defines the Colton blood group. Glut1 is a glucose and L-dehydroascorbic acid transporter. Kidd antigen protein is responsible for urea transporter. RhAG is a major gas transporter, probably of carbon dioxide (defines Rh blood group and the associated unusual blood group phenotype Rh null phenotype. The Kx and Diego blood group antigens are also associated with membrane transport The red cell membrane also plays an active role in cell adhesion. Examples of blood group antigen associated with cell adhesion include the; Lutheran, LW, XG and the Indian blood group antigen proteins. Examples of blood group antigen associated with membrane bound enzymes include the; Cartwright and Kell blood group antigen proteins. The red cell membrane plays a structural role. The following membrane proteins establish linkages with skeletal proteins and may play an important role in regulating cohesion between the lipid bilayer andmembrane skeleton, likely enabling the red cell to maintain its favorable membrane surface area by preventing the membrane from collapsing; ankyrin-based macromolecular complex - proteins linking the bilayer to the membrane skeleton through the interaction of their cytoplasmic domains with Ankyrin. The MNSs and Gerbich are associated with structural assembly. The Duffy blood group antigen play an active role as a chemokine receptor while the Cromer and Knops blood group antigen have been found associated with complement regulation.

Antibody

An antibody is a proteins occurring in body fluids produced by lymphocytes as a result of stimulation by an antigen and which can interact specifically with that particular antigen. Antibodies are immune system-related proteins called immunoglobulin. Each antibody consists of four polypeptides– two heavy chains and two light chains joined to form a "Y" shaped molecule and linked by disulphide bonds. There are two pairs of chains in the molecule: heavy and light. There are two classes (isotypes) of the light chain called kappa and lambda. Heavy chains have five different isotypes which divide the Igs into five different classes (IgG1-4, IgA1-2, IgD, IgM, and IgE). The amino acid sequence in the tips of the "Y" varies greatly among different antibodies. This variable region, composed of 110-130 amino acids, give the antibody its specificity for binding antigen. The variable region includes the ends of the light and heavy chains. Treating the antibody with a protease can cleave this region, producing Fab or fragment antigen binding that includes the variable ends of an antibody. Antibodies are immunoglobulin. The clases of immunoglobulins include; IgG which provides long-term immunity or protection, IgM which is the first antibody produced in response to an antigenic stimulus, IgA which are found in secretions and help protects against infections in urinary, gastro intestinal and respiratory tracts, IgE which are involved in allergic reactions and IgD which occur as surface receptor of B lymphocytes. The most clinically significant antibodies in transfusion medicine are IgM and IgG and to an extent IgA. IgG frequently cause in vivo haemolysis compared to Igm which does not cause invivo haemolysis except for ABO blood group antibodies. The clinical significance of a red cell antibody depends on the following:

- Ability of the red cell antibody to cause haemolysis in vivo
- Ability of the red cell antibody to cause a transfusion reaction

- Ability of the red cell antibody to cause haemolytic disease of the foetus and newborn (HDFN).

Structure of an Antibody

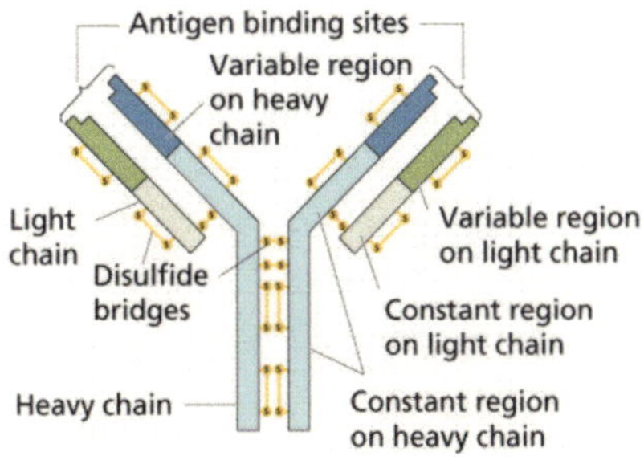

Parts of an antibody:

1. Heavy chains - made of alpha, gamma, delta, mu, or epsilon chains
2. Light chains - made of kappa or lambda chains
3. Disulfide bonds - hold chains together
4. Hinge region - allows antibody to flex to reach more antigen sites
5. Fab fragments - contains variable portion of antibody: antigen-binding sites

Antibody production. Antibodies are immunoglobulin used by the immune system to identify and neutralize foreign substances (antigen) such as bacteria and viruses. The antibody recognizes a unique part of the foreign target, termed an antigen. Each antibody contains a paratope that is specific for one particular epitope on an antigen, allowing these two structures to bind together with precision. Using this binding mechanism, an antibody can tag a microbe or an infected cell for attack by other parts of the immune system, or can neutralize its target directly (for example, by blocking a part of a microbe that is essential for its invasion and survival). Antibodies are produced via the humoral immune response mechanism. Antigens are processed by the antigen presenting cells (APC) which are macrophages. The processed antigen is presented by the APC together with a glycoprotein coded for by the Major Histocompaibility Complex (MHC) to a CD4+ (helper) T-lymphocyte. These in turn intearacts with other cells including interlukin-1 which stimulates the CD4+ cells to secrete cytokines and interferon which help to stimulate proliferation of more T lymphocytes resulting in the activation of B lymphocytes. The activated B cells differentiate into either antibody-producing cells called plasma cells that secrete soluble antibody or memory cells that survive in the body for years afterward in order to allow the immune system to remember an antigen and respond faster upon future exposures. The plasma cells synthesizes and secretes antibody molecule that is specific for the antigen structure that stimulated it's production. A variable number of B lymphocytes may be involved in each immune response. A number of plasma cells may be stimulated to secrete monospecific antibody which is aimed at a single antigenic specificity. The immune response is dependent on a number of factors such as; the amount of antigen introduced, the immune competence of the individual and the immunogenicity of the substance. The production of antibody involving circulating monocytes, T and B lymphocytes and tissue bound macrophages can result in either a primary or secondary immune response. The antibody molecule is made up of heavy and light chains held together by a non-covalent disulphide bond. There are five types of chains; gamma (G), MU (M), alpha (A), delta (D) and epsilon (E) which determines the 5 classes of immunoglobulin (IgG, IgM, IgA, IgD and IgE respectively). IgG is made up of 4 classes (IgG 1 to 4). The subtypes IgG 1 and 3 are most immune compared to 2 and 4. There are 2 types of light chains; kappa (K) and Lamd (L). Most blood grou antibodies are predominantly Igm, IgG and IgA and never IgD and E.

Summary of a primary immune response

- Immunisation by foreign substance (Antigen)
- Contact betwen antigen and antigen presenting cells (APC)
- Ingestion of antigen and MHC class 2 protein by APC
- Interaction between APC and CD4 lymphocites (recognising antigen)
- APC secrets IL-1 and CD4 secretes cytokine promote T cell proliferation
- Interaction between CD4 and Bcell growth factors
- B cell divides to produce identical daughter cells
- Daughter cells develop into plasma and memory
- Plasma cells secretes antibodies

Primary and secondary immune responses. Following an encounter with a foreign antigenic substances (several weeks and months), the body produces small amount of IgM antibodies. This constitutes a primary immune response. Once the IgM antibody has been produced some of the B cells (memory B cells) will survive in the body and remember that same antigen in subsequent future exposure leading to the production of antibody of the IgG class. This type of immune response produced by primed (memory) B lymphocytes (anamnestic or secondary immune response) following a second exposure to a second dose of the antigen produces a larger amount of IgG with less delay as in primary immune response. The antibody produced following a secondary immune response has a better affinity for the corresponding specifc antigen (Avidity).

Circumstances surrounding the production of red cells antibodies. Response to red cell antigen exposure: An individual can become exposed to the red cell of another person either throgh blood transfusion or pregnancy. Either of these exposure can result in antibody production if the red cell antigen introdued is foreign or the exposed individual lacks the introduced antigen. Such exposure stimulates the recipient immune system to produce immune alloantibodies. About 2-9% of patients produces immune antibodies. Transfusion of a red cell containing antigen which the receipinet lacks can stimulate the recipient to produce immune antibody against that antigen (for example transfusing Kell positive red cells to a Kell negative receipient). Feto maternal haemorrhage during pregnancy or delivery can introduce foetal red cells containing red cells antigen which the mother lacks into the maternal circulation and stimulate the mum to produce immune antibody against the foetal red cell antigen (example is feto maternal haemorrhage of Rhesus positive foetal red cells into a mum that is Rhesus negative).

Exposure to environmental antigen: Chemical structures (carbonhydrate) similar to red cell antigen are common in nature (food and surface of bacterial). Exposures of the body to these chemical structures can result in the production of antibodies. The anti-A, anti-B and anti A,B present in group B,A and O individuals respectively are thought to arise as a result to exposure to ABO like chemical substances which occur in nature. This happens at an early age because sugars that are identical to or very similar to the ABO blood group antigens are found throughout nature. This is based on the observation that animals kept in a sterile room from birth were shown to lack these antibodies.

Immunoglobulin subclasses. The classes of immunoglobulins can de divided into subclasses based on small differences in the amino acid sequences in the constant region of the heavy chains. All immunoglobulins within a subclass will have very similar heavy chain constant region amino acid sequences. IgG subclasses includes; IgG1 - Gamma 1 heavy chains, IgG2 - Gamma 2 heavy chains, IgG3 - Gamma 3 heavy chains and IgG4 - Gamma 4 heavy chains. The IgA subclasses includes; IgA1 - alpha 1 heavy chain and IgA2 - Alpha 2 heavy chains.

IgM immunoglobulin. IgM normally exists as a pentamer but it can also exist as a monomer. In the pentameric form all heavy chains are identical and all light chains are identical. IgM has an extra domain on the mu chain (CH4) and it has another protein covalently bound via a S-S bond called the J chain. This chain functions in polymerization of the molecule into a pentamer. IgM is the third most common serum Ig. IgM is the first Ig to be made by the fetus and the first Ig to be made by a virgin B cells when it is stimulated by antigen. As a consequence of its pentameric structure, IgM is a good complement fixing Ig. Thus, IgM antibodies are very efficient in leading to the lysis of microorganisms. As a consequence of its pentameric structure, IgM is a good complement fixing Ig. Thus, IgM antibodies are very efficient in leading to the lysis of microorganisms. As a consequence of its structure, IgM is also a good agglutinating Ig. Thus, IgM antibodies are very good in clumping microorganisms for eventual elimination from the body. IgM binds to some cells via Fc receptors.

IgG immunoglobulin. All IgG's are monomers (7S immunoglobulin). The subclasses differ in the number of disulfide bonds and length of the hinge region. IgG is the most versatile immunoglobulin because it is capable of carrying out all of the functions of immunoglobulin molecules. IgG is the major Ig in serum - 75% of serum Ig is IgG. IgG is the major Ig in extra vascular spaces. Placental transfer - IgG is the only class of Ig that crosses the placenta. Transfer is mediated by a receptor on placental cells for the Fc region of IgG. Not all subclasses cross equally well; IgG2 does not cross well. Fixes complement - Not all subclasses fix equally well; IgG4 does not fix complement. Binding to cells - macrophages, monocytes, and some lymphocytes have Fc receptors for the Fc region of IgG. Not all subclasses bind equally well. IgG2 and IgG4 do not bind to Fc receptors. A consequence of binding to the Fc receptors on PMNs, monocytes and macrophages is that the cell can now internalize the antigen better. The antibody has prepared the antigen for eating by the phagocytic cells. The term opsonin is used to describe substances that enhance phagocytosis. IgG is a good opsonin. Binding of IgG to Fc receptors on other types of cells results in the activation of other functions.

IgA immunoglobulin. Serum IgA is a monomer but IgA found in secretions is a dimer. When IgA is found in secretions is also has another protein associated with it called the secretory piece or T piece; IgA is sometimes referred to as 11S immunoglobulin. Unlike the remainder of the IgA which is made in the plasma cell, the secretory piece is made in epithelial cells and is added to the IgA as it passes into the secretions. The secretory piece helps IgA to be transported across mucosa and also protects it from degradation in the secretions. IgA is the 2nd most common serum Ig. IgA is the major class of Ig in secretions - tears, saliva, colostrum, mucus. Since it is found in secretions secretory IgA is important in local (mucosal) immunity. Normally IgA does not fix complement, unless aggregated. IgA can bind to some cells - polymorphonuclear leukocytes and some lymphocytes.

IgD immunoglobulin. IgD exists only as a monomer. IgD is found in low levels in serum; its role in serum uncertain. IgD is primarily found on B cell surfaces where it functions as a receptor for antigen. IgD on the surface of B cells has extra amino acids at C-terminal end for anchoring to the membrane. It also associates with the Ig-alpha and Ig-beta chains. IgD does not bind complement.

IgE immunoglobulin. IgE exists as a monomer and has an extra domain in the constant region. IgE is the least common serum Ig since it binds very tightly to Fc receptors on basophils and mast cells even before interacting with antigen. Involved in allergic reactions - As a consequence of its binding to basophils an mast cells, IgE is involved in allergic reactions. Binding of the allergen to the IgE on the cells results in the release of various pharmacological mediators that result in allergic symptoms. IgE also plays a role in parasitic helminth diseases. Since serum IgE levels rise in parasitic diseases, measuring IgE levels is helpful in diagnosing parasitic infections. Eosinophils have Fc receptors for IgE and binding of eosinophils to IgE-coated helminths results in killing of the parasite. IgE does not fix complement.

Functional parts of an immunoglobulin molecule.

An antibody (immunoglobulin) is a large Y-shaped protein used by the immune system to identify and neutralize foreign objects such as bacteria and viruses. The immunoglobulin molecule can be brokem down into its functional parts by the action of a proteolytic enzymes papain into 2 Fab fragments and one Fc fragment. The Fab fragment is made up of an intact light chain and the amino –terminal end of the heavy chain linked by a disulphide bondThe Fab portion is predominantly carbonhydrate and contains specific antigen binding ability (contain antigen binding site). The Fc (Fragment Crystalline) portion is made up of carboxy terminal portions of 2 heavy chains linked by disulphide bond. It is commonly associated with some IgG molecule and play a role in complement and macrophage binding.

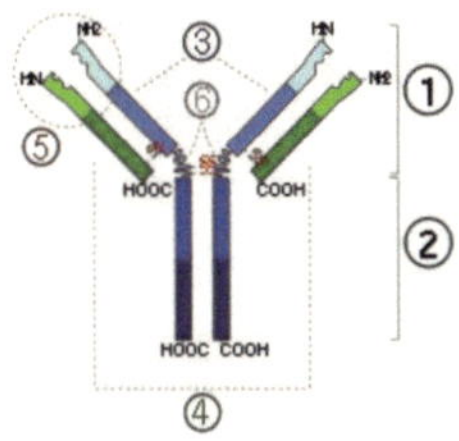

1. Fab region
2. Fc region
3. Heavy chain (blue) with one variable (VH) domain followed by a constant domain (CH1), a hinge region, and two more constant (CH2 and CH3) domains.
4. Light chain (green) with one variable (VL) and one constant (CL) domain
5. Antigen binding site (paratope)
6. Hinge regions.

Immunoglobulins are composed of four polypeptide chains: two "light" chains (lambda or kappa), and two "heavy" chains (alpha, delta, gamma, epsilon or mu). The type of heavy chain determines the immunoglobulin isotype (IgA, IgD, IgG, IgE, and IgM respectively). Light chains are composed of 220 amino acid residues while heavy chains are composed of 440-550 amino acids. Each chain has "constant" and "variable" regions.

Variable region. Variable regions are contained within the amino (NH2) terminal end of the polypeptide chain (amino acids 1-110). When comparing one antibody to another, these amino acid sequences are quite distinct. This region determines the specificity of an antibody and is composed of variable amino acids sequences.

Constant region. Constant regions, comprising amino acids 111-220 (or 440-550), are rather uniform, in comparison from one antibody to another, within the same isotype. This section determines the biological function such as complement activation, placenta transfer and the ability to bind to macropgages.

Hinge region. The hinge region is located within the constant section of the heavy chain and provides the heavy chain a degree of flexibility enabling it to change its shape. The hinge region allows the IgG immunoglobulin to maintain its T shape in serum or plasma and enable the antigen binding sites to be maximally distant from each other. The IgG molecule becomes a characteristically Y shaped on binding with an antigen allowing for greater accessibility of the constant region and facillites complement activation.

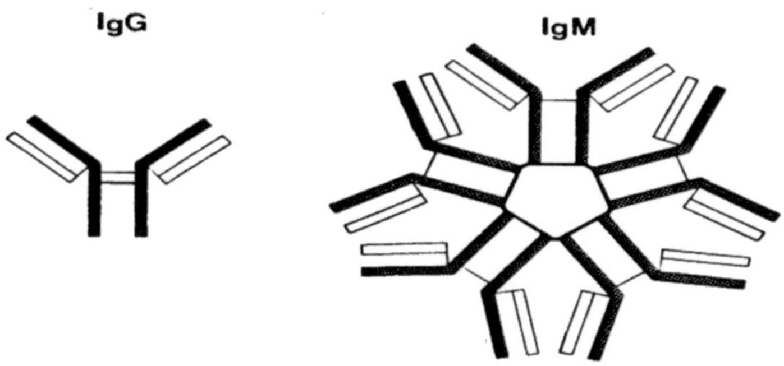

Structure of IgG and IgM immunoglobulin

Property	IgG	IgM
Capacity to cross the placenta	Yes	No
Capable of complement activation	Yes	Yes
Normal temperature of reaction	4-20°C	37°C
Number of subclasses	4	None
Approximate molecular weight	150,000	900,000
Number of antigen-binding sites	2	10
Size of antibody	Comprises of single immunoglobulin subunit (monomer)	Comprised of 5 immunoglobulin subunits (pentamer)

Table: Comparison between the properties of IgM and IgG immunoglobulin.

3. Blood Group Systems and ABO groups

Blood Group terminologies

There are terminologies used to represent different blood group antigens. Correct usage of these terminologies is critical to ensure that the correct information is recorded and transmitted. These terminologies include:

- Allerlic genes are represented as superscript. Examples as; Duffy A (Fy^a), B (Fy^b), Kidd blood group as (JK^a and JK^b), Lewis blood group antigen as (Le^a and Le^b).
- Positive and negative signs are often used to represent the presence or absence of red cell antigens. For examples; Fy (a+b -), K+. However in the ABO blood group system a positive and negative sign after the ABO blood group indicates the presence of not just the ABO group but the Rh (D) antigen. For example A+ indicates presence of antigen A and D.
- Short hand notations and subscript symbols and letter as well as subscript numbers are often used as nomenclature for the Rh blood group system. Examples are (r', r') or Ro, R1, R2 Rz).
- Antibodies are written as their antigen notations with the prefix anti-. Examples are; anti-D, anti –K, anti-Fy^a and anti –S).
- If a patient is grouped using single antibody specificity say anti-S and found positive. It is erroneous to assume that the patients is negative for the antithetical antigen s-. This assumption will only be correct if the patient red cells was also tested against an antibody with anti-s specificity.
- If a patient is positive for an alloantibody say anti-Le^a, it is wrong to assume that the patient is negative for antigen Le^a unless the patient red cells have been tested against anti- Le^a sera). Grouping a patient to establish negativity for a red cell antigen can sometimes be used to confirm the specificity of an alloantibody.
- ISBT numbers are now being used to produce uniformity in the terminology used to identify red cell antigens (eye readable and adaptable for computer use). Each red cell antigen is given a 6 unique digit number (first 3 representing the blood group system and the 2nd three the antigen itself). The table below shows the nomenclature including the ISBT number for the 9 most clinical significant blood group systems.

Blood group system	ISBT number	Common antigens	Phenotypic variations
ABO	001	A and B	A, A1, A2, B, AB,A1B, A2B and O
MNS	002	M, N, S and s	M+, M-, N+, N-, S+,S-,s+ & s-
P	003	P1 & P	P1 and P2
Rhesus (Rh)	004	C, c, D, E and e	C+, C-, c+, c-, D+, D-, E+ and e-

Lutheran	005	Lua and Lub	Lua+, Lua-, Lub+ and Lub-
Kell	006	K, k, Kpa, Kpb, Jsa and Jsb	K+, K-, k+, and k-.
Lewis	007	Lea and Leb	Lea-, Lea+, Leb+ and Leb-
Duffy	008	Fya, Fyb	Fya+ Fya-, Fyb+ and Fyb-
Kidd	009	Jka and Jkb	Jka+, Jka-, Jkb+, Jkb-

Table: Nomenclature for the most clinical significant blood group systems

The ABO Blood group system

The ABO blood group system first described by the Austrian scientist Karl Landsteiner in 1901 is the most clinically significant blood group system in human blood transfusion. Four major groups were characterized (A, B, AB and O). This characterization was based on the occurrence of two antigens (A and B) occurring singly as A or B, doubling as AB or the absence of both as O. The associated anti-A and anti-B antibodies are usually IgM antibodies, which are not present in the newborn at birth but, appear after the first 6 months of life by sensitization to environmental substances such as food, bacteria (Gram negative E. Coli), and viruses (Influenza). Anti-A and anti-B antibodies are not able to pass through the placenta barrier to the fetal blood circulation and seldom cause hemolytic disease of the foetus and newborn (HDFN). However, some group O-type mother can produce IgG-type ABO antibodies. which have the potential to cross the placenta barrier and cause a less severe HDFN. Majority of the hemolytic blood transfusion reactions observed in practice are caused by the clerical and technical errors associated the ABO blood group system (complement-mediated lysis) of the RBCs. Landsteiner discovered this system out of curiosity after observing that the serum/plasma of certain health individuals agglutinated the red cells of others. This led to the postulation of the theory that: individuals who have the A and B antigens on their red cells lack the corresponding antibodies in their plasma. Historically, while Landsteiner described A, B, and O antigens, Alfred von Decastello and Adriano Sturli discovered the fourth type (AB), in 1902. Ludwik Hirszfeld and von Dungern discovered the heritability of ABO blood groups in 1910–11. Felix Bernstein demonstrating the correct blood group inheritance pattern of multiple alleles at one locus in 1924 while Watkins and Morgan, in England, discovered that the ABO epitopes were conferred by specific sugars; N-acetylgalactosamine for the A-type and galactose for the B-type. The ABO blood group system is the most clinical significant system for the following reasons.

- The regular occurrence of ABO blood group antibodies in the plasma or serum of healthy persons who lack the corresponding antigens on their red cells.
- The ability of ABO antibodies to cause intravascular haemolysis in the circulation of recipient transfused with red cells antigen to which they have the corresponding antibody.

- The high frequency of the determinant A and B antigen in both Black and Caucasian population.

ABO Group	Phenotype	ABO blood group antigen present on red cells	ABO antibodies present in plasma/serum	Possible genotypes
A	A	A antigen	Anti-B	AA or AO
B	B	B antigen	Anti-A	BB or BO
AB	AB	A and B antigens	None	AB
O	O	None	Anti-A and anti-B	OO

ABO phenotypes and possible genotypes

Are ABO blood group antibodies really naturally occurring?

ABO blood group antibodies are universally present in the serum /plasma of healthy adults. As a result of this fact, these antibodies were thought to be naturally occurring. However from the definition of an antibody, it is clear that an antibody only occurs as a result of stimulation by an antigen. In reality, ABO antibodies in the serum are not formed naturally. Their production is stimulated when the immune system encounters ABO blood group like antigens in foods or in micro-organisms. This happens at an early age because sugars that are identical to, or very similar to, the ABO blood group antigens are found throughout nature. The ABO locus has three main alleleic forms: A, B, and O. The A allele encodes a glycosyltransferase that produces the A antigen (N-acetylgalactosamine is its immunodominant sugar), and the B allele encodes a glycosyltransferase that creates the B antigen (D-galactose is its immunodominant sugar). ABO blood group antibodies react optimally at 16-22°C. They bind complements. ABO blood group antibodies can be immune (IgG) if stimulated by pregnancy and incompatible blood transfusion. To buttress this the agument that ABO antibodies are naturally occurring;

- Animal studies have shown that animal kept in a sterile room from birth do not produce antibodies. This is an indication that antibody production results from exposure to environmental stimulus.
- Children at birth have no ABO antibodies. Neonates under the age of 6 months have little or no ABO group antibody. Any ABO blood group antibody detected at birth is likely to be maternaternal antibody that have been passively transferred via the placenta. ABO antibody levels reaches the adult level about the age of 5years, remaining relatively stable during adult life and then usually decline at old age.

Clinical significance of the ABO blood group system

Transfusion. Transfusion of ABO incompatible unit (such as transfusing a B patient with group A red cell, a group A patient with a group B red cells or transfusing a group O patient with a group A, B or AB red cells) to a patient has result in the activation of complements leading to life threatening acute intravascular haemolysis

Organ and bone marrow. The ABO blood group system is the most clinically significant organ transplantation medicine. ABO antigens are expressed on most blood cells, organs, and tissues and in most body fluids in a variety of tissue cells within the body. Some transplanted organs (kidney or liver) must be ABO compatible to prevent rejection.

Recipients Blood Group	Donor's Blood Group
O	O
A	A or O
B	B or O
AB	A, B, AB or O

Table: Organ Transplant and ABO blood group requirement

Pregnancy. ABO blood group antibodies are a common cause of Haemolytic Disease of the Foetus and Newborn (HDFN). This is a common occurrence when there is ABO blood group incompatibility between mother and developing foetus. This often occurs when mother is O (and has IgG anti-A,B) and baby is group A or B). The IgG anti-A,B in the maternal circulation is able to cross the placenta barrier and cause the coating and eventual destruction of the foetal red cell. The effect of ABO HDFN is often mild. Such baby may have a positive DAT at birth.

Universal donors and recipients phenomenom. Individuals who are blood group AB are called universal recipient: This is based on the notion that because they lack ABO blood group antibodies in their plasma, it should be safe for them to receive blood from blood donors who are group A, B and O. Similarly individuals who are group O lack ABO blood group antigens on their red cell and as such should be able to donate blood for use by other individuals of other ABO groups (A, B and AB). However there is one caveat to this universal donor/recipient phenomenon. This is the fact that the universal donor phenomenon only applies to packed RBCs, and not to whole blood products. This is because blood group O individuals have anti-A and anti-B antibodies in the serum. Some blood group O individuals have a high titre of this anti-A and B haemolysin that are capable of producing a hemolytic transfusion reaction when their whole blood is given to A, B and AB patients. Also blood group A, B and O whole blood containing high titre A and B haemolysin when given to group AB individuals (based on group AB being universal recipient) can cause complement activation resulting in hemolytic transfusion reaction. As a rule, all group O blood that are intended for use against ABO blood group barrier by A, B and AB individuals must be tested for high titre anti-A and B haemolysis. Only those that are negative should be used for group A, B and AB recipients. Those that are positive for anti A and B haemolysins should be reserved strictly for recipients who are group O. Blood group O individuals are said to be universal donors. Blood group O red cells can be given not only to group O individuals, but also to individuals who are group A, B and AB. However use of group O blood against the ABO blood group barrier to A, B and AB individuals should be with caution as some group O individual s are positive for high titres anti A and B haemolysins which are capable of causing the haemolysis of A and D cells of the recipients

RBC Compatibility chart

Recipient ABO blood group	Group O	Group A	Group B	Group AB
1st Choice	O *	A	B	AB
2nd Choice	A	AB	A **	A **
3rd Choice	B	B **	AB	B **
4th Choice	AB	-	-	-

Transfusion policy for Fresh frozen Plasma (FFP)

Key

** = Group O FFP must only be transfused to group O patients*

*** = All group A and B FFP intended for use against ABO blood group barrier (Group A FFP given to a group B patient or group B FFP given to an A patient) must be tested and found negative for high titre anti-A and B haemolysin.*

Red blood cell compatibility. The aim of red cell transfusion is for the management of anaemia. For red cell transfusion to achieve this aim, the transfused red cell must be able to survive the red cell life span of 120 days the recipients system to allow for enough time for the recipients haematopoietic system to start its own red cell production. Among other consideration, for a blood transfusion to be successful, units selected for crossmatch and transfused to recipients must be AB0 blood groups compatible with the donor unit. If they are not, the red blood cells from the donated unit will clump or agglutinate. The agglutinated red cells can clog blood vessels and stop the circulation of the blood to various parts of the body. The agglutinated red blood cells also can have their membrane damaged and its contents leak out in the body.

Plasma compatibility. Plasma –related products (fresh frozen plasma, cryoprecipitate and platelets) for transfusion should be selected with caution and should take into consideration the ABO blood groups of donors and recipients. In addition to donating to the same blood group; plasma from type AB can be given to AB, A, B and O. Plasma from types A, B and AB can be given to O. Recipients can receive plasma of the same blood group. The donor-recipient compatibility for blood plasma is the converse of that of RBCs. Plasma extracted from type AB blood can be transfused to individuals of any blood group. Individuals of blood group O can receive plasma from any blood group and type O plasma can be used only by type O recipients. Under normal circumstances, plasma from a group A donor should not be transfused to a B patient. Also plasma from a B donor should not be transfused to an A patient. However blood group A and B individuals can be transfused with B and A plasma respectively provided they have been test for high titre anti-A and anti-B haemolysis and found to be negative. Also all plasma intended for transfusion should be free from antibody D and other atypical antibodies.

Recipient ABO blood group	Group O	Group A	Group B	Group AB
1st Choice	O *	A	B	AB
2nd Choice	A	AB	A **	A **
3rd Choice	B	B **	AB	B **
4th Choice	AB	-	-	-

Transfusion policy for Fresh frozen Plasma (FFP)

Key

** = Group O FFP must only be transfused to group O patients*

** = All group A and B FFP intended for use against ABO blood group barrier (Group A FFP given to a group B patient or a group B FFP given to a group A patient) must be tested and found negative for high titre anti-A and B haemolysin.

Recipient ABO blood group	O	A	B	AB
1st Choice	O	A	B	AB
2nd Choice	A *	B *	A *	A * or B*
3rd Choice	B *	O *	O *	O *

Transfusion policy for Platelet concentrate

Key

** = All group A, B and O platelet concentrate intended for use against ABO blood group barrier (Group A platelet given to a group B O and AB patients and group B platelet concentrate given to a group A, O and AB patient as well as group O platelet concentrate given to an A, B and AB patients must be tested and found negative for high titre anti-A and B haemolysin.*

** = Due to the possibility that platelet concentrate may be contaminated with red cell, it is advisable to transfuse all Rhesus negative women of child bearing age with Rhesus negative platelet to prevent the risk of Rh sensitization and production of immune anti-D. Also platelet concentrate intended for transfusion to pregnant and immunocompromised (including HIV positive patient) must be CMV negative.

Blood grouping. The blood group of an individual can be determined in two ways. You can determine the ABO blood group antigens present on the red cells of the individuals by using potent monoclonal anti-A, Anti -B and anti-AB (cell, forward or front group). The principle is based on the principle that anti-A and B will agglutinate red cells containing the group specific A and B antigens. Alternatively you can determine the ABO blood group antibody present in the serum or plasma by add the patient serum or plasma to the red cells of known ABO antigen status (A1 and B). This is known as reverse/serum or back group). The principle is based on identifying the antibody present in the plasma based on their agglutination of the A1 and B cells. Plasma that agglutinates A1 contains anti-A while those that agglutinate B cells contain anti-B. ABO blood group antibodies are universally present in the serum /plasma of healthy adults. It is not possible to determine the back group of neonate until they are 6 months of age. This is due to the fact that ABO antibodies are not fully developed at this age (6 months). These 2 methods must be used together to routinely determine the ABO group of a patient because of the clinical significance of the ABO blood group system in transfusion and to avoid error in grouping as well as possibly identify rare and unusual ABO groups. The result obtained should reflect the results shown in the 2 tables below. If the back group is not in agreement with the forward group or the result obtained does not agree with the group recorded on the laboratory information management system (LIMS) / the patient notes or if there are unusual reactions, it must be investigated. It should first be repeated. If results remain inconclusive, a repeat sample must be requested before attempting to selects unit for transfusion. The ABO blood group antigens remain of prime importance in transfusion medicine—they are the most immunogenic of all the blood group antigens. The most common cause of death from a blood transfusion is a clerical error in which an incompatible type of ABO blood is transfused.

Red cell Sample	Anti-A	Anti-B	Anti AB	ABO Group
W	N	N	N	O
X	P	P	P	AB
Y	P	N	P	A
Z	N	P	P	B

Red cell grouping (Forward grouping)

Key:
P= Positive reaction
N= Negative reaction

Serum/plasma sample	A1 Cells	B cells	Antibody present	ABO Group
E	P	N	Anti A + B	O
F	P	N	Nil	AB
G	P	N	Anti-A	B
H	P	N	Anti-B	A

Serum grouping results (Backward grouping)

Key:
P= Positive reaction
N= Negative reaction

Common causes of ABO blood group anomalies. Common causes of ABO blood group anomalies include; technical errors, weak reacting antigen and antibody, effect of alloantibodies and autoantibodies, age related issues, previous transfusion or bone marrow transplant and other factors.

Technical errors. If red cell and serum sample is taken from the wrong patient. The forward and back group may be different from that on the LMIS or patient case note. If serum or antisera reagent was mistakenly not added the desired result will not be evident. If patient sample is haemolysed or plasma sample is denatured due to poor storage. Use of antisera reagent that has lost it potency due to suboptimal storage conditions can cause false result. Inadequate incubation time or incorrect incubation temperature. Use of time expired products (irrespective of whether reagent is still potent or not, ABO blood grouping reagents must not be used after the manufacturers stated expiry date). Antigen and antibody reaction occur in optimal proportion. In an agglutination test, a person's serum (which contains antibodies) is added to a test tube which contains antigen (red cells). Occasionally, it is observed that when the concentration of antibody is high, there is no agglutination and then, as the sample is diluted, agglutination occurs. The lack of agglutination at high concentrations of antibodies is called the prozone effect. Lack of agglutination in the prozone is due to antibody excess resulting in very small complexes that do not clump to form visible agglutination.

Weak reacting antigen and antibody. Red cell that has fewer antigenic determinants is likely to react less strongly with the corresponding antibody compared to one with more antigenic determinants. Also the titre of ABO blood group antibody tends to diminish in old age and as such will result in a weaker than expected reactions in the serum/back group.

Effect of an alloantibody and autoantibody. Presence of an alloantibody or autoantibody can produce non-specific reactions during forward and back groups. For patients who have an alloantibody with a positive DAT, the autoantibody coating the red cells may need to be eluted first to allow the ABO group to be effectively determined.

Age-related issues. It is not possible to determine the back group of neonate until they are 6 months of age. This is due to the fact that ABO antibodies are not fully developed at this age (6 months). ABO antibody levels reaches the adult level about the age of 5 years, remaining relatively stable during adult life and then usually decline at old age and may affect serum/back group.

Previous transfusion or bone marrow transplant. Previous transfusion or marrow transplant with ABO compatible rather than specific red cells or marrow can cause some considerable challenges in ABO group determination. Such information must always be included in the patient case note and on the LIMS.

Other Factors. Other factors that can cause anomaly during blood group determination include; disease conditions (cancers and agammaglobulinaemia), Chimerism phenomenom, genetic abnormalities, presence of rare or low incidence ABO groups and sub-groups and staff carrying out test not adequately trained and certified competent to do test.

Acquired (Pseudo) B phenomenom. Difficulty is sometimes experienced in determining the ABO group in some patients. It is commonly seen in group A individual who react as AB. These patients are often grouped as AB with a weakly reacting B component, while their serum contained anti-B agglutinins. The saliva also characteristically does not contained B substance. It is now known to be caused by the enzymatic (enzyme produced by Escherichia coli) breakdown (deacetylation) of group A antigen (N acetyl-D-galactosamine) to galactosamine which is similar in structure to group B antigen immunodominant sugar (D-galactose). This enzymatic change is often brought about by some bacteria in-vivo in patients with gastrointestinal septicaemia. It can also occur if the red cells reagent is infected with bacteria (in-vitro). This phenomenon can result in a patient's red cell being polyagglutibable (being agglutinated by all human sera including serum form a blood group B individual. This occurrence has also been observed in patients with bowel carcinoma.

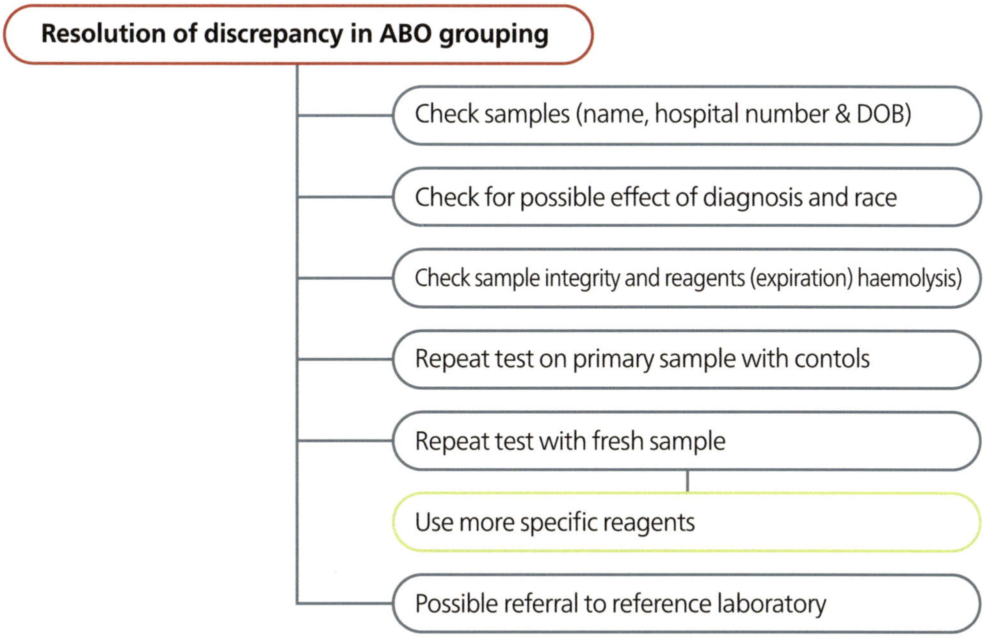

Approach to resolution of discrepancy in ABO grouping

Subgroups of Group A and B. The A blood type contains about twenty subgroups, of which A1 and A2 are the most common (over 99%). These sub groups exist as a result of genetic variations which often results in weaker and variable reactions of the A antigen with the group specific A antibody. A1 makes up about 80% of all A-type blood, with A2 making up the rest. These two subgroups were first described by von Dungern and Herszfeld. Individuals who are group A2 has fewer antigenic determinants (antigen sites) compared to A1 individuals (250,000 versus 1,000,000 per cell respectively). The antibody A found in group B contains inseparable anti- A and A1 antibodies. While the anti-A reacts with both A1 and A2 red cells, the anti-A1 reacts only against A1 cells. The A1 gene is dominant over A2 gene. Both A1 and A2 are codominant with B. Individuals who are phenotypically A1 will have the genotype A1A1, A1O or A1A2. Some 1-8% of A2 individuals and 22-35% of group A2B individuals produce a naturally occurring clinically insignificant cold reacting anti-A1.

ABO Groups	Phenotype	Possible genotype
A	A_1	A_1A_1, A_1A_2, A_1O
B	B	BB and BO
AB	A_1B and A_2B	A_1B and A_2B
O	O	OO

Possible phenotypes and genotypes based on subgroups of A

Phenotype	Caucasian	Black	Indian	Oriental	Australian Aborigine	Native Americans
A_1	33	19	26	27	56	0
A_2	10	8	3	Rare	0	0
A_1B	3	3	9	5	0	0
A_2B	1	1	1	Rare	0	0

Racial variations in the distribution of the subgroups of A

Other subgroups of A include A_3, A_4 (A_X).

Subgroup A_3. Occur in 1 out of 1000 of group A individuals. Produces a mixed field reaction with polyclonal anti-A and anti-AB. Occur as a result of fewer A antigenic determinants on A_3 red cells. Monoclonal anti sera often produces a strong and complete reaction with A_3 red cells. A_3 individuals have anti-B in their sera and may occasionally produce anti-A_1. All reacted strongly with anti-H lectin.

Subgroup A_4 or A_X. 1 in 40,000 to 77,000 groups A individuals are A_4 or A_X. A_4 or A_X individuals have very few A antigenic determinants (5,000) on their red cells. Cells are only agglutinated by monoclonal anti-A and some anti A, B sera as well as some polyclonal anti-A, B sera but not by polyclonal anti-A. Group A_4 or A_X individuals often have anti-B and occasionally anti-A_1 in their sera. Show a strong agglutination with anti-H lectin.

Subgroups of B. Subgroups of B are rare but occur predominantly among Africans, Chinese and Indian population where the frequency of B antigen is high. Occur as a result of fewer B antigenic determinants on the red cells of these individuals resulting in a weak and variable reaction with anti-B. Examples of weak group B include B_3, B_X, B_m and B_{el}. Red blood cells in the B_{el} subgroup show no agglutination with anti-B or anti-A, B antisera. B antigen is only detected by adsorption with polyclonal group A sera. B_{el} can be differentiated from B_m by saliva testing, which only detects only the H antigen.

ABO blood group discripancies. Any deviation fromthe expected pattern of antigen on red cells and the opposite antibodies in plasma or serum constitute a discrepancy and **must** be investigated before any attempt is made to select units for crossmatching. All ABO blood grouping discrepancies **must** be investigated and resolved. In receipients the discrepancies must be resolved before any blood component is transfused. If not resolved before blood is needed, transfuse group O blood. If there is a discrepancy in the Rh type also, group O Negative must be tenasfused until discrepancy is resolved. In donor the discrepancies must be resolved before any blood is labeled with a blood type. The general rules involved in resolution of blood group discripancies include:

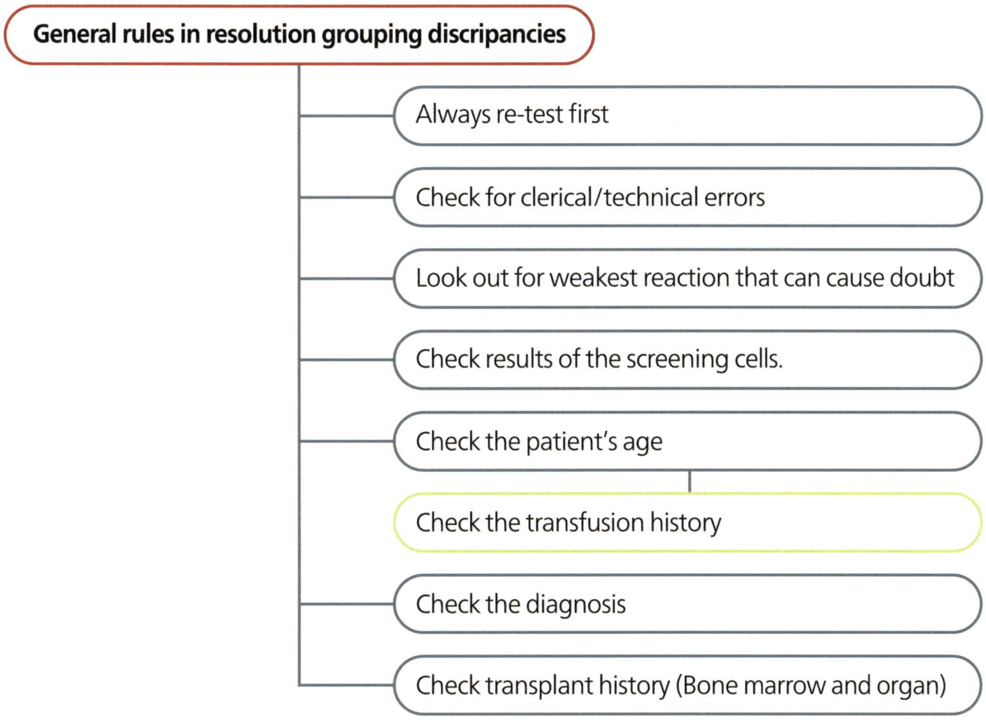

Types of discripancies

Clerical errors (Transcription errors). Clerical errors are the most common types of error that cause discripancies in blood group result. To avoid such errors the following must be taken into consideration. Record the results as you read each tube. Always check which tube you are reading and record the results immediately. Make sure you are recording the results on the right worksheet. One way to prevent this error is to minimize the times you are working with more than one patient or donor at a time. Recording results in the wrong spot on worksheet could occur when you put some of the serum results in the cell typing area or vice versa. Be sure you have techniques that will prevent you from performing this error (Appriopriate labelling).

Technical errors. There are a number of technical errors that can occur in blood grouping. They include; Sample mix-up such as wrong serum tube, failure to add serum or reagent can lead to technical errors where no reaction is occurring where one is expected (remember for both ABO and Rh always add your reagent antisera and serum before adding cells), addition of wrong reagent such as screening cells, which are O, instead of A_1 and B cells, can lead to significant technical errors, use of suboptimal red cell suspension (few cells in suspension), use of contaminated reagents could result in either false negative or false positive results depending on whether the reagent added neutralized or added to the reactivity of the original reagent. Over centrifugation can lead to you reading the reaction as positive while there is still a button on the bottom of the tube or your shaking to dislodge the button broke up the agglutination reaction, warming the test could result in a false negative reaction since ABO antibodies are IgM that react better in the cold, failure to control the reagent before use, inappriopriate storage of antisera and red cell reagents, too many cells in your cell suspension can lead to decreased or negative reactions since there are too many cells for the number of antibodies present in the reagents. Remember we want to be in the zone of equivalence for our reactions, failure to detect weak results can occur if you are not watching the reactions while you are shaking them out or if you shake too hard, failure to detect hemolysis can be a definite problem. Remember a positive reaction can be hemolysis as well as agglutination since the antigen-antibody reaction can bind complement. When complement is bound it can lead to hemolysis that is also an indication of a positive reaction and dirty glassware can cause the cells to artificially clumping of cells.

Foward group (Cell group)			Back Group (Serum group)		Possible reason for discripancy
Anti-A	Anti-B	Anti –A, B	A1 Cell	B Cell	
4	0	4	0	0	Age-related weak or no back group/ failure to add serum
4	4	4	0	4	Pseudo B phenomenom (? Septicaemia of colon by gram negative organism)
4	4	4	4	4	Strong positive DAT/infected red cell reagents
0	4	4	0	0	Age-related weak or no back group/ failure to add serum

Table: Examples of common discripancies in ABO blood grouping

Problems associated with red cell testing. There are a number of problems that can occur with the red cell testing including, mixed-field agglutination, weak or missing antigens, unexpected antigen and polyagglutinable cells.

Cell of forward grouping		Serum or backward grouping	
Anti-A	Anti-B	A1 cells	B cells
Mixed-field agglutination			
MF	0	0	4+
Polyagglutinable cells			
0	0	0	4+
Weak or missing antigen			
0	0	0	4+
Unexpected antigen			
4+	2+	0	4+

Table: Common causes of Discripancies in red cell grouping

Problems with serum grouping. Problems can occur in serum grouping. It is important to investigate the problem to determine if it is actually a true discrepancy between the ABO cell type and the ABO serum test. Problems with serum testing are more common than problems with cell typing. This is either manifest as an extra antibody present or an expected antibody missing. The steps to follow to resolve a discrepancy in serum grouping include the following:

1. Check birth date since newborns and the elderly are more likely to demonstrate this discrepancy. Newborn antibodies are not present until at least 6 months. As individuals ages they may also lose their ability to maintain their antibody levels. Therefore, the very elderly have decreased antibody levels.
2. Check diagnosis since patient conditions such as; immune deficiencies, chemotherapy, radiatiotherapy and bone marrow transplantation may affect serum grouping.

Add two more drops of serum just in case you forgot to add them the first time and centrifuge. If negative then incubate in cold (4-18°C) 15-30 minutes. Include autocontrol to rule out interference from natural anti-I when incubating at (4-18°C).

Cell grouping		**Serum grouping**	
Anti-A	Anti-B	A1 Cell	B Cell
Extra Antibody			
4+	0	2+	4+
Missing Antibody			
4+	0	4+	0

Descripancies in serum grouping

Forward or cell grouping			**Back or serum grouping**	
Anti-A	Anti-B	Anti-A,B	A1 Cells	B Cells
4	0	4	0	0
0	4	4	0	0
0	0	0	0	0

An extreme example of no reaction in the reverse typings.

S/no	**Cell/forward grouping**		**Back/serum grouping**		**Autocontrol**	**Reaction condition**
	Anti-A	**Anti-B**	**A1 Cell**	**B Cell**		
1.	0	0	2+	2+	0	Group O at 4°C. Anti-A and Anti-B enhanced
2.	0	0	2+	2+	2+	Group O at 4°C. Auto-Anti-I enhanced

3.	4+	0	0	2+	0	Group A at 4°C. Anti-B enhanced
4.	4+	0	0	2+	0	Anti-I enhanced along with anti-A and incubated at 18°C

Examples of interference from natural anti-I
Key
At 4°C Anti-A and Anti-B enhanced since they are saline, cold-acting antibodies as seen in this example for an O individual.
Compare this with a 4°C Auto-Anti-I enhanced would have a positive autocontrol.
Group A or Group B can serve as its own negative control. 4°C Anti-B enhanced
If anti-I enhanced along with anti-B, can re-set up and incubate at 18°C. As seen in this example of 18°C: Anti-B enhanced, anti-I nonreactive

Presence of unexpected Anti-A

The presence of Anti-A_1 should be suspected when the antibody is reactive against the A cells but not the screening cells at immediate spin as seen in the example below.

Cell Grouping		Serum Grouping	
Anti-A	**Anti-B**	**A1 Cell**	**B Cell**
4+	0	2+	4+
Antibody screen			
Screening cells	Immediate Spin	AHG	
Screening Cell I	0	0	
Screening Cell II	0	0	
Autocontrol	0	0	

Naturally anti-A_1 occurs in subgroups of A or is passively-transfused from Group O platelets and other blood products.

How to Resolve the Issue of Unexpected Anti-A:

1. Check recent transfusion history for group O products, (especially platelets) that would explain the presence of this antibody.
2. Test patient cells with lectin-A_1. Subgroups will be negative with this reagent but A_1cells will be positive.
    - Lectin + A1 cell = 4+
    - Lectin + A subgroups cells = 0
3. Test patient serum with three A1 cells and three A2 cells and if it is an anti-A1. Anti-A1 will react only with the A1 cells but not with the A2 cells. The following reactions will occur:
    - Anti-A1: serum + A1 cells = +

- Serum + A2 cells = 0

4. In the case of passive Anti-A from Group O platelets the reactions would be the following:

    - Serum + A1 cells = Positive
    - Serum + A2 cells = Positive

Unexpected A and B antibody in patients with a positive antibody screen. You may have a positive reaction with the reagent A_1 or B cell that is due to a room-temperature antibody reacting with an antigen other than A or B on the cells. For example, if the patient had an anti-N that was showing up at room temperature according to the antibody identification process, you would then type for N on the reagent cells used for the reverse typing. If anti-N is causing your problem, then the cells should have N antigen present.

Red cell grouping		Serum grouping	
Anti-A	Anti-B	A1 Cell	B Cell
4+	0	2+	4+
	Immediate spin antibody screening		
Screening Cell I		2+	
Screening Cell II		0	
Autocontrol		0	

Table: Unexpected A antibody in patients with a positive antibody screen

How to Resolve the Issue of Unexpected Anti-A that is probably another antibody due to the results of the Antibody Screening:

1. Identify the antibody by performing an identification panel at room temperature.

2. Pre-warm away (use caution) the effect of this antibody by doing the reverse typing with prewarmed serum and reagent cells.

3. Type reagent A_1 or B cell for the corresponding antigen once the antibody is identified.

Rouleaux formation giving unexpected agglutination in serum grouping. Rouleaux can give unexpected agglutination in all serum tests. Rouleaux may also give false positive cell typing if strong enough and cells are insufficiently washed. This phenomenon is due to alteration in serum protein concentration such as:

Diseases associated with Rouleaux

- Multiple myeloma
- Macroglobulinemia
- Liver disease (decreased albumin)
- Patients on volume expanders (crystalloids dextran)

Also seen in patients who have had volume expanders such as crystalloids (dextran)

Characteristics of rouleaux. Rouleaux are stacks of red blood cells (RBCs) which form because of the unique discoid shape of the cells in vertebrate body. The flat surface of the discoid RBCs give them a large surface area to make contact and stick to each other; thus, forming a rouleau. They occur when the plasma protein concentration is high, and because of them the ESR (erythrocyte sedimentation rate) is also increased. This is a non-specific indicator of the presence of certain diseases. Conditions which cause rouleaux formation include infections, Multiple myeloma, inflammatory and connective tissue disorders, and cancers. It also occurs in diabetes mellitus and is one of the causative factors for microvascular occlusion in diabetic retinopathy. The presence of acute phase proteins, particularly fibrinogen, interacts with sialic acid on the surface of RBC and allows the formation of rouleau. Anaemia, by altering the ratio of RBC to plasma, increases rouleaux formation and accelerates sedimentation. Rouleaux formation is retarded by albumin proteins. To resolve rouleaux-related problems, you do saline replacement technique: Re-centrifuge the test tube. Draw off serum without disturbing cell button. Add two drops of saline. Resuspend. Rouleax disperses in saline why true agglutination remains intact.

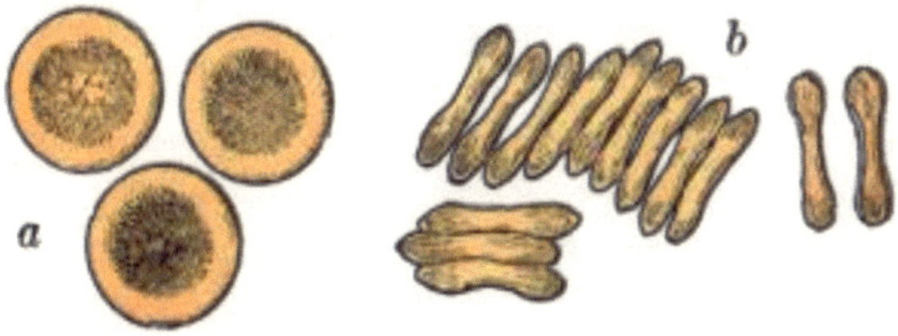

Typical mammalian erythrocytes: (a) Normal red cells (b) Red cells forming rouleaux.

Mixed-field agglutination. In transfusion medicine, mixed-field (MF) reaction refers to reactions during cell grouping where 2 distict populations of red cells are present. Agglutinated cells are admixed with unagglutinated cells. The presence of two or more cell population is known as chimerism. MF agglutination is an important cause of ABO typing and genotype discripancies. Most times the cause of MF should be investigated prior to giving a blood transfusion. Mixed-field agglutination is seen as large or small agglutinates with many unagglutinated cells. Usually mixed-field agglutination means a mixed cells population (agglutinated and non-agglutinated cell population). There are 2 types of chimerism:

False chimerism: By far the most common cause of mixed-field agglutination is false chimerism artificially induced through transfusion of identical donor red cells or through a stem cell transplant. For example, a type B individual who has received massive transfusion of group O donor red cells may show mixed field agglutination with anti-B sera whereby his own group B red cells are agglutinated, while the group O donor red cells in his circulation are unagglutinated.

True chimerism: A true chimerism is a rare sporadic phenomenon whereby an individual has a dual cell population derived from more than one zygote. This may result from intrauterine exchange of erythrocyte precursors between twins (twin chimerism) or two fertilized eggs fuse into one individual. Twin chimerism results from mixing of blood between two twin fetuses through placental blood vessel anastomoses, leading to engraftment of hematopoietic stem cells from one twin within the marrow of the other. Each twin ends up with two distinct cell populations of varying proportions. The causes of mixed-field agglutination can be:

1. Mixed cell populations resulting from massive transfusion of another blood group such as an A individual receiving "O" red blood cell donor units due to inadequate supply of group A donor unit. Such O blood used against ABO blood group barrier must be tested for high titre (HT) beta haemolysis and found negative.
2. Bone marrow transplant patients may have both some of their original type of cells and the type of the bone marrow transplant.

3. Weak subgroups of A_3 traditionally give a mixed field reaction.
4. Chimerism due to intrauterine exchange of erythrocyte precursors between twins or 2 fertilized eggs fuse into one individual.
5. Exchange transfusion in HDFN when a group A or B baby whose mother is O is giving an O exchange transfusion.
6. Cause of mixed field agglutination **must** be investigated before attempting to transfuse a patient. It is also worthwhile to check the patient's transfusion records and clinical history.

Weak or missing antigen. Weak or missing antigen may be due to the following; very weak subgroup of A or B, loss of transferase in acute leukemia, massive transfusion of group O and bone marrow transplant.

Anti-A	Anti-B	A1 Cell	B Ccell
0	0	0	4+

Table: Example of a weak or missing antigen

How would you resolve a weak or missing antigen?

1. Obtain recent transfusion history and any clinical history of bone marrow transplant.
2. Read forward grouping microscopically.
3. Use anti-A,B and incubate at 4-22°C at least 15 minutes.
4. Use monoclonal antisera that is known to react with antigens like A_x and B_x
5. Perform specialized tests if the above steps do not resolve the problem.
6. Specialized tests would include absorption/elution techniques and saliva studies.

Acquired B antigen. Acquired B antigens are seen in problems with the colon or infections with Gram-negative rods. Bacterial enzymes modify the A antigen to a B antigen and the patient forward types as an AB but reverses as an A.

Example of acquired B antigen reaction

Anti-A	Anti-B	A1 Cell	B Cell
4+	2+	0	4+

Resolution of a possible acquired B antigen

1. Set-up an autocontrol. The patient's own anti-B will not agglutinate their own AB cells.
2. Check clinical history for evidence of colon problems or Gram-negative rods.

3. Check monoclonal anti-B product inserts since some will not react with B acquired antisera

4. Acidify some reagents anti-B to pH 6 and re-test. Modified (acquired) B antigens will not react in the acidified antiserum but normal B antigens will still react

Polyagglutinable red cells. Most monoclonal anti-A and anti-B will show problems with polyagglutinable cells if it is a problem with the cell membrane that leads to the agglutination. The most likely causes of due to the following; Wharton's Jelly found in cord blood and strong positive direct antiglobulin test due to a cold agglutinin. In the case of the strong positive DAT, it would appear to be an AB in the forward type and an O on reverse.

Forward (Cell group)			Back (Serum group)	
Anti-A	Anti-B	Anti-A+B	A_1 Cell	B Cell
2+	2+	2+	4+	4+

Polyagglutinable RBCS with forward group appearing as group AB and serum group as O

Wharton's Jelly. Wharton's jelly (substantia gelatinea funiculi umbilicalis) is a gelatinous substance within the umbilical cord, largely made up of mucopolysaccharides (hyaluronic acid and chondroitin sulfate). It also contains some fibroblasts and macrophages. It is derived from extra-embryonic mesoderm. Wharton's jelly can cause some challenges particularly when determing the blood groups of neonates because of it's potential to make red cells of newborn polyagglutinable. Wharton's jelly can coats newborn cord cells and the child's type may appear AB. Reverse grouping would have been able to resolve such anomaly. However we do not do a reverse on newborn blood since they have not made any anti-A or anit-B yet. If the baby types as an AB re-check by washing cells several times and re-testing since you need to make sure you have removed the Wharton's Jelly and the baby is truly an AB. Better yet always wash cord blood 3-4 times in saline before determining the bloog group of the baby.

Ethnic variation in distribution of ABO blood groups. For example, early European races are characterized by a very low type B frequency, and a relatively high type A frequency while the Asian races are characterized by a high frequency of types A and B. The frequency with which Blood types are observed is determined by the frequency with which the three alleles of the ABO gene are found in different parts of the world. Variation in this allele frequency of the ABO gene reflects the social tendency of populations to marry and reproduce within their national, regional, or ethnic group. As people throughout the world intermingle to a greater degree, the distribution of the different Blood types will continue to become more uniform. Blood Type O - Type O Blood, which is known as the standard form of Blood types is widely distributed over the whole world uniformly, where populations have mixed.

Ethnic variation in ABO blood group distribution

Ethnic Groups	Group O (%)	Group A (%)	Group B (%)	Group AB (%)
Nigerians	58.2	21	17	2
South Africans	45	40	11	4
Kenyan	60	19	20	1
Arabs	34	31	29	6
United Kingdom	47	42	8	3
French	43	47	7	3
Germans	41	43	11	5
Indians	37	22	33	7
US (Blacks)	49	27	20	4
US (Whites)	45	40	11	4

Disease pre-disposition. Compared to non-O group (A, AB, and B) individuals, O group individuals have a 14% reduced risk of squamous cell carcinoma and 4% reduced risk of basal cell carcinoma. It is also associated with a reduced risk of pancreatic cancer. The B antigen links with increased risk of ovarian cancer. Gastric cancer has reported to be more common in blood group A and least in group O.

The ABO antigen production and the peculiar role of the H substance. The genes for the ABO system are on chromosome 9. The A, B and H gene codes for a different enzyme (glycosyl transferase) which acts on different sugars on the polypeptide or lipid (precursor substance) to produce a unique antigen. The A and B antigens are defined by specific sugars attached to a chain of oligosaccharide which protrude from the red cell membrane. The H substance is produced by the action of the H gene (HH or Hh). The H antigen is an essential precursor to the ABO blood group antigens. The H locus is located on chromosome 19. It encodes the enzyme fucosyl transferase which transfers the sugar L-fucose to the terminal sugar of the membrane galactose. This is known as the H antigen. The H antigen is the structure found in group O and is also the precursor required for the addition of the A and B antigens. Two genes regulate the production of the H antigen on red cells (FUT1) and other tissues (FUT2). The A allele encodes a glycosyltransferase that bonds α-N-acetylgalactosamine to D-galactose end of H antigen, producing the A antigen. The B allele encodes a glycosyltransferase that joins α-D-glucosamine bonded to D-galactose end of H antigen, creating the B antigen. Group O is amorphic and thus contain the highest amount of H substance. Groups A, B and AB have less H substance since a significant portion has been converted to A and or B antigens. The A1 is more effective in the conversion of H substance compared to A2. Thus A2 individuals have more H substance compared to A1. AB individuals have little or no H substance as a considerable amount of it has been converted to A and B antigens. A1 and A1B are capable of sometimes producing anti-H because of the insignificant amount of H substance on their red cell membrane. Such antibodies are usually cold reacting naturally acquired non-clinically significant and may sometimes be detected by a sensitive IAT antibody screen at 37°C.

Decreasing amount of H substance: O, A^2, B, A^1, A^1B

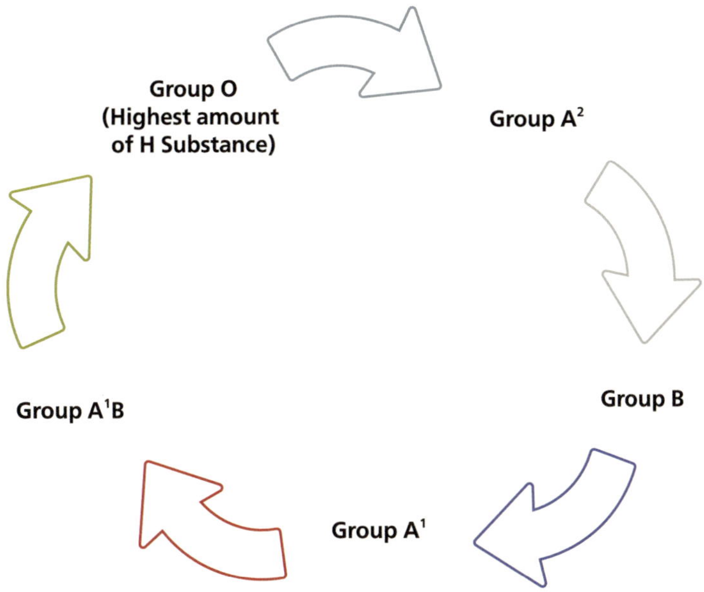

Gene	Gene product present	Carbonhydrate present
A	α-3-N-acetyl-D-galactosaminyltransferase	N-acetyl-D-galactosamine
B	α-3-D-galactosaminyltransferase	D-galactose
H	α-2-L-fucosyltransferase	L-fucose

Table: Gene products and carbohydrate expression on the H, A and B gene

ABH Secretor status. ABO and H antigens are not only present in the red cell membrane but also in most other cells of the body where they exist as glycolipds. Approximately 80% of the population secrete A, B and H substances of the same specificity as that found on the red cells in their serum/plasma (as glycoproteins) and in certain other body fluids such as saliva. These A, B and H are produced and secreted by the mucous gland (secretion). These individuals (secretors) have the secretor (Se) gene. These individuals who have the genotypes (SeSe or Sese) are known as secretors. These people secrete water-soluble blood group substances in their saliva and other body fluids. Group A individuals secretes A substance and a small amount of H, group B secretes B (and H) substance, group O secretes H substance only, and group AB secretes A, B, and a small amount of H. These substances can act as interference during red cell grouping. It is extremely important to wash red cell in saline before grouping to prevent these water soluble serum and plasma antigens from inhibiting the test and produce false negative reaction. There are laboratory test to determine if a person is a secretor. This test is based on the principle of **Agglutination Inhibition.** The presence of agglutination means a negative test, and no agglutination is interpreted as a positive result. The test is divided into phases; antibody neutralization and agglutination inhibition.

Antibody Neutralization. Saliva is mixed with commercial antiserum (Anti-A, Anti-B or Anti-H) and allowed to incubate briefly. If the patient is a secretor, the soluble blood group antigens in the saliva will react with and neutralize the antibodies in the commercial antiserum. It is necessary, however, to dilute the commercial antiserum so that its antibody titer more closely matches the antigen level in the saliva.

Agglutination Inhibition. When commercial RBC of the appropriate blood group are then added to the test mixture, there should be no free antibody to agglutinate them if the patient is a secretor, because the antibodies have already reacted with the blood group antigens in the saliva (neutralization). The will be no reaction (no agglutination) which indicates that the patient is positive for secretor status. However if the patient is a non-secretor, there will be no blood group antigens in the saliva; the antibodies in the antiserum will not be neutralized and will be free to react when the test cells are added. Therefore, agglutination is a negative test for secretor status.

Reagents, equipment used for determining the secretors status of patient

1. Clean tube to collect saliva
2. 16 x 100 mm Pyrex test tube
3. Disposable pipettes
4. Boiling water bath
5. 12 x 75 mm tubes
6. Reagent Anti-A, Anti-B or Anti-H, diluted to give about 2+ reactions.
7. Reagent A_1 cells, B cells or O cells (Screening cells)
8. Centrifuge
9. Lighted agglutination viewer

Procedure

1. Collect 2 to 3 ml saliva in a clean tube. Use paraffin wax or clean rubber bands to stimulate secretions (do not use chewing gum to prevent contamination).
2. Place in a boiling water bath for 10 minutes. This process inactivates enzymes that might otherwise destroy blood group substances.
3. Allow to cool briefly and then transfer to a 12 x 75 mm tube.
4. Centrifuge for at least 5 minutes.
5. Label three 12 x 75 mm test tubes (A test, B test and H test)
6. Label three more tubes (A Control, B Control and H Control)

7. The aim of these controls (step 6 and 7) is to as dilution controls to ensure that the anti-sera are not diluted beyond its capacity to agglutinate red cells containing the corresponding group specific antigens.
8. Add one drop of the appropriate dilute antiserum to each tube (one drop dilute anti-A to the A cell and A control, one drop dilute anti-B to the B cell and B control and one drop anti-H to the H cell and H control)
9. To each test tube containing anti-A, B and H, add one drop of clear saliva.
10. To each control tube, add one drop of saline.
11. Mix and incubate at room temperature 10 minutes.
12. Add one drop of the appropriate reagent red cells to each tube (A_1 cells for the A test and control, B cells for the B test and control and Screening cell I or II for the H test and control).
13. Mix and incubate at room temperature 10 minutes.
14. Centrifuge test and control tubes in the centrifuge lightly for 2-3 minutes.
15. Using the lighted agglutination viewer, read, grade and record the reactions.
16. The control tube should have agglutination for the test to be valid.

Result interpretation. Agglutination in all of the patient test tubes indicates a negative result for secretor status. If any one of the patient test tubes is not agglutinated, this indicates a positive test for secretor status, and the tube showing the non-agglutination should indicate the ABO secretor status of the patient.

Bombay Phenotype (Oh). Individuals with the rare Bombay phenotype (hh) do not express antigen H on their red blood cells. As H antigen serves as precursor for producing A and B antigens, the absence of H antigen means the individuals do not have A or B antigens as well (similar to O blood group). However, unlike blood group O individuals, the H antigen is absent on their red cells while the corresponding specific anti-H isoantibodies to antigen H as well as to both A and B antigens are present in their serum/plasma. This antibody is so called naturally acquired and acts as both an agglutinin and a haemolysis and produces a strong reaction at 20°C and 37°C. This antibody is clinically significant since only compatible unit from a Bombay phenotype donor (Oh) can be transfused. If these patients receive blood from a group donor, the anti-H antibodies in the recipient's serum/plasma will bind to H antigen on RBC of donor blood and destroy the RBCs by complement-mediated lysis. Therefore Bombay phenotype individuals can only receive blood only from Bombay phenotype (hh) donors. The Bombay phenotype although more predominant in people of Bombay (0.007%) is not restricted only to the Indian subcontinent. Anti-H (lectin) reagents can be prepared from the seeds of a common gorse bush (Ulex europaeus). Ulex europaeus gorse is a common gorse and an evergreen shrub in the family Fabaceae, native to western Europe from the northerly point of the United Kingdom south to Portugal, and from the westerly point of the Republic of Ireland east to Galicia in Poland and Ukraine. Lectin extracted from seeds of this species binds to and is remarkably specific for and is the standard method for identification of H-substance (absent in the hh antigen system) on human red blood cells. The vast majority of humans express H-substance, which is the basis for the ABO blood group system, but a few rare individuals ("Bombay phenotype") do not--and a chemical isolated from Ulex europaeus is used to identify these individuals.

Group	Grouping sera (Back group)					Auto	Red cell (Forward group)			
	Anti-A	Anti-B	Anti- A,B	Anti-A1	Anti-H		A1	A2	B	O
O	N	N	N	N	P	N	P	P	P	N
Bombay phenotype (Oh)	N	N	N	N	N	N	P	P	P	P

Blood grouping results from a group O and Bombay phenotype individual
Key:
P= Positive reaction
N= Negative reaction

ABO haemolytic disease of the newborn (ABO HDN). In ABO haemolytic disease of the newborn maternal IgG antibodies with specificity for the ABO blood group system pass through the placenta to the fetal circulation where they can cause haemolysis of foetal red blood cells which can lead to foetal anaemia and HDN. In contrast to Rh disease, about half of the cases of ABO HDN occur in a firstborn baby and ABO HDN does not become more severe after further pregnancies. The ABO blood group system is the best known surface antigen system, expressed on a wide variety of human cells. For Caucasian populations about one fifth of all pregnancies have ABO incompatibility between the fetus and the mother, but only a tiny minority develop symptomatic ABO HDN. The latter only occurs in mothers of blood group O because they can produce enough IgG antibodies to cause hemolysis. Although very uncommon, cases of ABO HDN have been reported in infants born to mothers with blood groups A and B.

Causes of ABO HDN

Environmental exposure: Anti-A and anti-B antibodies are usually IgM and do not pass through the placenta, but some mothers "naturally" have IgG anti-A or IgG anti-B antibodies, which can pass through the placenta. Exposure to A-antigens and B-antigens, which are both widespread in nature, usually leads to the production of IgM anti-A and IgM anti-B antibodies but occasionally IgG antibodies are produced.

Foetal-maternal transfusion: Some mothers may be sensitized by foetal-maternal transfusion of ABO incompatible red blood and produce immune IgG antibodies against the antigen they do not have and their baby does. For example, when a mother of genotype OO (blood group O) carries a fetus of genotype AO (blood group A) she may produce IgG anti-A antibodies.

The father will either have blood group A, with genotype AA or AO, or more rarely, have blood group AB, with genotype AB.

Blood transfusion: It would be very very rare for ABO sensitization to be caused by therapeutic blood transfusion as a great deal of effort and checking is done to ensure that blood is ABO compatible between the recipient and the donor.

Other moderating factors: In about a third of all ABO incompatible pregnancies maternal IgG anti-A or IgG anti-B antibodies pass through the placenta to the foetal circulation leading to a weakly positive direct Coombs test for the neonate's blood. However, ABO HDN is generally mild and short-lived and only occasionally severe because:

1. IgG anti-A (or IgG anti-B) antibodies that enter the foetal circulation from the mother find A (or B) antigens on many different foetal cell types, leaving fewer antibodies available for binding onto foetal red blood cells.
2. Foetal RBC surface A and B antigens are not fully developed during gestation and so there are a smaller number of antigenic sites on foetal RBCs.

Diagnosis: Routine antenatal antibody screening blood tests (indirect Coombs test) do not screen for ABO HDN. IgG anti-A or IgG anti-B antibodies are found in the pregnant woman's blood, they are not reported with the test results, because they do not correlate well with ABO HDN. Diagnosis is usually made by investigation of a newborn baby who has developed jaundice during the first day of life.

Treatment: Neonatal jaundice caused by ABO HDN is usually successfully treated with phototherapy, unless the ABO HDN is uncommonly severe. Treatment of moderate or severe HDN caused by ABO antibodies is similar to that for Rh disease.

Inheritance of ABO Blood Groups. The ABO blood group antigens are encoded by one genetic locus, the ABO locus which is located on chromosome 9 and has three alternative (allelic) genes- A, B, and O. Each individual has a pair of chromosome 9 (one inherited from each parent). A child receives one of the three genes from each parent, giving rise to six possible genotypes and four possible blood phenotypes. The O gene is an amorph (produces no antigenic products) and it is recessive to the A and B genes which are both co-dominant. Each individual inherit two ABO genes (one from both parents). It is the combination of these 2 genes that determine an individual ABO groups. The A phenotype is produced by the genotype AA or AO, the B phenotype by BB or BO while the AB and O phenotypes are produced respectively by the AB and OO genotype. The ABO blood group antigen do not exhibit a dosage effect (the reaction produced by a A or B person who has the genotype AA or BB has the same strength as a person who has genotype AO or BO. The genotypes AA/AO and BB/BO are only distinguishable by family studies and molecular genetics techniques (DNA analysis).

Blood group	Red cell antigen (phenotype)	Genes present (Genotype)
A	A	AA or AO
B	B	BB or BO
AB	A and B	AB
O	None	OO

Table: Possible phenotypes and genotypes of ABO blood group system

Genetics in transfusion medicine. Inheritance of ABO blood groups is based on Mendelian principles of inheritance. The basic principles is based on the following:

1. Each parent contributes 1/2 of the genetic information.
2. The genetic information is contained on chromosomes composed of DNA
3. Humans have 23 pairs of chromosomes (22 matched (autosomal) chromosomes and 1pair of sex chromosomes (females have 2 X chromosomes and males an X and a Y chromosome).

Genetic aspects of blood groups. Genes are the units of inheritance within the chromosomes. At each location, or loci, on the chromosomes there are possibilities of different forms of the genes, these different forms are called alleles. (For example the ABO Blood Group System, there are A^1, A^2, B, and O as common alleles. or allelic genes). When the inherited alleles are the same the person is homozygous such as OO, when the individual inherits 2 different alleles such as AO, they are heterozygous for both the A and O genes. On occasion we will see examples of dosage where some antibodies will react more strongly with homozygous cells than with heterozygous cells. For example, an anti-E that reacts as a 3+ with EE cells and only 1+ with Ee cells. A Punnett Square is used to determine the inheritance possibilities for a particular mating. For example if the mother's genotype (genes) are AO and the father's genotype (genes) are BO, you would have the following Punnet square possibilities. In this example there three heterozygous possibilities AB, AO, and BO and one homozygous possibility OO.

Blood group system	Common Genes	Located on Chromosome
ABO	A, B, O	9
MNSsU	M, N, S,s,U	4
P	P1	22
Rh	D, C, E, c, e	1
Kell	K, k, Kpa, Jsa,Kpb, Jsb	7
Lewis	Le, le	19
Duffy	Fya, Fyb, Fy3	1
Kidd	Jka, Jkb	18
Xg	Xga	X

Examples of Chromosome locations for common Blood Groups

Dad ➦ Mom ↓	B	O
A	AB	AO
O	BO	OO

Punnett Square showing the inheritance of ABO blood groups

In the above Punnett Square, the AB genotype will have both A and B antigens, therefore the phenotype are AB since both are expressed. AO and BO genotypes will demonstrate only the A and the B antigens respectively and therefore the phenotypes are A and B respectively. The individual that is OO will have the O phenotype. A and B genes are dominant, or co-dominant, and the O gene is recessive. The dominant genes will be expressed if present. Recessive genes will only be expressed if they are homozygous. Most Blood Group genes are co-dominant and therefore will be expressed if present.

Mitosis and Meiosis. Two kinds of cell division exist (mitosis and meiosis). Mitosis is cell division that leads to two identical cells that has the same number of paired chromosomes. (In humans there are 23 pairs or 46 chromosomes). Meiosis is the cell division that occurs when gametes (sperm and eggs) are formed and will not have pairs of chromosomes. (In humans there will be 23 chromosomes in the sperm that will match up with the 23 chromosomes in the egg when fertilization occurs to form the gametocyte.). The sex of the child is determined by the X and Y chromosomes. Males provide either X or Y chromosome and females provide only provide X chromosomes. Genes that are found only on the X chromosome are said to be sex-linked. Genes found on the other 22 pairs of chromosomes are autosomal.

Other Concepts Relating to Blood Group Genetics. Certain characteristics that make blood genetics useful for the field of human genetics includes the following; simple and unquestionable pattern of inheritance, possibility to test or determine the phenotypes readily, the fact that more than 1 allele occurring fairly frequently and the fact that environmental factors does not affect the expression of the genes. Some discoveries that were found in blood genetics include; multiple alleles seen in ABO system and linkage between the secretor genes with the Lutheran genes on the same chromosome

Linkage: Linkage between the secretor genes with the Lutheran genes on the same chromosome was already noted. We now know that the D gene is closely linked to the Cc and Ee genes. The most frequently inherited Rh positive set of genes is CDe and the most frequent Rh negative gene is cde or ce since d is an amorph. The MNSs genes are also linked, MS, NS, Ms, Ns leading to a difference between the expected frequency and the observed frequency.

Silent genes: Silent mutations are DNA mutations that do not result in a change to the amino acid sequence of a protein. They may occur in a non-coding region (outside of a gene or within an intron), or they may occur within an exon in a manner that does not alter the final amino acid sequence. As indicated already there are some amorph blood group genes that exist and lead to none expression of a blood antigen. The following are some examples of silent genes.

Blood group gene	Blood group system	Homozygous phenotype
H	ABO	O_h or Bombay
R	Rh	Rh_{null}
K°	Kell	K_{null}
Lu	Lutheran	Lu(a-b-)
Jk	Kidd	Jk(a-b-)
Fy	Duffy	Fy(a-b-)

Examples of silent gene phenomenom

Blood Group Nomenclature

1. Genes encoding the expression of blood group antigens are written in italics (or underlined if italics are not available). If the antigen name includes a subscript (A_1, the encoding gene is expressed with a superscript (A^1)
2. Antigen names are designated by a superscript or a number (eg, Fy^a, Fy: 1) are written in normal (Roman) script. Superscript letters are lowercase.
3. When antigen phenotypes are expressed using single letter designation, results are usually written as + or -, set on the same line as the letter(s) of the antigen: K+ k-.
4. To express phenotypes of antigens designated with a superscript letter, that letter is placed in parentheses on the same line as the symbol defining the antigen: Fy (a+).
5. For antigens designated by numbers, the symbol defining the system is notated in capital letters followed by a colon, followed by the number representing the antigen tested. Plus signs do no appear when test results are positive (K: 1), but a minus sign is placed before negative test results: K: 1, K:-1. If tests for several antigens in one blood group have been done, the phenotypes is designated by the letter(s) of the locus or blood group system followed by a colon, followed by antigen numbers separated by commas: K: -1, 2, -3, 4. Only antigens tested are listed.

Term Description	Correct Terminology	Incorrect Terminology
Phenotype	Fy(a+)	Fya+, Fy(a+), Fya(+), Fya+, Fya(+), Duffya+
Phenotype	Fy(a+b-)	Fya+b-, Fy(a+b-), Fya(+)b(-), Fya(+)b(-)
Antibody	Anti-Fya	Anti Fya, Anti-Duffy
Antigen	K	Kell (name of system)
Antibody	anti-k	Anti-Cellano

Term Description	Correct Terminology	Incorrect Terminology
Phenotype	K:1, K:-1	k1+, K:1+, K(1), K:(1), K1-, K:1-, K1-negative
Phenotypes	A Rh+, B Rh-	A+ (means positive for A antigen) B- (means negative for B antigen)
Phenotype	M+N-	M(+), MM (unproven genotypes)
Phenotype	Rh:-1, -2, -3, 4,5	Rh: -1, -2, -3, +4, +5, Rh: 1-,2-,3-, 4+,5+

Table: Examples of Correct and Incorrect Terminology

Public versus Private Genes: Public Genes are found in most of the population. In the Kell Blood Group System, the Kp^b is found in close to 100% of the population. Genes that are very rare are referred to private genes. Kp^a is very rarely found (2.3% in whites and almost never in African Americans) and therefore close to being a private gene.

Paternity Testing: Parental testing is the test carried out to determine whether two individuals have a biological parent-child relationship. A paternity test establishes genetic proof as to whether a man (putative) is the biological father of an individual, and a maternity test establishes whether a woman is the biological mother of an individual. Though genetic testing is the most reliable standard, older methods also exist and includes; red cell testing for the following blood group systems (ABO, MNSs, Rh, Duffy, Kidd, Kell), analysis of various other proteins and enzymes, or using human leukocyte antigen antigens (HLA antigens). The current techniques for paternal testing are using polymerase chain reaction (PCR) and restriction fragment length polymorphism.

Role of ABO blood groups in paternity dispute. Although blood types can offer clues about paternity (and were used for paternity tests until the late 20th century), it is not consistent enough for definitive paternity test results. Human blood types stem from dominant/recessive genes similar to Mendel's rule. Dominant blood types include A and B while type O is recessive. Alleles for type A and type B blood are co-dominant which means that, when both are present, the resulting blood type is AB. Type O is am amorph meaning that it's expression is suppressed if inherited along with dorminant A and B alleles. The table below illustrates possible blood types that can be expressed in a child from the mating of parents with blood types A, B, AB, and O (If the mother's and father's blood types are known). The inheritance of ABO blood groups is based on Mendel's rule. The application of Mendel's rule in paternity dispute is based on 2 laws:

1. For ABO blood group type to occur in a child, it **must have been inherited from one or both parents**. This law indicates that
    - Two blood group O parents cannot give birth to an A, B or AB child.
    - Two blood group AB parents cannot give birth to an O child.
    - A blood group A and O parent cannot give birth to a B child.
    - A blood group B and O parents cannot give birth to a group A child.

2. A blood group AB parent **cannot** give birth to a group O child.

   - An O child will have the genotype OO. This indicates that the child must have inherited an O from both parents.
   - In a mating between a blood group AB and group O parents, the AB parent must always contribute either A or B for every mating and the O parent will alway contribute O. When A and O is inherited from both parent, the child will be group A.
   - When B and O are inherited from both parents, the child will be blood group B.
   - A and B are co-dominant over O. When O and A or O and B is inherited from both parents by a child the A and B are dominant while the O (amorph) is recessive and not expressed.

Mother's blood group	Father's blood group				
	A	B	AB	O	
A	A or O	A,B or O	A, B or AB	A or O	Child's blood group must be
B	B or O	B or O	A, B or AB	B or O	
AB	A, B or AB	A, B or AB	A, B or AB	A, B	
O	A or O	B or O	A or B	O	

Table: Child's possible phenotype if the mother's and father's ABO blood types are known

Mother's blood group	Child's blood group				
	A	B	AB	O	
A	A, B, AB or O	B or AB	B or AB	A, B, or O	Father's blood group must be
B	A or AB	A, B, AB or O	A or AB	A, B, or O	
AB	A, B, AB or O	A, B, AB or O	A, B, or AB	A, B, AB or O	
O	A or AB	B or AB	Not possible	A,B or O	

Biological fathers's possible phenotype if the mother's and child's ABO blood types are known.

4. Anticoagulation and preservation in transfusion

An anticoagulant is a substance that prevents coagulation; that is, it stops blood from clotting. Some chemical compounds are used in blood transfusion bags to prevent blood from clotting. Various anticoagulant-preservative solutions have been formulated for better red cell preservation. Correct proportion of this anticoagulant to blood is crucial for effective anticoagulation.

Short-term Storage. Routine blood storage is limited to 21 days at 1°- 6°C when treated with acid citrate -dextrose (ACD), citrate phosphate-dextrose (CPD) or citrate-phosphate-double dextrose (CP2D) and 35 days when treated with citrate-phosphate-dextrose-adenine (CPDA1) **(5 weeks for whole blood and 6 weeks for RBC)**, and involves refrigeration but usually not freezing. There has been increasing controversy about whether the age of blood is a factor in transfusion efficacy, specifically on whether older blood directly or indirectly increases risks of complications. Studies have not been consistent on answering this question, with some showing that older blood is indeed less effective but with others showing no such difference; nevertheless as storage time remains the only available way to estimate quality status or loss is a first-in-first-out inventory management approach is standard presently.

Long-term Storage. Long-term storage is relatively uncommon, compared to short-term storage. Cryopreservation of red blood cells is done to store rare units for up to 10 years. The cells are incubated in a glycerol solution which acts as a cryoprotectant ("antifreeze") within the cells. The units are then placed in special sterile containers in a freezer at very cold temperatures. The exact temperature depends on the glycerol concentration.

Examples of commonly used anticoagulants in transfusions include:
Whole blood

1. Acid Citrate Dextrose (ACD)
2. Citrate phosphate Dextrose solution (CPD)
3. Citrate phosphate dextrose adenine. (CPDA-1)

Frozen red cell

1. High glycerol solution
2. Low glycerol solution

Citrate Based Anticoagulants. The commonly used citrate based anticoagulant - preservative solutions is: Acid Citrate Dextrose (ACD): The most widely used ACD solution has the following components;Trisodium citrate 22. Og, citric acid (monohydrate) 8.0 g, Dextrose (monohydrate) 24.6 g and distilled water to make upto one litre. Citrate Phosphate Dextrose Adenine (CPDA): For each 450 ml, whole blood, 67.5 ml of ACD solution is required.

Mechanism of action. Citrate is a calcium chelator. It prevents coagulation of blood as well as retards glycolysis. Dextrose improves red cell viability, provides energy for ATP synthesis and decreases rate of hydrolysis of phosphorus. Citric acid prevents glucose caramalization during autoclaving and provides optimal pH with citrate for red cells. ACD Solution preserves ATP level, helps maintain red cells shape, prevents haemolysis and maintains pH. Shelf life of whole blood or red cells collected in ACD and stored at 4°C ± 2°C is 21 days. Citrate phosphate dextrose (CPD) decrease acidosis and improves ATP synthesis. Shelf-life of whole blood stored in CPD at 4°C ± 2°C is 28 days. Citrate Phosphate Dextrose Adenine (CPDA) helps to maintain high ATP levels. Blood collected in CPDA is safe, well tolerated and has a shelf-life of 35 days when stored at at 4°C ± 2°C.

Optimal Additive Solution (OAS) for Preservation of Red Cells. Different types of additive systems are now in use to allow for the optimum preservation of red cells. These solutions contain saline, adenine and glucose and are added to the red cells after separating them from plasma. Blood is collected into a multiple bag system including one plastic bag containing 100 ml of optimal additive solution. After collection the whole blood is centrifuged and maximum amount of plasma along with the buffy coat is expressed into a transfer bag for further processing. Red cells are now suspended by running down the optimal additive solution (100 ml) to the main bag containing red cells. Currently available additive solutions are:

- CPD-SAG. CPD-SAG (Citrate phosphate dextrose - saline, adenine, glucose). In this besides CPD as the primary anticoagulant, a satellite bag contains the additive solution - 100 ml physiological saline with adenine and glucose. CPD-SAG causes undesirable amountof haemolysis.
- CPD-SAGMAN. (Citrate phosphate dextrose -saline, adenine, glucose, mannitol). In this the additive solution also has mannitol to prevent lysis of red cels. The 24 hr post transfusion survival is better with the additive.
- CPD-ADSOL. (Citrate phosphate dextrose Adenine- saline, glucose, mannitol. This additive solution is similar to CPD-SAGMAN but has greater quantities of glucose, adenine and mannitol. It has better red cell preservation and 24 hr post-transfusion survival. The shelf life with this solution can be increased to 42-49 days. Advantages of optimal additive solutions include:

Advantages of red cells additive solutions

- Provides red cells with nutrients that optimizes function
- Enhances viscosity of blood and ease of transfusion
- Optimize yield of plasma for fractionation
- Removal of unwanted buffy coat
- Optimum storage of red cells from 28 days (CPDA) to 35 days
- Avoidance of unnecessary plasma transfusion

Red cell lesions

The various changes that occur within both the RBC and storage media during ex vivo preservation have been collectively termed the RBC "storage lesion" These alterations can be extensive and are primarily classified into three broad categories: biochemical, biomechanical, and immunologic. Storage of red blood cells in preservative medium is associated with metabolic, biochemical and molecular changes to erythrocytes collectively referred to as the "storage lesion." In addition to corpuscular injury, bio-reactive substances including cytokines and lipids accumulate in the medium during storage. Storage related changes can have potential clinical implications for red blood cell transfusion. The term "storage lesion" has been traditionally used to describe the progressive degradation of red cell structure and function that occurs during conventional red cell storage. These changes include a reduction in red blood cell deformability, altered red blood cell adhesiveness and aggregability. Bioactive compounds with pro-inflammatory effects also accumulate in the storage medium. These changes reduce post transfusion viability of red blood cells. The clinical effects beyond post transfusion viability are uncertain, but a growing body of evidence suggests that the storage lesion may reduce tissue oxygen availability, have pro-inflammatory and immunomodulatory effects, and influence morbidity and mortality One of the most notable changes during RBC storage is the rapid fall in 2,3-DPG. 2, 3-DPG is an allosteric modifier of hemoglobin which plays a critical role in the release of oxygen at the end-organ. Levels of 2, 3-DPG has been shown to fall quickly during the storage of RBC, becoming undetectable within 2 weeks. This observation has raised concern that despite improved oxygen delivery with transfusion, stored RBCs may not release sufficient oxygen to the tissues. While biologically plausible, there appears to be little clinical consequence from this dramatic fall in the DPG as multiple authors have failed to find a meaningful effect from the transfusion of RBCs deplete in DPG. In part, this lack of affect may result from the quick recovery of 2, 3-DPG following transfusion. Normalization of 2, 3-DPG levels begins within hours of transfusion and is completely restored within 48 to 72 hours.

ATP reduction. The second well-described biochemical change of potential significance is a time-dependent reduction in intracellular RBC ATP. Due to its central role in cellular metabolism, adequate levels of ATP are essential for innumerable cellular processes. Examples include the maintenance of Na+-K+ ATPase activity, RBC membrane stability, glucose transport, oxidative stress defense mechanisms, membrane phospholipids distribution, and regional vasodilation under hypoxic conditions. Raat and colleagues have shown marked reductions in ATP levels during RBC storage. The fall in ATP levels appear most pronounced in blood stored for greater than weeks. While ATP depletion can result in the characteristic deformation changes seen with prolonged RBC storage. These morphologic changes are readably reversed with normalization of ATP levels. Importantly, these levels normalize quickly after RBC transfusion. Additionally, more gradual reductions in intracellular ATP results in erythrocyte shape changes, increased osmotic fragility, and decreased deformability levels do not appear to correlate well with these morphologic changes.

Red cells 2, 3 Di -phosphoglycerate level decreases. One of the most notable changes during RBC storage is the rapid fall in 2, 3-DPG. 2,3DPG is an allosteric modifier of haemoglobin which plays a critical role in the release of oxygen at the end-organ. Levels of 2, 3-DPG has been shown to fall quickly during the storage of RBC, becoming undetectable within few weeks. While structural changes are observed on the red cell surface as storage time increases, biochemical changes also occur intracellularly, with decreases in enzymes and stored energy concentrations that affect red blood cell function. The metabolite and enzymatic regulator of hemoglobin, 2, 3-diphsophoglycerate (2, 3 DPG), has been shown to decrease to near non-detectible levels within two weeks of storage. The decreased concentration in 2, 3-DPG leads to significant increases in hemoglobin's affinity for oxygen, which ultimately decreases oxygen delivery to the peripheral tissues upon re-infusion, because oxygen will not unbind from hemoglobin. The red cell devoid of 2, 3-DPG can recover its normal levels within 72 hours after infusion, and no irreversible effect in the function of the red cell has been observed. Given the delay to complete recovery of ideal enzymatic function and oxygen unloading in the peripheral tissue, the desired augmentation of oxygen delivery following transfusion is not immediate, but rather potentially delayed until 2,3-DPG levels are normalized.

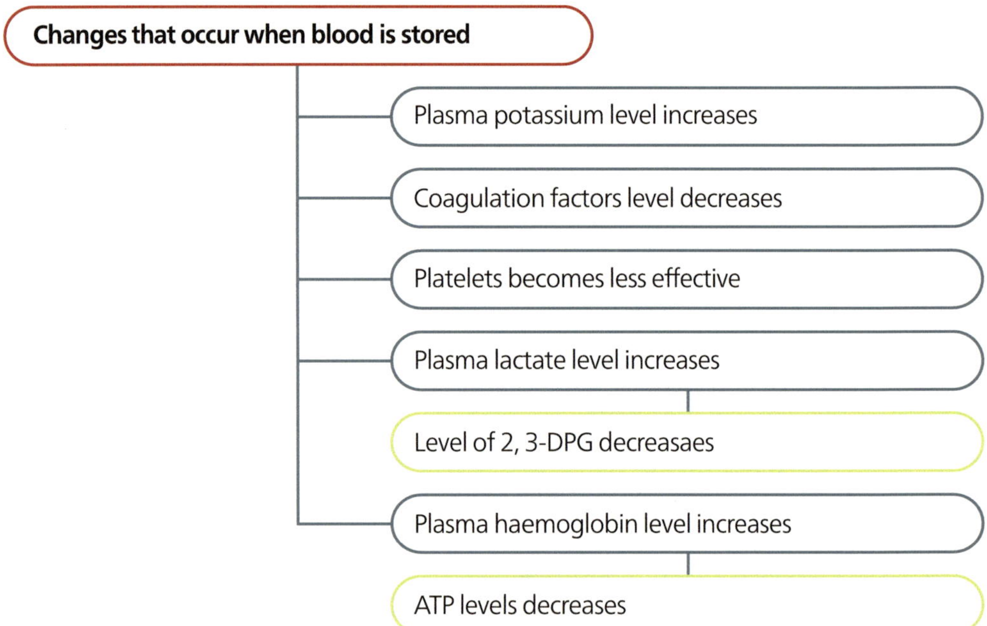

Days of storage	CPDA whole blood at day zero	CPDA whole blood at 35 days	Red cell concentrate at day zero	Red cell concentrate at 35 days
% viable cell 24 hours post transfusion	100	79	100	71
pH at 37°C	7.2	6.98	7.55	6.71
ATP level (% of initial value)	100	56 (± 16)	100	45 (± 12)
2,3-DPG (% of initial value)	100	<10	100	<10
Plasma potassium level (mEq/L)	3.9	27.3	5.1	78.5
Plasma sodium level (mEq/L)	168	155	169	111
Plasma haemoglobin (mg/dl)	1.7	46.1	7.8	658

Biochemical changes of blood stored in CPDA

5. Blood donation testing

A blood donation occurs when a person voluntarily has blood drawn and used for transfusions or made into medications by a process called fractionation. In the developed world, most blood donors are unpaid volunteers who give blood for a community supply. In poorer countries, established supplies are limited and donors usually give blood when family or friends need a transfusion or for commercial reasons. Many donors donate as an act of charity, but some are paid and in some cases there are incentives other than money such as paid time off from work.

Characteristics of a blood donor

1. Age: A donor is an adult male or female between the ages of 17-65 years

2. Frequency of donation: The interval between donations of a unit of whole blood is 16 weeks. The minimum interval is 12 weeks. Normally not more than 3 donations should be collected from a donor during any 12 months period.

3. Volume of donation: A donation of 450mls ± 10% collected into a blood bag containing plus 63 mL of anticoagulant is required to ensure that the final red cell component meets specification.

4. Weight: The minimum weight for donation is 50kg (7 stone 12lb). Donors less than 50kg are more likely to suffer adverse reactions (dizzyness and fainting) after a standard donation.

5. Haemoglobin level: The haemoglobin level should be determined each time a potential donor presents. The acceptable lower limit for venous blood are 135g/L for male and 12.5g/L for female donors.

6. All donation are tested for ABO and Rh D group. All units should be tested for Rh types (C, c, E, e) and for presence of alloantibodies to avoid the transfusion of potent IgG reactive atypical antibodies in donor plasma. Each donor unit that are group O, A and B should also be tested for the presence for high titre A and B haemolysin and labelled as high titre (HT) positive or negative. Only those that HT negative should be transfused against ABO blood group barrier.

Potential donors are evaluated for anything that might make their blood unsafe to use. The screening includes testing for diseases that can be transmitted by a blood transfusion, including HIV and viral hepatitis. The donor is also asked about medical history and given a short physical examination to make sure that the donation is not hazardous to his or her health. The amount of blood drawn and the methods vary. The collection can be done manually or with automated equipment that only takes specific portions of the blood. Most of the components of blood used for transfusions have a short shelf life, and maintaining a constant supply

Screening. Donors are typically required to give consent for the process. If a potential donor does not meet these criteria, they are deferred. This term is used because many donors who are ineligible may be allowed to donate later. Blood banks in the United States may be required to label the blood if it is from a therapeutic donor, so some do not accept donations from donors with any blood disease. The donor's race or ethnic background is sometimes important since certain blood types, especially rare ones, are more common in certain ethnic groups. Historically, donors were segregated or excluded on race, religion, or ethnicity, but this is no longer a standard practice.

Recipient safety. Donors are screened for health risks that might make the donation unsafe for the recipient. Some of these restrictions are controversial, such as restricting donations from men who have sex with men for HIV risk. Autologous donors are not always screened for recipient safety problems since the donor is the only person who will receive the blood. Donors are also asked about medications such as dutasteride since they can be dangerous to a pregnant woman receiving the blood. Donors are examined for signs and symptoms of diseases that can be transmitted in a blood transfusion, such as HIV, malaria, and viral hepatitis. Screening may extend to questions about risk factors for various diseases, such as travel to countries at risk for malaria or variant Creutzfeldt - Jakob disease (vCJD). These questions vary from country to country. For example, while blood centers in Québec, Poland, and many other places defer donors who lived in the United Kingdom for risk of vCJD, donors in the United Kingdom are only restricted for vCJD risk if they have had a blood transfusion in the United Kingdom.

Donor safety. The donor is also examined and asked specific questions about their medical history to make sure that donating blood is not hazardous to their health. The donor's hematocrit or hemoglobin level is tested to make sure that the loss of blood will not make them anemic, and this check is the most common reason that a donor is ineligible. Pulse, blood pressure, and body temperature are also evaluated. Elderly donors are sometimes also deferred on age alone because of health concerns. The safety of donating blood during pregnancy has not been studied thoroughly and pregnant women are usually deferred.

Obtaining the blood

There are two main methods of obtaining blood from a donor.

1. The most frequent is simply to take the blood from a vein as whole blood. This blood is typically separated into parts, usually red blood cells and plasma, since most recipients need only a specific component for transfusions. A typical donation is 450 milliliters (or approximately one US pint) of whole blood, though 500 milliliter donations are also common. Historically, blood donors in India would donate only 250 or 350 milliliters and donors in the People's Republic of China would donate only 200 milliliters, though larger 300 and 400 milliliter donations have become more common.

2. The other method is to draw blood from the donor, separate it using a centrifuge or a filter, store the desired part, and return the rest to the donor. This process is called apheresis, and it is often done with a machine specifically designed for this purpose. This process is especially common for plasma and platelets.

Site preparation and drawing blood. The blood is drawn from a large arm vein close to the skin, usually the median cubital vein on the inside of the elbow. The skin over the blood vessel is cleaned with an antiseptic such as iodine or chlorhexidine to prevent skin bacteria from contaminating the collected blood and also to prevent infections where the needle pierced the donor's skin. A large needle (16 to 17 gauge) is used to minimize shearing forces that may physically damage red blood cells as they flow through the needle. A tourniquet is sometimes wrapped around the upper arm to increase the pressure of the blood in the arm veins and speed up the process. The donor may also be prompted to hold an object and squeeze it repeatedly to increase the blood flow through the vein. A mechanical tray agitates the bag to mix the blood with anticoagulants and prevent clotting.

Whole blood. The most common method is collecting the blood from the donor's vein into a container. The amount of blood drawn varies from 200 milliliters to 550 milliliters depending on the country, but 450-500 milliliters is typical. The blood is usually stored in a flexible plastic bag that also contains sodium citrate, phosphate, dextrose, and sometimes adenine. This combination keeps the blood from clotting and preserves it during storage. Other chemicals are sometimes added during processing. The plasma from whole blood can be used to make plasma for transfusions or it can also be processed into other medications using a process called fractionation. This was a development of the dried plasma used to treat the wounded during World War II and variants on the process are still used to make a variety of other medications.

Apheresis, Plasmapheresis, and Plateletpheresis. Apheresis is a blood donation method where the blood is passed through an apparatus that separates out one particular constituent and returns the remainder to the donor. Usually the component returned is the red blood cells, the portion of the blood that takes the longest to replace. Using this method an individual can donate plasma or platelets much more frequently than they can safely donate whole blood. These can be combined, with a donor giving both plasma and platelets in the same donation. Platelets can also be separated from whole blood, but they must be pooled from multiple donations. From three to ten units of whole blood are required for a therapeutic dose. Plateletpheresis provides at least one full dose from each donation. Plasmapheresis is frequently used to collect source plasma that is used for manufacturing into medications much like the plasma from whole blood. Plasma collected at the same time as plateletpheresis is sometimes called concurrent plasma. Apheresis is also used to collect more red blood cells than usual in a single donation and to collect white blood cells for trnsafusion.

Recovery and time between donations. Donors are usually kept at the donation site for 10–15 minutes after donating since most adverse reactions take place during or immediately after the donation. Blood centers typically provide light refreshments or a lunch allowance to help the donor recover. The needle site is covered with a bandage and the donor is directed to keep the bandage on for several hours. Donated plasma is replaced after 2–3 days. Red blood cells are replaced by bone marrow into the circulatory system at a slower rate, on average 36 days in healthy adult males. In one study, the range was 20 to 59 days for recovery. These replacement rates are the basis of how frequently a donor can give blood. Plasmapheresis and plateletpheresis donors can give much more frequently because they do not lose significant amounts of red cells. The exact rate of how often a donor can donate differs from country to country. For example, plasmapheresis donors in the United States are allowed to donate large volumes twice a week and could nominally give 83 liters (about 22 gallons) in a year, whereas the same donor in Japan may only donate every other week and could only donate about 16 liters (about 4 gallons) in a year. Red blood cells are the limiting step for whole blood donations, and the frequency of donation varies widely depending on the type of donor and local policies. For example, adult men in Hong Kong can donate once every three months, women every four months, and youth aged sixteen or seventeen only every six months. In Canada and the United States it is 56 days for any type of donor.

Complications. Donors are screened for health problems that would put them at risk for serious complications from donating. First-time donors, teenagers, and women are at a higher risk of a reaction. One study showed that 2% of donors had an adverse reaction to donation. Most of these reactions are minor. A study of 194,000 donations found only one donor with long-term complications. In most developed countries, a blood bank is required to report any adverse effect/ death that might possibly be linked to a blood donation. Examples of complications associated with blood donatiion include:

1. Bruising of the arm from the needle insertion is the most common concern as well as bruising three days after donation.

2. Hypovolemic reactions can occur because of a rapid change in blood pressure.

3. Fainting is generally the worst problem encountered. The process has similar risks to other forms of phlebotomy.

4. Donors sometimes have adverse reactions to the sodium citrate used in apheresis collection procedures to keep the blood from clotting. Since the anticoagulant is returned to the donor along with blood components that are not being collected, it can bind the calcium in the donor's blood and cause hypocalcemia. These reactions tend to cause tingling in the lips, but may cause convulsions, seizure, hypertension, or more serious problems. Donors are sometimes given calcium supplements during the donation to prevent these side effects. In apheresis procedures, the red blood cells are often returned. If this is done manually and the donor receives the blood from a different person, a transfusion reaction can take place. Manual apheresis is extremely rare in the developed world because of this risk and automated procedures are as safe as whole blood donations.

5. A number of less common complications of blood donation are known to occur. These include; arterial puncture, delayed bleeding, nerve irritation, nerve injury, tendon injury, thrombophlebitis, and allergic reactions.

Storage, supply and demand. The collected blood is usually stored as separate components, and some of these have short shelf lives. There are no storage solutions to keep platelets for extended periods of time, though some are being studied as of 2008. The longest shelf life used for platelets is seven days. Red blood cells, the most frequently used component, have a shelf life of 35–42 days at refrigerated temperatures. This can be extended by freezing the blood with a mixture of glycerol but this process is expensive, rarely done, and requires an extremely cold freezer for storage. Plasma can be stored frozen for an extended period of time and is typically given an expiration date of one year and maintaining a supply is less of a problem. The limited storage time means that it is difficult to have a stockpile of blood to prepare for a disaster. The subject was discussed at length after the September 11th attacks in the United States, and the consensus was that collecting during a disaster was impractical and that efforts should be focused on maintaining an adequate supply at all times. Blood centers in the U.S. often have difficulty maintaining even a three day supply for routine transfusion demands.

Information on blood product label

- Component name and volume
- The blood component producer's name*
- The donation number*
- The ABO group
- The RhD group stated as positive or negative*
- The optimum temperature of storage
- The blood pack lot number*
- The date of collection
- The expiry date of the frozen component*
- Information on use over period after thawing

Labelling of blood products

Key: * = in eye-readable)

6. Apheresis principle and practice

Apheresis is a process in which the blood of a donor or patient is passed through an apparatus that separates out one particular constituent and returns the remainder to the circulation. It is thus an extracorporeal therapy. The process of apheresis involves removal of whole blood from a patient or donor. Within an instrument that is essentially designed as a centrifuge, the components of whole blood are separated. One of the separated portions is then withdrawn and the remaining components are retransfused into the patient or donor.

Method. Depending on the substance that is being removed, different processes are employed in apheresis. If separation by density is required, centrifugation is the most common method. Other methods involve absorption onto beads coated with an absorbent material and filtration. The process involve the introduction of whole blood into a chamber that is spinning, and the blood separates into components (P = plasma; PRP = platelet rich plasma; WBC = leukocytes; RBC = red blood cells) by gravity along the wall of the chamber. The component to be removed can be selected by moving the level of the aspiration device at the right. In this example, plasma is being removed. The centrifugation method can be divided into two basic categories; continuous flow centrifugation (CFC) and intermittent flow centrifugation

Continuous flow centrifugation (CFC). Continuous flow centrifugation (CFC) historically required two venepunctures as the "continuous" means the blood is collected, spun, and returned simultaneously. Newer systems can use a single venipuncture. The main advantage of this system is the low extracorporeal volume (calculated by volume of the apheresis chamber, the donor's haematocrit, and total blood volume of the donor) used in the procedure, which may be advantageous in the elderly and for children.

Intermittent flow centrifugation. Intermittent flow centrifugation works in cycles, taking blood, spinning/processing it and then giving back the necessary parts to the donor in a bolus. The main advantage is a single venipuncture site. To stop the blood from coagulating, anticoagulant is automatically mixed with the blood as it is pumped from the body into the apheresis machine.

Centrifugation Variables. The centrifugation process itself has four variables that can be controlled to selectively remove desired components. The first is spin speed and bowl diameter, the second is "sit time" in centrifuge, the third is solutes added, and the fourth is not as easily controllable: plasma volume and cellular content of the donor. The end product in most cases is the classic sedimented blood sample with the RBC's at the bottom, the "buffy coat" of platelets and WBC's (lymphocytes/granulocytes (PMN's, basophils, eosinophils/monocytes) in the middle and the plasma on top.

Types of apheresis

Disinfect, insert the cannula, pull out the cannula, dress the wound. The blue pressure cuff is controlled by the platelet apheresis machine in newer models. There are numerous types of apheresis. Blood taken from a healthy donor can be separated into its component parts during blood donation, where the needed component is collected and the "unused" components are returned to the donor. Fluid replacement is usually not needed in this type of collections. There are large categories of component collections:

1. Plasmapheresis. Plasmapheresis is useful in collecting FFP (fresh frozen plasma) of a particular ABO group. Commercial uses aside from FFP for this procedure include immune globulin products, plasma derivatives, and collection of rare WBC and RBC antibodies.

2. Erythrocytapheresis. Erythrocytapheresis is the separation of erythrocytes from whole blood. It is most commonly accomplished using the method of centrifugal sedimentation. This process is used for red blood cell diseases such as sickle cell crises or severe malaria. The automated red blood cell collection procedure for donating erythrocytes is referred to as 'Double Reds' or 'Double Red Cell Apheresis.

3. Plateletpheresis (thrombapheresis, thrombocytapheresis). Plateletpheresis, like it sounds, is the collection of platelets by apheresis; while returning the RBC's, WBC's, and component plasma. The yield is normally the equivalent of between six and ten random platelet concentrates. Quality control demands the platelets from apheresis be equal to or greater than 3.0×10^{11} in number and have a pH of equal to or greater than 6.2 in 90% of the products tested and must be used within five days.

4. Leukapheresis (white blood cells). Leukopheresis is the removal of PMN's, basophils, eosinophils for transfusion into patients whose PMN's are ineffective or traditional therapy has failed. There is limited data to suggest the benefit of granulocyte infusion. The complications of this procedure are the difficulty in collection and short shelf life (24 hours at 20 to 24°C). Since the "buffy coat" layer sits directly atop the RBC layer, HES, a sedimenting agent, is employed to improve yield while minimizing RBC collection. Quality control demands the resultant concentrate be 1.0×10^{10} granulocytes in 75% of the units tested and that the product be irradiated to avoid graft-versus-host disease (inactivate lymphocytes). Irradiation does not affect PMN function. Since there is usually a small amount of RBC's collected, ABO compatibility should be employed when feasible.

5. Stem cell harvesting. Cells are harvested to use in bone marrow transplant.

7. Blood component preparation

Preparation of blood component

With the widespread implementation of component therapy and the need to maximise the une of a donated unit to meet the clinical need of a number of patients, the demand of specific blood component has arisen. The aim of component therapy is to meet the specific deficiency in several patient using a unit of whole blood that hitherto would have wasted if given as a whole to a single patient. The production of blood component has been facilitated by the following:

1. Availability of large volume centrifugation techniques

2. The availability of sterile multi-blood packs

3. Availability of strile tube connecting devices.

Blood component are produced to ensure that a concentrated form of a clinically efficient product is available to patient and to ensure that patient is exposed to a relative small volume rather than the large volume of whole blood. It also facilitate the optimal storage (storage temperature and shelf life) of the different components of whole blood. Donated blood is usually subjected to processing after it is collected, to make it suitable for use in specific patient populations. Collected blood is then separated into blood components by centrifugation: red bllod cells, plasma, platelets, albumin protein, clotting factor concentrates, cryoprecipitate, fibrinogen concentrate, and immunoglobulins. Red cells, plasma and platelets can also be donated individually via a more complex process called apheresis. Blood separation is accomplished by centrifugation at high force (3-4000g). This result in the sedimentation of suspended solid particles (blood cells) from a liquid by gravity. The rate of sedimentation is a function of liquid viscosity, particle density, particle size, concentration of the solution (fraction of dissolved solids), and the force of gravity. This strategy maximizes the benefit derived from each individual unit while minimizing the risk to each recipient. The separation is achived using automated presses. The disadvange however is that there is the potential to infect several patients who are transfused with components produced from a unit of whole blood particularly if the unit is contaminated with a TTI'S. This risk is more pronounced with fractionated plasma products produced from a pool of several donors.

Collection pack. The blood component collection pack has a leucodepletion filter attached such that as the blood is collected into the primary pack all the leucocytes are selective filtered leaving the whole blood in the primary pack free of leucocytes. There are 2 types of pack configurations available; Whole Blood Filter (WBF) and the Bottom and Top (BAT) pack. Leukoreduction is a process in which the majority of white blood cells are removed from blood components. Reducing donor leukocytes helps;

1. Prevent non-haemolytic transfusion reaction

2. Prevent alloimmunization to HLA antigen

3. Prevent the transmission of leukocyte-borne viruses such as cytomegalovirus (CMV).

Whole Blood Filter (WBF). In this type of pack, the filter is close to the primary collection pack. It allow the whole blood to be filtered free of lleucocyte before it is separated into the various component. The advantage of this method is that the component produced from the whole blood from the primary pack does not need further leucodepletion. This method is commonly used to prepare red cell concentrate and plasma products. Red cell concentrate is produced by removing most of the plasma from the primary tube and an additive solution, formulated to support erythrocyte metabolism, is added to the remaining red cells. Example of additive solution designed to optimise red cell preservation include saline solution containing added adenine, glucose and mannitol (also called SAGM, SAGMAN, Adsol or optimal additive solution). The disadvantage of this pack type is that a significant number of platelet are filtered along with the leucocytes. Most modern leucodepletion filter selectively filters leucocytes withput removing platelet. An example of this type of filter is the Imuflex®-WB-SP. It is a quadruple blood bag system (CPD/S.A.G.M.) with an integrated leukocyte removal whole blood filter saving platelets, designed to produce three leukocyte-depleted blood components: red cells, plasma and platelets.

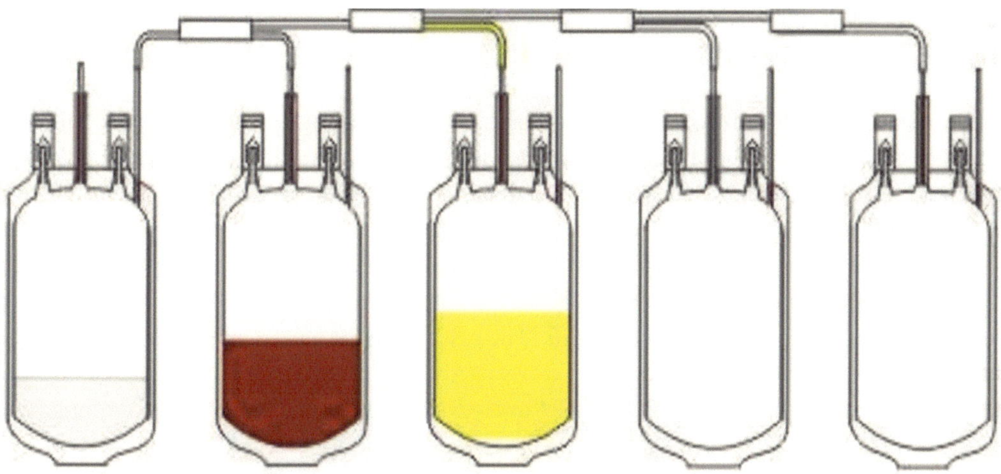

Figure: An example of a leucocyte depletion filter blood pack

Botton and Top (BAT) pack. This method is used for platelet preparation. In this type of pack there is tubing coming out from the top and bottom. Separation of component is done before leucodepletion to allow for platelet to be extracted. The disadvantage of this pack is that each component needs to be leucodepleted separately. This method can be used to prepare red cells, plasma and platelets.

Preparation of Red cell concentrate. If red blood cell and plasma components are required, then the donation is collected into a multiple bag system with an integral whole blood filter for leukoreduction. First, whole blood is filtered to to reduce the number of leukocytes. Next, the filtered whole blood unit is centrifuged using carefully controlled centrifugation speeds and temperatures to separate the red cells from the plasma. Approximately 190-260 mL of donor plasma is expressed into the first satellite bag (the maximum amount of plasma is removed). The plasma can be used to prepare Fresh Frozen Plasma (FFP), Frozen Plasma (FP) or cryoprecipitate and cryosupernatant plasma. Then AS-3 (Nutricel®) solution is added to the red cells to produce AS-3 red cells, LR (Leukocyte reduced by filtration). The AS-3 RBC LR unit is sealed and stored at 1-6ºC for 42 days. Cells are commonly re-suspended in SAG-M which has a shelf life of 35 days. The advantages of producing SAG-M red cells incude:

1. Adenine maintains red cell metabolism and promote survival during storage
2. Manitol help reduce the degree of storage –related haemolysis
3. SAG-M enhances the flow rate of blood close to that of whole blood.

Red cells intended for prolonged storage can be stored frozen in glycerol at -80°C. This method is useful for rare blood groups such as Vel negative, Fy(a-b-) and others as well as for patient with alloantibody to a high incidence antigen. The role of glycerol is as a cryoprotectant. It enters the cells and bind water molecule in the cell and prevent water loss. The glycerol is removed by washing when thawed prior to use. Thawed and washed red cells should be transfused immediately or stored at 4°C ± 2°C and transfused with 5 days.

Preparation of Fresh Frozen Plasma. Fresh Frozen Plasma is plasma that is frozen within 8 hours of collection. It may be prepared from a whole blood donation (by separating the red cells and plasma collected) or from an apheresis collection. Frozen Plasma is plasma that is frozen within 24 hours of collection. Leucodepleted whole blood donation is centrifuged (3-4000g) to separate red cells from plasma. Approximately 190-260 mL of donor plasma is expressed (automated press or plasma ectractor) into the first satellite bag. The RBC unit is sealed and stored at 1 – 6°C for its shelf-life. The plasma can be stored as FP or FFP that can be further processed to cryoprecipitate and cryosupernatant plasma using the attached satellite container. Plasma is stored frozen by the manufacturer at temperatures less than minus 20°C for up to 12 months. FFP can be stored at -18°C or colder for up to 12 months and thawed FFP is stored at 1-6°C for up to 24 hours.

Preparation of Cryoprecipitate. Cryoprecipitated Antihemophilic Factor (AHF, also known as Cryoprecipitate or Cryo) is made from one unit (225 - 250 mls) of Fresh Frozen Plasma. Cryoprecipitate is the insoluble portion of plasma that precipitates when a unit of Fresh Frozen Plasma is thawed between 1 - 6° C. The excess plasma is removed from the precipitate, creating Cryoprecipitate Poor Plasma (Cryo-Poor Plasma.). To make Cryoprecipitate, a full unit (225 - 250 mls) of Fresh Frozen Plasma with at least one integrally attached satellite bag is needed. When harvesting the Fresh Frozen Plasma from the unit of Whole Blood, allow the plasma to flow into one satellite bag. Seal off the two bags, but leave the line between the two bags open. Freeze the unit of plasma as specified in the procedure for Fresh Frozen Plasma. The plasma must be frozen solid before the subsequent steps to make cryoprecipitate are carried out. Separation of cryoprecipitate and cryoprecipitate-Poor Plasma. Allow the unit of Fresh Frozen Plasma to thaw at 1 - 6° C. This process takes approximately 8 hours. Harvest the cryoprecipitate using one of the two following methods. When the plasma becomes slushy, place the thawed plasma in a plasma extractor. Express the liquid plasma in to the integrally attached satellite bag. The satellite bag containing liquid plasma should contain 90% of the original volume of the Fresh Frozen Plasma or allow the Fresh Frozen Plasma to completely thaw. Centrifuge the FFP using a heavy spin. The cryoprecipitate will precipitate and adhere to the sides of the bag. Express 90% of the supernatant in to the attached satellite bag. Using either method, the Cryoprecipitate Poor Plasma is expressed into the satellite bag and the cryoprecipitate remains in the bag that originally held the Fresh Frozen Plasma. Expiration is one year from the date of phlebotomy (not from the date of preparation.) Freeze the Cryoprecipitate and the Cryo Poor Plasma within 1 hour of preparation. Both products should be stored at -18° C or lower.

Preparation of Platelet Rich Plasma. Platelet Rich Plasma is made from one unit of Fresh Whole Blood. To prepare Platelet Rich Plasma, a unit of Fresh Whole Blood with at least one integrally attached satellite bag is needed. The unit of Fresh Whole Blood should be maintained at 22 - 25° C and processed immediately in order to harvest viable platelets. Centrifugation at room temperature (20-24° C) is required to prevent the platelets from aggregating. A "light spin" is used to keep the platelets suspended in plasma. Approximately 190-260 mL of donor plasma is expressed through a filter into the first satellite bag to produce platelet-rich plasma (PRP). The RBC unit and additive pack are separated from the PRP and sent for preparation of AS-3 RBC LR. Following filtration, the RBC unit is sealed and stored at 1-6° C for 42 days. The PRP is centrifuged at room temperature using a "hard spin" to concentrate the platelets. All but approximately 50 mL of plasma is expressed into the second satellite bag. The supernatant (platelet poor) plasma is stored at temperatures of less than -20° C as Fresh Frozen Plasma, LR for up to 12 months. The plasma may also be shipped as recovered plasma for further manufacture.

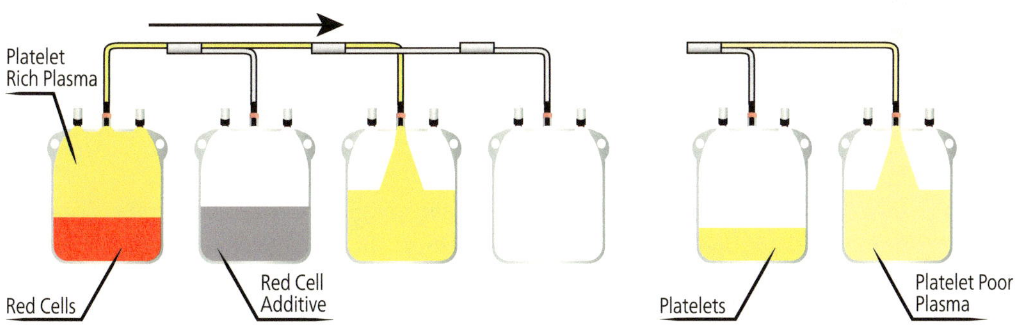

Leucocytes (Granulocytes). Leucocyte (granulocyte) blood products are required for the treatment of patient with haematological malignancies (leukaemia) as well as patients with chronic bacteria infection and life threatening septicaemia. A dose of about 2 x 10^9 cells is indicated.A fresh unit of whole blood contain about 1.5 x 10^9 cells. Leucocyte can also be collected using apheresis technique. Buffy coat collected durig the preparation of platelet concentrate can also be used if granulocytes are not available.

Component	Properties	Storage temperature/shelf life
Whole blood (leucodepleted)	Volume= 450mls, Hb= >40g/unit	4°C ± 2°C/ 35 days for in CPDA
Red cell concentrate	Volume = 280mls, Hb= >40g/unit	4°C ± 2°C /35 days for in CPDA and SAG-M
Saline washed red cells	Variable volume.Hb > 40g/unit.Residual protein < 0.5g/unit	4°C ± 2°C/24 hours
Thawed washed red cells	Variable volume.Hb ≥ 36g/unit	4°C ± 2°C/5 days
Platelet concentrate	Variable volume (160ml).Platelet ≥ 240 x 10^9/L	In platelet agitator/22°C ± 2°C
Fresh frozen plasma	CPDA plasma volume > 150ml. Separated and frozen with 8 hoursof collection. FV111c concentration >0.7IU/ml.	2 years at ≤ -30°C
Cryoprecipitate (pooled)	Each unit produced from 5 single unit of CPDA. Volume 150-250ml. Fibrinogen >700mg/unit and FV111c concentration < 350iu/unit	2 years at ≤ -30°C
Granulocytes (apheresis)	Variable citrated plasma volume. Granulocyte per unit >15 x 10^9/L	

Properties of blood components

Donor Safety. Single use kits - Apheresis is done using single-use kits, so there is no risk of infection from blood-contaminated tubing or centrifuge. Immune system effects - "the immediate decreases in blood lymphocyte counts and serum immunoglobulin concentrations are of slight to moderate degree and are without known adverse effects. Plasticizer exposure. Apheresis uses plastics and tubing, which come into contact with the blood. The plastics are made of PVC in addition to additives such as a plasticizer, often DEHP. DEHP leaches from the plastic into the blood, and people have begun to study the possible effects of this leached DEHP on donors as well as transfusion recipients.

Use in therapy. The various apheresis techniques may be used whenever the removed constituent is causing severe symptoms of disease. Generally, apheresis has to be performed fairly often, and is an invasive process. It is therefore only employed if other means to control a particular disease have failed, or the symptoms are of such a nature that waiting for medication to become effective would cause suffering or risk of complications. Apheresis techniques are used as a form of therapy in certain disease conditions.

Plasmapheresis: within the plasma are contained antibodies and antigen-antibody complexes that may contribute to the deleterious effects of autoimmune diseases. Removal of the plasma (and replacement with saline solution) will help to reduce circulating antibodies and immune complexes. In rare circumstances, excess blood proteins are present that may cause circulatory problems. Examples of these diseases include:

1. Waldenstrom's macroglobulinemia
2. Myasthenia gravis
3. Guillain-Barré syndrome
4. Hyperviscosity Syndromes
5. Paraproteinemia
6. Cryoglobulinemia
7. Goodpasture's syndrome

Plateletpheresis: In essential thrombasthenia, polycythemia vera and rarely in myeloproliferative disorders, the platelet count can be very high (thrombocytosis). Removal of platelets can help to avoid complications of thrombosis and bleeding.

Leukapheresis: in some cases of leukemia with very high white blood cell counts, removal of the excess leukocytes may help to prevent complications of thrombosis.

Stem Cell Harvesting: the small number of circulating bone marrow stem cells can be harvested to use in transplantation procedures.

8. Challenges of Blood transfusion in Africa

Globally, approximately 80 million units of blood are donated each year. Of this total, 2 million units are donated in sub-Saharan Africa, where the need for blood transfusions is great because of maternal morbidity, malnutrition, and a heavy burden of infectious diseases such as malaria. Alarmed by the chronic shortage of safe blood and blood products particularly in low- and medium-income countries, mindful that preventing the transmission of HIV and other blood borne pathogens through unsafe blood and blood-product transfusions requires the collection of blood only from donors at the lowest risk of carrying such infectious agents and recognizing that voluntary, non-remunerated blood donation is the cornerstone of a safe and adequate national blood supply that meets the transfusion requirements of all patients has lead to the World Health Assembly resolutions WHA28.72 3 and WHA58.13 4 urging member states to develop national blood transfusion services based on voluntary non- remunerated blood donation. The collection of blood only from voluntary, non-remunerated blood donors is an important measure for ensuring:

- The safety
- Quality
- Availability and accessibility of blood transfusion.

Innovative ways to recruit and retain voluntary donors in sub Saharan Africa include; celebration of the gift of blood donation, recognition of voluntary blood donors, increasing public awareness of voluntary non-remunerated blood donation, educating the public on the importance of regular voluntary non-remunerated blood donation, educating the public on the benefits of voluntary non- remunerated blood donation to recipients, promoting healthy living – nutrition, exercise and lifestyle and provision of non-cash motivation to encourage people to donate blood. Blood safety remains an issue of major concern in transfusion practice in most countries in sub Saharan Africa because;national blood transfusion services and policies are often lacking, appropriate infrastructure including trained personnel and financial resources are often inadequate to support the running of a voluntary non-remunerated donor transfusion service and predominance of family replacement and commercially remunerated blood donors, rather than regular benevolent, non-remunerated donors who give blood as a result of altruism. Despite recommendations that all blood donors should be voluntary and non-remunerated, replacement donors are common throughout sub-Saharan Africa (SSA). The primary steps of setting up a national blood transfusion programme should include; the enactment of a national policy for the blood transfusion service with time-bound programme, setting up of a centrally coordinated, structured and organized blood transfusion service for a country/state under a defined authority, development of a transfusion service based on an organized voluntary blood donor programme and the enactment of a national policy on the screening of blood for transfusion-transmissible infections (TTI'S) appropriate to the region, setting up an appropriate and evidence based use of available blood and blood products, employment and retention of qualified personnel to head and manage the blood transfusion service.

In many countries in sub Saharan Africa majority and sometimes none of these steps are in place. There is lack of political will and open-mindedness to innovative ways to improve supply and safety of blood from voluntary donors. The resultant effect of this is failure in the stewardship of blood and blood products with a resultant effect of a high incidence of transmission transmissible infection. Blood transfusions remain a substantial source of HIV and other TTI'S in sub-Saharan Africa especially among women with pregnancy-related complication and children with malaria and malnutrition –associated anaemia. The use of a culturally and socially adapted environment to make the gift of blood a pleasurable and festive experience can generate a new pool of blood donors and spontaneously repeating donations. Education is an essential part of a donor recruitment strategy. There are 3 basic goals for a donor education motivation and recruitment campaign;

1. To promote changes in the public's knowledge, attitudes and beliefs so that they understand why blood donation is a vital.

2. Life saving service to the community, to promote changes in people's behaviour so that they become willing to donate blood on a regular, voluntary basis
3. To advocate for non-remunerated blood donation to ensure that potential donors understand the importance of safe blood so that they do not donate blood if they are in poor health or at risk for transfusion transmissible infections.

There are several cultural and awareness –related challenges associated with blood donors and their distributions in sub Saharan Africa. Some controversy exists about there being insufficient voluntary donations. Countries in SSA need to find ways of maintaining sufficient blood supply from voluntary non-remunerated donors and improving blood safety from the available replacement donors. In brief, the reasons why replacement donors remain the main source of blood in SSA include;

1. It costs less to procure and fits well with the African culture of extended family support.
2. The mentality of altruism through the voluntary donation of blood is not as accepted in SSA like it is in most developed countries.
3. Only an insignificant number of eligible donors actually donate blood voluntarily in most sub Saharan African countries.
4. There is no optimistic feeling of altruism in most African settings. Several issues influence donor motivation and perceptions in SSA.

There are several prejudices and misconceptions which affect principle altruism in SSA; cultural differences and lack of information, fear of knowing one's HIV serologic status, fear of being infected with diseases, erroneous belief that donating blood can decrease one's libido, cause weight loss, cause high blood pressure or even lead to death. More effort is required in the drive for education, motivation and recruitment of regular donor. In most studies in Africa there is male gender dominance in blood donation programmes. The reason for this male gender predisposition to blood donation is based on;the erroneous belief that men are healthier than women, the general belief that women make monthly blood donations to nature through their menstrual cycle and other factors such as pregnancy and breastfeeding further restrict many women from donating blood in SSA. Interestingly this pattern seems to differ significantly from what obtains in some developed countries of Europe. In 2003 female blood donors represented 40% in Austria, 49·7% in France, 50% in Norway and 55% in Great-Britain blood donor population.

9. Blood donation and donor types

Blood donations are divided into groups based on who will receive the collected blood. An allogeneic (also called homologous) donation is when a donor gives blood for storage at a blood bank for transfusion to an unknown recipient. A directed donation is when a person, often a family member, donates blood for transfusion to a specific individual. Directed donations are relatively rare when an established supply exists. A replacement donor donation is a hybrid of the two and is common in developing countries such as Nigeria. In this case, a friend or family member of the recipient donates blood to replace the stored blood used in a transfusion, ensuring a consistent supply. When a person has blood stored that will be transfused back to the donor at a later date, usually after surgery, that is called an autologous donation. Blood that is used to make medications can be made from allogeneic donations or from donations exclusively used for manufacturing. The actual process varies according to the laws of the country, and recommendations to donors vary according to the collecting organization. The World Health Organization gives recommendations for blood donation policies, but in developing countries many of these are not followed. For example, the recommended testing requires laboratory facilities, trained staff, and specialized reagents, all of which may not be available or too expensive in developing countries. An event where donors come to give allogeneic blood is sometimes called a blood drive or a blood donor session. These can occur at a blood bank but they are often set up at a location in the community such as a shopping center, workplace, school, or house of worship.

Voluntary Donors

Safe blood donors are the cornerstone of a safe and adequate supply of blood and blood products. The safest blood donors are voluntary, non-remunerated blood donors from low-risk populations. Donors who give blood voluntarily and for altruistic reasons have the lowest prevalence of HIV, hepatitis viruses and other blood-borne infections, as compared to people who donate for family members or in lieu of payment. Despite this, family/replacement and paid donors, which are associated with a significantly higher prevalence of transfusion-transmissible infections (TTIs) including HIV, hepatitis B, hepatitis C, syphilis and Chagas disease, still provide more than 50% of the blood collected in developing countries. WHO advocates and recommends to its Member States to develop national blood transfusion services based on voluntary non-remunerated regular blood donation in accordance with World Health Assembly resolution 28.72, which was adopted in 1975. The key to recruiting and retaining safe blood donors is:

- Good epidemiological data on the prevalence (and incidence, where possible) of infectious markers in the general population to identify low-risk donor populations.

- Effective donor education, motivation and recruitment strategy to recruit new voluntary non-remunerated blood donors from these populations.

- A pleasant experience during blood donation, good donor care and effective communication between blood centre staff and blood donors are all important factors for the retention of safe blood donors.

WHO has developed a set of simple guidelines designed to assist those responsible for blood donor recruitment in resource poor settings to develop and implement a programme to improve communication with blood donors. These guidelines provide approaches for setting up a communication programme – organizing, collecting information, and developing plans; as well as providing ideas that individual centres might consider for recruiting, educating and retaining safe donors. Elements and activities in promoting voluntary non-remunerated blood donation include;

1. National blood donor programme for the education, recruitment and retention of low-risk blood donors, including community-based voluntary blood donor organizations and youth programmes;

2. Appointment of an officer responsible for the national blood donor programme to include donor education, motivation, recruitment and retention;

3. Training of donor recruitment and donor care staff in donor education, motivation, recruitment, selection and retention;

4. Development of partnerships with nongovernmental organizations, such as national Red Cross and Red Crescent societies, voluntary blood donor organizations, national service organizations and the media

5. Identification of donor populations at low risk for transfusion-transmissible infections and development of strategies to promote positive attitudes towards voluntary blood donation;

6. Development of donor education and recruitment materials;

7. Educational and media campaigns in workplaces, communities and educational institutions;

8. Establishment and maintenance of a database/register of donor records;

9. Guidelines and protocols for donor selection and deferral, donor confidentiality and donor care;

10. Guidelines on the management of donor sessions and blood collection;

11. Monitoring of TTIs in donor population;

12. Training of staff in pre- and post-donation counseling;

13. Donor notification and referral for counseling;

14. Monitoring and evaluation of the blood donor programme

Family replacement donors. Developing countries face considerable obstacles to ensuring a safe blood supply and safe blood transfusions. There is a tendency for developing countries not to have enough available blood so they depend on family blood donors. Family replacement donor is one who gives blood when it is required by a member of the donor's family or community. The disadvantages of this method of blood donation include; patients or their relatives are under intense strain when their relatives are on admission in hospital. Being expected to provide replacement donors puts additional responsibility and stress on them, there is undue pressure on members of the family to give blood, even when they know that donating blood may affect their own health or that they may be potentially at risk of transmission of transfusion-transmissible. It is difficult for a country's transfusion needs to be met solely relying on family replacement donations. The World Health Assembly recommended that reliance on replacement donations should be phased out due to their association with an increased risk of transfusion-transmitted infections. There is the challenge of transfusion need of recipient not being met because blood given may not necessarily be replaced in type or quantity. This leaves relatives who cannot find suitable donors with no other option than to seek commercial remunerated high risk blood donors. Blood donated by certain relatives particularly spouses of women of child bearing ages can put their wives/partners potentially at risk of producing antibodies to clinically significant antigen that the husband and the developing foetus may have but which the wife lacks.

Commercial-remunerated donors. Blood safety remains an issue of major concern in transfusion practice in most countries in sub Saharan Africa. This is further aggravated by the predominance of commercially remunerated blood donors, rather than regular benevolent, non-remunerated donors who give blood as a result of altruism. Previous reports in most countries in sub-Saharan Africa have indicated a high prevalence of transfusion transmissible infections among commercially remunerated blood donors. Blood and blood products from commercial remunerated donors are unsafe for various reasons;

1. They often come from the poorest sectors of the economy, may be poor in health.

2. Are more likely to give blood more often than recommended for financial gains.

3. Are also at a higher risk of being undernourished and having a transfusion-transmissible infection from high risk behaviours like maintenance of multiple sex partners, intravenous drug abuse and unprotected sexual intercourse.

Autologous Transfusion

Three main techniques for autologous transfusion are; Predeposit Autologous Donation (PAD), Acute Normovolaemic Haemodilution (ANH), and Perioperative Cell Salvage (PCS). Autologous blood transfusion is; extremely safe, crossmatching is not required, iso-immunisation to foreign protein is excluded, fear of transfusion transmissible disease can be ignored.

Some of the complications associated with allogenic blood are immunological, and are thought to be responsible for; increase in tumour recurrence after surgical resection, increased post-operative infection rates, increased progression of HIV infection and multiorgan failure. These sequelae can be reduced by the use of syngeneic or autologous blood. Experiences in many sub Saharan African countries has shown that autologous transfusion can help prevent the use of allogenic blood.

10. Advantages of autologous blood over allogeneic blood

The global medical community has increasingly moved from allogenic blood towards autologous infusion in which patients receive their own blood. The reasons for this movement include:

1. Providing safe blood for transfusion remains a challenge despite advances in preventing transmission of hepatitis B, hepatitis C, AIDS/HIV, West Nile virus(WNV), and transfusion-transmitted bacterial infection. Human errors such as misidentifying patients and drawing blood samples from the wrong person present much more of a risk than transmissible diseases.

2. Additional risks include transfusion related acute lung injury (TRALI), a potentially life-threatening condition with symptoms such as dyspnea, fever, and hypotension occurring within hours of transfusion.

3. Transfusion-associated immunomodulation, which may suppress the immune response and cause adverse effects such a small increase in the risk of post operative infection.

4. Other risks such as variant Creutzfeldt-Jakob disease (vCJD), an invariably fatal disease.

5. Allogenic blood shortages coupled with the challenges of an aging population and fear of being able to meet the future blood transfusion need relying solely on allogenic blood.

6. Another impetus for autologous transfusion is the position of Jehovah's Witnesses on blood transfusions. For religious reasons, Jehovah's Witnesses will not accept any allogeneic transfusions from a volunteer's blood donation, but may accept the use of autologous blood salvaged during surgery to restore their blood volume and homeostasis during the course of an operation.

Perioperative RBC salvage. Perioperative RBC salvage or Intraoperative bloods salvage (IBS) entails the collection and reinfusion of blood lost during or after surgery. Shed blood is aspirated from the operative field into a specially designed centrifuge. Citrate or heparin anticoagulant is added, and the contents are filtered to remove clots and debris. Devices used can vary from simple, inexpensive, sterile bottles filled with anticoagulant to expensive, sophisticated, high-speed cell washing devices. ABT seems a feasible, effective and secure method that could be implemented in sub Saharan African countries. It may be a solution to the problems of shortage of blood products and transfusion safety. However training and motivation are necessary for its successful implementation. Intraoperative blood salvage (IBS) is used extensively after blunt abdominal trauma, but when blood is contaminated by enteric contents its use has been considered contraindicated. Blood component sequestration refers to a specific technique in which blood is collected intraoperatively, but then subjected to various procedures, including apheresis, centrifugation and blood component separation. From a defined volume of whole blood, platelet concentrate, plasma and packed red blood cells are separated and then used as needed during the surgical procedure. The main difference between ANH or "whole blood sequestration" and blood component sequestration is cost. The latter requires sophisticated apheresis or autotranfusion equipment.

Indication

1. Cardiothoracic and vascular surgery, in which blood usage has traditionally been high. Several processes have been developed to assist in salvaging the patient's own whole blood in the perioperative setting.
2. Coronary artery bypass grafts (CABG).
3. Valve replacement.
4. Surgical repair of the great vessels.

Several medical devices have been developed to assist in salvaging the patient's own blood in the perioperative setting. These are used frequently; cell processors and salvage devices that wash and save red blood cells (cell washers or RBC-savers), direct transfusion of salvaged red cells and ultrafiltration of whole blood. Regardless of manufacturer, there are many types of cell processors. Cell processors are red cell washing devices that collect anticoagulated shed or recovered blood, wash and separate the red blood cells (RBCs) by centrifugation, and reinfuse the RBCs. RBC washing devices can help remove byproducts in salvaged blood such as; activated cytokines, anaphylatoxins and other waste substances that may have been collected in the reservoir suctioned from the surgical field. The various RBC-savers also yield RBC concentrates with different characteristics and quality. Direct transfusion is a blood salvaging method associated with cardiopulmonary bypass (CPB) circuits or other extracorporeal circuits (ECC) that are used in surgery such as coronary artery bypass grafts (CABG), valve replacement, or surgical repair of the great vessels. Following bypass surgery the ECC circuit contains a significant volume of diluted whole blood that can be harvested in transfer bags and re-infused into patients. Residual CPB blood is fairly dilute ([Hb] = 6–9 g/dL; 60–90 g/L) compared to normal values (12–18 g/dL; 120–180 g/L) and can also contain potentially harmful contaminants such as activated cytokines, anaphylatoxins, and other waste substances that have been linked to organ edema and organ dysfunction and need a diuretic to reverse.

Hemofiltration or ultrafiltration devices constitute the third major type of blood salvage appearing in operating rooms. In general, ultrafiltration devices filter the patient's anticoagulated whole blood. The filter process removes unwanted excess non-cellular plasma water, low molecular weight solutes, platelet inhibitors and some particulate matter through hemoconcentration, including activated cytokines, anaphylatoxins, and other waste substances making concentrated whole blood available for reinfusion. Hemofilter devices return the patient's whole blood with all the blood elements and fractions including platelets, clotting factors, and plasma proteins with a substantial Hb level. An example of whole blood ultrafiltration device in clinical use is the Hemobag. These devices do not totally remove potentially harmful contaminants that can be washed away by most RBC-savers. The key is that coagulation and homeostasis are immediately improved with the return of concentrated autologous whole blood.

Preoerative Autologous Donation (PAD). The risks of infection transmitted by transfusion of allogeneic blood components and association of allogeneic blood with increase in tumour recurrence after surgical resection, increased postoperative infection rates and multiorgan failure has resulted in growing patient demand for alternatives to allogeneic blood transfusion and an increase in the advocacy for;increased use of intraoperative autologous transfusion and continuing developments in surgical techniques resulting in reduced blood requirements. Preoperative autologous donation (PAD) is the most popular and widely used of the autologous options, which also include preoperative hemodilution and blood salvage. Interest in all forms of autologous transfusion, particularly PAD, mushroomed in response to the AIDS epidemic, beginning as early as 1983. By 1993, when participation in PAD peaked, approximately 6 percent of all blood collected in the United States was collected for autologous use. PAD entails repeated preoperative phlebotomy, 4 - 5 weeks before surgery, during which time 4 or 5 units of in-date blood can be collected with ease. This technique has several advantages; reduces exposure to allogeneic blood, it avoids many of the risks of transfusion, especially immunisation to red cell/platelets/ HLA antigens and the transmission of infection, the most obvious benefit of PAD for the donor/patient is freedom from concern about infectivity of the blood, assuming that the donor is not bacteremic at the time of donation and/or there are no clerical errors resulting in the inadvertent transfusion of the wrong unit of blood, the patient is also protected against hemolytic, febrile or allergic transfusion reactions; alloimmunization to erythrocyte, leukocyte, platelet or protein antigens; and graft-versus-host disease (GVHD). An additional benefit is that erythropoiesis may be stimulated by repeated phlebotomies, thereby enabling the patient to regenerate hemoglobin at an accelerated rate after surgery. PAD major drawbacks are that autologous blood is considerably more expensive than allogeneic blood. The use of pre-operative autologous blood donation (PAD) is not recommended unless the clinical circumstances are exceptional. Exceptional circumstances may include:

1. Rare blood groups where allogeneic difficult to obtain

2. Children with scoliosis

3. Patients at serious psychiatric risk if blood transfusion is thought to be likely to cover their elective surgery
4. Patients considered for the procedure must be candidates for elective surgery, where blood transfusion is expected to be needed.
5. The admission and operation days must be guaranteed.
6. Sufficient time to enable optimal collection of the blood must be allowed prior to surgery but should not exceed the licensed time for storing the collected blood component.
7. Sufficient time should be given from the date and time of the ultimate PAD collection prior to surgery for the patient to make a full circulatory and volaemic recovery.
8. Patient should be judged by a competent clinician to be able to tolerate the repeated loss of the predetermined volume of blood at each collection.
9. Patient should be provided with adequate information concerning the eligibility criteria for PAD and the reasons behind such criteria by the physicians providing the PAD service
10. Should be considered for supplementation with erythropoietin
11. Should present with the following haemoglobin (Hb) before embarking on PAD
    - Men, 110 to 145 grams per liter (g/L)
    - Women, 130 to 145 g/L
12. For each individual case, there should be a clear reason for preferring PAD to allogeneic blood as PAD is not indicated for most patients not fulfilling the above criteria.
13. PAD is not recommended for children younger than 10 years, mainly because of technical difficulties (large bore needle in veins of limited size) and it can be difficult to gain sufficient co-operation.
14. Candidates who meet the criteria for PAD but who are positive for relevant markers of transfusion-transmissible infection present safety issues for staff collecting and processing the donations and also potential for administrative and other errors.
15. Although iron therapy prior to PAD has little effect on subsequent transfusion needs in individuals who are iron replete, there are advocates of iron therapy during PAD on a priori grounds.

Acute normovolaemic haemodilution (ANH). Acute normovolaemic haemodilution (also called acute normovolaemic haemodilution, acute isovolemic hemodilution, acute normovolemic anemia, intraoperative autolgous donation, hemospasia and controlled exsanguination) is a form of autologous donation performed preoperatively in the operating theatre or anaesthetic area. It is usually restricted to patients in whom substantial blood loss (> 1 litre or 20% of blood volume) is predicted. Whole blood (1.0 - 1.5 l) is removed, and simultaneously intravascular volume is replaced with crystalloid or colloid, or both, to maintain blood volume. The anticoagulated blood is then reinfused during or shortly after surgical blood loss has stopped in reverse order of collection. ANH is associated with reduced surgical hemorrhage and reduced allogeneic blood transfusion. Acute, since it is conducted relatively rapidly; normovolemia, since the volume of the patient's blood is maintained normal by the hemodilution, which occurs as a result of the asanguinous fluid infusion. ANH enjoys considerable popularity in Europe, but has waned recently in the United States and Canada. It is probably one of the most misunderstood perioperative blood conservation techniques. When utilized correctly, ANH is an extremely helpful modality. However, when used incorrectly, it has limited efficacy.

Basic Principles of ANH. The technique essentially employs two steps. Firstly whole blood is collected from a patient via gravity into blood bags containing anticoagulant on the day of surgery before anticipated surgical blood loss. Secondly as blood is collected, asanguinous fluid must be infused to maintain normovolemia or euvolemia. This is accomplished with either crystalloid (normal saline, lactated Ringer's solution) or colloid (albumin, hetastarch). The development of hemodilution has a variety of implications for both the patient and the practitioner. Hemodilution is associated with; reduced blood viscosity, reduced afterload and increased cardiac output, the hemoglobin (Hb) concentration of the patient's blood is reduced secondary to hemodilution, any blood lost via the surgical field in the form of hemorrhage, contains relatively less Hb, other advantages of ANH include provision of a fresh supply of coagulation factors and platelets. Once reinfused, these procoagulant components are thought to augment a patient's inherent coagulation function and surgical hemorrhage might be reduced perioperatively.

Patient Selection. Not every patient is eligible for ANH. Not every surgical procedure requires ANH. Patients undergoing surgical procedures associated with minimal blood loss clearly will not benefit from ANH. In selecting patients for ANH, one should take into consideration the following; Patient's overall condition, presence or absence of anemia, presence of comorbid conditions and the type of surgery and the surgeon's skills.

Indications for ANH. Contrary to current thinking, any surgical procedure in which there is a potential for significant surgical blood loss is suited to ANH. This include; cardiac surgery - on of off-pump procedures, minimally invasive techniques, general surgery - major bowel or cancer resections, neurosurgery - major back procedures, orthopedic surgery - major back, joint replacement procedures, thoracic surgery - lobectomy, pneumonectomy, urologic surgery - prostatectomy, cystectomy, nephrectomy and vascular surgery including major reconstructive vascular surgery.

Contraindications. There are a few absolute contraindications to ANH, in which ANH cannot be used under any circumstances. These include; presence of severe sepsis, respiratory failure, myocardial pumps failure, hemorrhagic shock secondary to trauma and severe anemia. Less severe degrees of anemia become a relative contraindication to ANH. Patients with mild forms of anemia might be eligible for ANH; however, the volume of blood that may be collected will be less, since baseline Hb or hematocrit is reduced. Other relative contraindications include; severe respiratory disease, end-stage renal disease, coronary artery disease with or without a history of myocardial infarction (MI), congestive heart failure and history of a cerebrovascular accident (stroke).

Procedure

1. In order to perform ANH, blood collection bags that contain anticoagulant (CPDA) are needed.
2. Most practitioners perform ANH after the induction of anesthesia, prior to the commencement of surgery. Performing ANH prior to the induction of anesthesia, with the patient awake, is performed in some centers. Advantages include having an abundance of time and the ability to assess the hemodynamic consequences in the absence of any anesthetic effects.
3. An adequate site for blood collection must be planned for. Peripheral venous lines are popular, but are associated with problems; venous valves, tubing resistance, sludging, need for an intravenous catheter of at least 18 gauge size, arterial lines may be used - here, arterial pressure serves as a pressure head that pumps the blood into the collection bag. The disadvantage of arterial lines is that the ability to monitor arterial blood pressure is lost. Central lines remain the most reliable and effective means of blood collection. They may be placed anywhere, although internal jugular and subclavian lines are the most popular.
4. Calculation of the volume of blood to be collected. The following information should be collated to facillitate the calculation of volume to be drawn; the patient's weight (kg) is needed in order to calculate the estimated blood volume (EBV). This reflects the total circulating blood volume. The total circulating blood volume is approximately 70 mLs/ kg for females and 75 mLs/ kg in males. Therefore, a 90 kg male patient might be expected to have an EBV of 90 X 75 mLs = 6750 mLs. The baseline, initial or starting Hb concentration or hematocrit and the target Hb for hematocrit for ANH. This is typically a value that reflects a level of Hb or hematocrit that is safe and tolerated by the patient without adverse effects. The Volume of Blood that may be sequestered is calculated using the formula: ANH = Baseline

Hb or hematocrit - target Hb or hematocrit/ Average Hb or hematocrit X EBV. For example, take a male patient weighing 90 kg with a starting Hb of 14 g/dl. We elect that an Hb of 10 g/dl is a safe, end-point for ANH. The volume of blood that may be sequestered = 14-10/12 X 6750 = 2,250 mLs.

5. Standard blood collection bags contain CPD anticoagulant typically have tubing and a needle attached. The needle may be detached and various connectors welded or interposed in the tubing, so that they may connect to a port in the intravenous line.

6. Commencement of whole blood sequestration. The stopcock or port is opened and blood should be seen flowing into the blood collection bag tubing from the patient. The blood collection bag is placed on the ground or on an agitator.

7. Asanguinous fluid is administered concurrently with the blood collection process; asanginous fluid must be administered, in order to manintain normovolemia. ANH assumes that for each mL of blood collected, one mL of fluid is administered. Crystalloid is particularly unique, in that following infusion, a sizeable proportion of that volume moves out of the circulation into the perivascular spaces.

8. Storage of whole blood. Once a whole blood bag is full, it must be disconnected, the tubing sealed, the bag labeled and kept in a safe location at room temperature (20 degrees C) for up to 6 hours. After 6 hours, this blood product should be refrigerated at 4°C ± 2°C.

9. Reinfusion of whole blood. Timing of whole blood reinfusion is an important aspect in the blood management and conservation approach. Blood should be reinfused as surgical conditions dictate. During rapid uncontrolled surgical hemorrhage whole blood might be needed to restore blood volume. If surgical hemorrhage is slow and protracted, whole blood would be needed to restore Hb levels to normal and correct a surgical anemia. When whole blood is collected with ANH, each subsequent unit becomes progressively more dilute. When blood is reinfused, it is recommended that the last collected unit be infused first.

Monitoring. The following basic hemodynamic parameters should be monitored during the conduct of ANH; heart rate, systemic blood pressure, pulse oximetry, capnography (is the monitoring of the concentration or partial pressure of carbon dioxide (CO2) in the respiratory gases. Its main development has been as a monitoring tool for use during anaesthesia and intensive care). Capnography provides information about CO2 production, pulmonary (lung) perfusion, alveolar ventilation, respiratory patterns, and elimination of CO2 from the anaesthesia breathing circuit and ventilator, central venous pressure, pulmonary arterial pressure, cardiac output, and transesophageal echocardiography (TEE).

Efficacy of ANH: ANH efficacy may be defined in terms of an outcome variable or surrogate marker. Some examples include; the volume of autologous RBCs that was saved or "spared", the reduction in the allogeneic blood transfusion rate, the maximal allowable or actual volume of perioperative surgical blood loss andpotential or realized economic savings.

Challenges associated with ANH

1. Safety of the iatrogenic production of anemia: ANH produces an anaemic syndrome which often leads to the conclusion that it may be potentially unsafe in certain patient/disease categories, since tissue hypoxia or ischemia may result. The recommended target Hb for ANH ranges from 7 g/dl for the healthy patient to 10 g/dl for patients with associated cardiac, respiratory or neurologic disease.

2. Bleeding Diasthesis: ANH is also thought to contribute to a bleeding diathesis during surgery. Since coagulation factors are sequestered from the patient, subsequent surgical hemorrhage may be compounded by a dilutional thrombocytopenia or hypofibrinogenemia.

11. Transfusion transmissible infectious diseases

Blood donor testing

The donor's blood type must be determined if the blood will be used for transfusions. The collecting agency usually determines the ABO (A, B, AB, or O) and Rh D blood type (positive or negative) of the donor and will screen for presence of antibodies to prevent the passive introduction of donor alloantibody to patient. Such passively transferred alloantibody can react with patient red cells and other transfused donor unit if they contains antigen to which the alloantibody is specific. All group O donors should ideally be tested for the presence of high titre anti-A and B haemolysin. About 5-10% of all group O donor units have high titre anti-A and B. Transfusion of group O donor units containing high titre anti-A and B to non O patients (A and B) potentially cause life threatening haemolytic transfusion reaction. Ideally patient should receive blood of their own ABO blood group. However in most developing countries where blood is scarce, group O units (universal donors) can be transfused to non O patients (A,B and AB). The universal rule is that all O blood containing high titre anti A and B haemolysin should be reserved for group O patients and only units negative for high titre anti A and B should be given to non O patients. Testing for high titre anti A and B test is carried out as follows:

Testing for high titre anti A and B haemolysin

1. Centrifuge 5mls of donors whole blood sample and separate the plasma

2. Prepare 1:56 dilution of the donor plasma with saline
3. Prepare a 5% suspension of A_2B red cells in saline
4. Add 2 drops of donor 1:56 diluted plasma to 1 drop of 5% A_2B red cells suspension
5. Centrifuge lightly and observe for agglutination
6. Agglutination indicates presence of high titre anti A and B

The ABO and RH groups are determined using monoclonal anti A, B and D. The anti-A used must be capable of detecting the weaker groups of antigen A (A_x). A_x is a rare form of antigen A that show a weak expression of the A antigen. In hospitals where only forward ABO groups are done and where the Anti-A used for forward grouping is not capable of detecting $A_{x,}$ these patients may be erronously grouped as O. If such donor units are transfused to group O patients with potent IgG anti-A, there is the risk of increased red cell destruction. The anti-D used for Rh D grouping must be capable of also detecting the weaker form of the D antigen as well as partial (variant) D types (DIV, DV and DVI). For example if partial D type (DVI) is wrongly grouped as Rh negative and transfused to Rh negative women of child bearing age, they potentially can produce immune anti-D which can potentially cause HDFN in subsequent D positive pregnancies. Some selected units may also be tested for CMV antibody as well as Rh and Kell phenotype to enable the selection of appriopriate units for patients that require CMV negative units (HIV, fetus requiring Intra Uterine Transfusion and immunosuppressed patients), haemoglobin S negative units (sickle cell negative red cells for sickle cell patients neonates and patients with certain other haematological conditions) as well as those patients that have developed alloantibodies as a result of previous transfusion and pregnancy and requires specific antigen negative red cells; Rh (C, c, E, e), M, S, s, Duffy (Fy^a and Fy^b), Kidd (Jk^a and Jk^b) and Kell negative units. Some units may also need to be irradiated. All blood for neonatal use and for haematology patient on purine analogues will need irradiated blood products to prevent the possibility of graft versus host disease (GvHD). In most developed countries there is universal leucodepletion of all donor units by using leucodepletion filter. Leucodepletion can help protect donated blood from CMV infection.

More testing, including a crossmatch, is usually done before a transfusion. Group O is often cited as the "universal donor" but this only refers to red cell transfusions. For plasma transfusions the system is reversed and AB is the universal donor type. WHO recommends that, at minimum, all donated blood to be used for transfusion should be screened for HIV, hepatitis B, hepatitis C and syphilis? Complete and accurate data on the screening of donated blood are not available from many developing countries because; blood services are not coordinated, many countries do not have reliable testing systems because of staff shortages; lack of basic laboratory services, poor quality test kits or their irregular supply. Most blood is tested for diseases, including some STDs. The tests used are high-sensitivity screening tests and no actual diagnosis is made. The blood is usually discarded if these tests are positive, but there are some exceptions, such as autologous donations. The donor is generally notified of the test result. Donated blood is tested by many methods, but the core tests recommended by the World Health Organization are these four; Hepatitis B Surface Antigen (HbsAg), Antibody to Hepatitis C Virus (HCV), Antibody to HIV, usually subtypes 1 and 2 and Serologic test for Syphilis. A variety of other tests for transfusion transmitted infections are often used based on local requirements. Additional testing is expensive, and in some cases the tests are not implemented because of the cost. These additional tests include other infectious diseases such as West Nile Virus. Sometimes multiple tests are used for a single disease to cover the limitations of each test. For example, the HIV antibody test will not detect a recently infected donor, so some blood banks use a p24 antigen or HIV nucleic acid test in addition to the basic antibody test to detect infected donors during that period. Cytomegalovirus is a special case in donor testing in that many donors will test positive for it. The virus is not a hazard to a healthy recipient, but it can harm infants and other recipients with weak immune systems. The potential risk of TTI's can be reduced by the following measures:

1. A strict donor selection process
2. Improved donor testing methods using Nucleic Acid Testing (NAT-PCR)
3. Reducing inappriopriate transfusion by using the indication coding system
4. Increased use of alternatives to allogeneic blood (autologous transfusion, oral and intravenous iron as well as erythropoietin treatment).
5. Using infective agent reduction and viral inactivation techniques such as leucodepletion and methylene blue treatment and solvent-detergent treatment of plasma products.

Syphilis. Through the years, a great controversy had arisen over the need for syphilis testing of blood donors. Although the American Association of Blood Banks (AABB) initially dropped its recommendation that donors be tested for syphilis in 1978, the Food and Drug administration (FDA) of the United States keeps on this requirement. This decision was reinforced by the HIV epidemic. It is now recommended in most countries that surrogate testing including syphilis should be done to prevent those at risk from donating blood. However cost of transfusion- transmissible infection testing is a major challenge to the provision of safe blood and blood products in sub Saharan Africa. Treponemics, non treponemics, immunochromatographics or nucleic acid testing is affordable and can significantly contribute to blood transfusion safety as in most resource poor countries. Most contries uses the TPHA test for syphilis.

Malaria. Malaria is endemic in many tropical and subtropical regions of the world. Over 300 million people worldwide are infected, with 1 million fatalities annually. The causative agent of malaria is Plasmodium, which has 4 species, namely the following; Plasmodium falciparum, P. Malariae, P. Ovale and P. Vivax. Malaria is spread mainly through mosquito bites, but cases have been reported about transfusion-transmitted malaria. The risk of spread depends on the prevalence of the disease. In highly endemic areas prevalence of malaria is high among donors. In areas with low malara prevalence, donors who are recent travelers or who are immigrants from endemic areas are potential sources for transmission of the infection. The FDA recommends that donors with a history of malaria be deferred for 3 years after becoming asymptomatic. Provided that donors are asymptomatic, travelers to endemic areas are deferred for 1 year in most developed countries. Malaria is a real public health problem in Africa. In spite of this fact, there is no consensus for measures to prevent post-transfusion malaria in endemic areas. Malaria remains a rare but serious complication of transfusion because of the asymptomatic persistence of parasites in some donors. In non-endemic countries, the predominant strategy of deferral or cellular component discard from "high risk" donors is effective in minimizing the incidence but wasteful. In endemic countries where recipients are commonly immune, transfusion strategies focus on chemoprophylaxis for the donor and recipient or ensure that blood collected in highly endemic regions is not transfused to patients from areas of low endemicity. Cheap and inexpensive giemsa-stained blood films examination can be a readily available minimal alternative to other more expensive malaria screening methods particularly in low income countries in sub Saharan Africa. The risk of introducing an unsafe-potentially dangerous transfusion-transmitted malaria is often lethal particularly Plasmodium falciparum infection. The administration of antimalarials to transfusion recipients may help to prevent transmission. Nonetheless, no matter what strategy is adopted, it is likely that cases of transfusion-transmitted malaria may still occur, so malaria must always be considered in any patient with a febrile illness post-transfusion.

HCV. Screening donated blood for hepatitis C virus (HCV) is important for HCV prevention and is routinely practiced in most countries. The risk of HCV transmission through the transfusion of unscreened blood has led to be the systematic screening of blood donors in many settings in sub Saharan Africa. HCV is recognized as the primary cause worldwide of transfusion-associated non-A-non-B viral hepatitis and is endemic in West Africa. HCV antibody is detected 70 days after infection. NAT testing can detect HCV viral RNA in infected donors as low as 10 days following infection. Its use can significantly reduce the risk of the window phase. HCV is a spherical, enveloped, single-stranded RNA virus belonging to the Flaviviridae family. The World Health Organization (WHO) estimates 170 million individuals worldwide are infected with HCV. HCV is predominantly transmitted by means of percutaneous exposure to infected blood. In developed countries, most new HCV infections are related to intravenous drug abuse and are found because of intensive screening. The screening of blood donors for the HCV antibody has decreased the risk of transfusion-associated HCV infection significantly. The use of polymerase chain reaction (PCR) in some countries has further reduced the risk of acquiring HCV from blood transfusions to 1 in 230,000 donations. Blood transfusion was a major risk for acute HCV infection in the past. The screening of blood donors by donor history and elevated serum alanine aminotransferase (ALT) caused a striking reduction of non-A, non-B posttransfusion hepatitis. Detection of HCV infection by MP-NAT is the standard of care in most developed countries for the detection of the viral RNA. The HCV MP-NAT has reduced the window period for the detection of infection by 80-90%

when compared with HCV testing by detection of antibodies. Hepatitis C–positive donors are permanently deferred from blood donations.

HIV. HIV is a member of the Lentivirus family of retroviruses. It is the causative agent of acquired immunodeficiency syndrome (AIDS). Blood transfusion continues to be an important route of transmission of HIV particularly in developing countries among young children and pregnant women following transfusion for malaria associated anaemia and pregnancy-related complications. HIV antibody is detectable 40 days after infection. HIV RNA is detectable in blood after 15-20 days after infection. HIV antigen is detectable by 20 days post infection. Most countries now use dual HIV antibody/antigen test to further prevent the likelihood of transfusing HIV infected unit during the window phase of infection. The window phase is the period between infection until the first detectable marker is observed. However during this period, antibody screen is negative but the blood is potentially infective. Most HIV antibody test are ELISA (enzyme linked immunosorbent assay). NAT testing has been introduced in most countries for the direct detection of the HIV virus by specific nucleic acid amplification. This method can detect infection in blood donors significantly earlier in the window phase of infection than conventional serological assays. Examples of NAT test includes the TMA or Transcription Mediated Amplification (sample preparation, amplification and detection phases) and the PCR test (Polymerase Chain Reaction). The PCR test involves 4 major steps (Extraction, reverse transcription, amplification and detection). HIV-positive individuals are permanently deferred from blood donations.

HBV. HBV is a Hepadna virus that is capable of withstanding extreme temperatures and humidity. Hepatitis B is a worldwide healthcare problem, especially in developing areas. An estimated one third of the global population has been infected with HBV. Approximately 300 million people are lifelong carriers, and only 2% spontaneously seroconvert annually. HBV is transmitted hematogenously and sexually. The outcome of this infection ranges from complicated viral-host interactions that result in either an acute symptomatic disease, an asymptomatic disease, or a chronic carrier state. Later consequences are cirrhosis and the development of hepatocellular carcinoma (HCC). Hepatitis B surface antigen (HBsAg) detection is a routine in many parts of the world. However, some chronic carriers have such a low viral load that screening by HBsAg may not be able to detect the infection in the donor. To overcome this obstacle, many blood banks in several countries also attempt to detect antibody against the hepatitis B core antigen (anti-HBcAg or anti-HBc). The core antibody develops early in the course of the infection and remains positive even in patients with low-level viremia. NAT has tremendous potential in this area of transfusion medicine. Hepatitis B–positive donors are permanently deferred from giving blood. The HBV is highly contagious and transmission of HBV occurs via percutaneous or permucosal routes, and infective blood or body fluids introduced at birth, through sexual contact or by contaminated needles. Transfusion-transmitted HBV infection is increasingly becoming a major mode of transmission of HBV in high-prevalence areas in sub-Saharan Africa.

Cytomegalovirus. Cytomegalovirus (CMV) belongs to the herpes group of viruses. The organism's transmission is prevented by transfusing leukocyte-depleted blood products, which is consistent with the fact that CMV is a leukocyte-associated pathogen. The organism is a major concern when it comes to transfusing immunocompromised hosts. For this reason, all immunocompromised patients are given CMV-seronegative or leukocyte-depleted blood products.

12. Complications of blood transfusion

Transfusions of blood products are associated with several complications, which can be broadly categorized as immunologic transfusion reactions, or non-immunologic complications. Immunologic reactions include acute hemolytic reactions, delayed hemolytic reactions, febrile non-hemolytic reactions, allergic reactions, and post transfusion purpura (PTP). Non-immunologic complications include infections; transfusion associated cardiac overload (TACO), transfusion-related acute lung injury (TRALI), and hypothermia and transfusion transmissible infections (TTI'S). The risks of complications usually increase with increasing frequency and volume of transfusion.

Immunologic reactions

Acute haemolytic reactions. Acute haemolytic reactions occur with transfusion of red blood cells, and occur in about 0.016 percent of transfusions, with about 0.003 percent being fatal. This is usually due to ABO incompatibility between donor and recipients (for example a group A and B red cells given in error to an O recipient) resulting in the destruction of donor red cells by the group specific antibodies in the recipient. Usually this type of reaction occurs as a result of clerical error resulting from a sample mismatch at venepuncture or patient misidentification during the bed side check. The anti A and /or anti B in the recipient plasma often react with A or B antigens on the donors red cells resulting in intravascular haemolysis. Signs and symptoms usually occur after 5-10 mls of donor red cells have been transfused. Patients may feel agitated, flushed, feel pain in the venepuncture site, show pain in the abdomen. Other symptoms include; fever, hypotension chills, chest pain, back pain, bleeding from wound and venepuncture site, increased heart rate and shortness of breath, haemglobinuria, disseminated intravascular coagulation and acute renal failure. It is often important to note that another patient may be potentially at risk due to a reciprocal error. When suspected, transfusion should be stopped immediately, and blood sent for tests to evaluate for presence of hemolysis. Laboratory investigation should include; a fall in haemoglobin, rise in lactate dehydrogenase, positive direct antihuman globulin test (DAT) and a serological incompatibility should be observed between the post transfusion sample from the patient and the donor sample. Treatment is usually supportive and is aimed at preventing kidney injury resulting from the deposition of haemoglobin pigment on the kidney resulting in nephropathy.

Delayed haemolytic reactions. Delayed haemolytic transfusion reaction occurs more frequently (about 0.025 percent of transfusions) and is due to the same mechanism as in acute haemolytic reactions. Patients in most cases may have been previously immunised by a red cell antigen or by a previous pregnancy and the antibody may have fallen to an undetectable level. If the antigen is encountered again in a subsequently transfusion, the subsequent encounter can become a booster dose and the antibody level is boosted by this secondary immune response causing extravascular haemolysis. A delayed haemolytic reaction occurs when a patient develops an antibody directed against an antigen on transfused red cells. The antibody may cause shortened red cell survival, with clinical features of fever, jaundice and lower than expected haemoglobin following transfusion. Most delayed haemolytic reactions produce few symptoms and may go unrecognised. Delayed haemolytic reaction can be minimized by performing an antibody screen as part of pre-transfusion testing for all prospective transfusion recipients. When an antibody is detected, it must be identified and appropriate antigen negative blood provided. Sometimes antibodies fall below detectable limits and may not be detected by pretransfusion testing. There may also be a rise in the LDH level, positive post transfusion DAT, spherocytes in the peripheral blood film, incompatible IAT post transfusion crossmatch and antibody screen and fever and mild to severe renal failure. Treatment is generally not needed, but due to the presence of recipient antibodies, future compatibility may be affected.

Non-haemolytic febrile transfusion reactions (NHFTR). Non-haemolytic febrile transfusion reactions are due to anti-leucocyte antibodies in a previously transfused or pregnant patient reacting with the leucocytes in donor unit. It can also arise from the release of cytokines in stored platelets causing an inflammatory response in the patient. Occur in 1-2% of recipients. Symptoms include fever, shivering and general discomfort associated with less that 1°C rise in baseline temperature or <38 °C is generally observed. Patient must be monitored for escalating symptoms. A fever of > 1°C above the baseline or > 38 °C particularly when there is no apparent pre-existing infective cause is a trigger to stop the transfusion. Transfusion of leucodepleted unit minimizes the incidence of NHFTR which occur in 1% of all transfusion and in up to 45% of multi transfused patients who receive non-leucodepleted units. Management includes slowing the transfusion and giving 1g paracetamol. Perform more frequent observations and monitor patient for additional /escalating symptoms. If symptoms do not resolve after 30 minutes with these measures, stop the transfusion. A febrile reaction in a neutropenic patient should have a blood culture and intravenous meropenim started.

Allergic reactions. Urticaria reaction occurs as results of immediate (class1) hypersensitivity reaction resulting from IgE antibodies in patients reacting with transfused plasma protein in the donor. Urticaria reaction occurs commonly with FFP and platelet transfusion. Symptoms include urticaria, pruritis, and wheal and flare reaction and rashes usually occur within minutes of the start of the transfusion and may sometimes be delayed. Swelling of lips or mouth or severe hypotension indicates a more serious reaction and may proceed to anaphylactic shock. A few patients that are IgA deficient develop antibodies to IgA. Some of these patients (0.13%) experience severe anaphylaxis if exposed to IgA-containing blood in donor unit. Signs and symptoms include hypotension, dyspnoea, stridor, wheezing, angioedema, pruritis and urticaria. Laboratory investigation should include the determination of IgA and anti IgA level. Mast cell tryptase may be useful in differentiating between allergic and anaphylactic reactions. Blood gases and chest X-ray may be required if patient becomes hypoxic.

Transfusion associated graft versus host disease (TGVHD). Engraftment of donor lymphocytes into an immunocompromised patient can result in TGVHD. The donor leukocyte (graft) often proliferates in the host patient causing a rejection of a variety of the host tissues. It often occurs when non-irradiated red cell or platelet units are transfused to certain immunocompromised patients such as those treated with purine analogues such as; recipients of blood from biologically related (directed) or HLA matched donors', Intrauterine and all subsequent transfusion and exchange transfusion recipients, patients with congenital cellular immunodeficiency, patients receiving granulocyte transfusions, patients with Hodgkin's Disease, peripheral blood stem cell (PBSC) and bone marrow transplant recipients, patients with aplastic anaemia receiving immunosuppressive therapy and patients treated with purine analogue drugs such as fludarabine. TAGVD can be minimised by transfusing such patients with gamma irradiated red cells, whole blood, granulocytes and platelet. Irradiation inactivates donor leucocytes and thus helps minimize the incidence of TGVHD. Signs and symptoms include; fever, skin rash, diarrhoea, hepatorenal failure and pancytopenia (fall in haemoglobin, white cells and platelet count occurring 4-30 days after transfusion). Laboratory investigation will show pancytopenia on a full blood count, impaired renal and liver function test and skin biopsy and PCR may demonstrate the presence of donor DNA.

Post transfusion purpura (PTP). Post transfusion purpura is rare immune-mediated thrombocytopenias often occurring in parous women. Severe thrombocytopenia and bleeding usually develop 5-9 days post transfusion. This complication often occurs after transfusion containing platelets that express a surface protein HPA-1a. Recipients who lack this protein develop sensitization to this protein from prior transfusions, and develop thrombocytopenia about 7–9 days after subsequent transfusions. Platelet counts are often very low. Alloantibodies against Human Platelet Antigen HPA1a are detectable in the patient's plasma. Platelet transfusion should be avoided. However if there is life threatening hemorrhage, HPA1A negative platelet is often preferred to platelet from a random donor. Treatment is with intravenous immunoglobulin, and recipients should only receive future transfusions with washed cells or HPA-1a negative cells. PTP may also occur as a result of sequestration of micro aggregates of fibrin, leucocytes and platelets in the spleen. These aggregates are often formed as the length of storage of donated blood increases. This risk is often minimised by use of filters during transfusion.

Transfusion-associated acute lung injury (TRALI). Transfusion-associated acute lung injury (TRALI) is an increasingly recognized adverse event associated with blood transfusion. TRALI is typically associated with plasma components rather than packed red blood cells (RBCs), though there is some residual plasma in RBC units. TRALI is a syndrome of acute respiratory distress, often associated with fever, non-cardiogenic pulmonary edema, and hypotension, which may occur 0.05% of recipients. It is usually due to the presence of anti-leucocyte antibodies in the plasma of donor unit which react with recipient leucocytes causing a severe inflammatory reaction in the patient lungs. Symptoms can range from mild to life-threatening rapid onset dyspnoea and non-productive cough. Chest x-ray often shows bilateral infiltrates (white-out appearance). There is often a normal central venous pressure and raised pulmonary wedge pressure. Patients are often not hypervolaemic and do not have a cardiac or infective cause. The occurrence of acute respiratory disease syndrome occurring within a few hours of transfusion should trigger a suspicion of TRALI. Mortality rate from this condition is less than 10%. TRALI has been consistently associated with anti-HLA antibodies. Patients will often require HLA/HNA antibody screen, HLA typing, blood gases and chest X-ray and a lymphocytotoxic/granulocyte crossmatch. The implicated donor unit should be screened for HLA/HNA antibodies. Because these types of antibodies are commonly formed during pregnancy, several transfusion organizations have decided to use only plasma from men for transfusion.

Non-immunologic complications

Transfusion-associated cardiac overload (TACO). TACO is a common complication simply due to the excessive and rapid infusion of blood products. This is especially the case in elderly recipients with heart failure and recipients with underlying cardiac or kidney disease. Plasma transfusion is especially prone to causing volume overload due to its hypertonicity. Signs and symptoms include dyspnoea, tachypnoea, tachycardia, pulmonary oedema, anxiety, cyanosis, sweating, cardiac irregularities, hypotension or hypertension and raised jugular venous pressure.

Iron Overload. The human body has no active mechanism for the excretion of iron. Iron homeostasis thus relies on the amount that is absorbed from the small intestine. During normal physiology, the amount of iron absorbed (1-2 mg/d) is lost by sloughing of intestinal mucosa and skin, as well as small amounts in the urine and bile. The day-to-day iron requirements, as iron is needed by virtually all body cells and especially erythrocytes, are met by recycling between various compartments. In some patients, noticeably those with thalassemia major, sickle cell disease, myelodysplastic syndrome, aplastic anemia, hemolytic anemia, and refractory sideroblastic anemia, who may become transfusion-dependent and receive excess iron with each transfusion (that the body has no means to excrete), iron gradually accumulates in various tissues, causing morbidity and mortality. The accumulation of iron from the transfused units can cause tissue damage in the liver, heart and endocrine system. This risk can be minimized by the use of chelating agents such as desferrioxamine, deferiprone or deferasirox which help to eliminate the unwanted iron.

Hypothermia. Hypothermia can occur with transfusions with large volume of cold blood products. Core body temperature can go down as low as 32 °C and can produce physiologic disturbances and cardiac arrest. This can be prevented by warming the blood to ambient temperature prior to transfusions. Rapid infusion of large volumes of stored blood contributes to hypothermia in infants particularly during exchange or massive transfusion. Appropriately maintained blood warmers should be used during massive or exchange transfusion.

Citrate toxicity. Citrate is an anticoagulant. It is a component of citrate phosphate dextrose adenine (CPDA) used in the preservation of stored blood intended for transfusion. It is usually rapidly metabolised by the liver. Rapid administration of large quantities of stored blood may cause hypocalcaemia and hypomagnesaemia when citrate binds calcium and magnesium. This can result in myocardial depression or coagulopathy. Patients most at risk are those with liver dysfunction or neonates with immature liver function having rapid large volume transfusion. Slowing or temporarily stopping the transfusion allows citrate to be metabolised. Replacement therapy may be required for symptomatic hypocalcaemia or hypomagnesaemia.

Hypocalcemia can also occur with massive blood transfusions due to the complex of citrate with serum calcium.

Infectious complications

Bacterial Contamination. Blood products can rarely be contaminated with bacteria with possible subsequent life threatening infection, also known as transfusion transmitted bacterial infection. Bacteria may be introduced into the pack at the time of blood collection from sources such as donor skin, donor bacteraemia or equipment used during blood collection or processing. Bacteria may multiply during storage. Gram positive and Gram negative organisms have been implicated. Bacterial contamination of blood can be detected in some cases by inspecting the blood products prior to transfusion. Some but not all bacterially contaminated products can be recognised (clots, clumps, or abnormal colour). Maintaining appropriate cold chain management of red cells in a monitored blood bank refrigerator is important. Transfusions should ideally not proceed beyond the recommended infusion time (4 hours). Platelets are more frequently implicated than red cells. The reason platelets are more often contaminated than other blood products is that it is often stored at room temperature. Platelet stored for greater than 5 days are more prone to contamination. Signs and symptoms may include hyper-pyrexia, rigors, nausea, hypotension, circulatory collapse, vomiting, diarrhoea and abdominal pain. Management involves an immediately stop of the transfusion and notification of the hospital blood bank. After initial supportive care, blood cultures should be taken and broad-spectrum antimicrobials commenced. Diagnosis of transfusion transmitted bacteria is made when there is a positive blood culture in the recipient and the identification of same contaminant in the donor blood. Patients may need to be managed with intravenous antibiotics. The estimated residual risk of contamination of blood products with bacterial agents is 1 in 5,000 for platelets and 1 in 30,000 for red blood cells. It has been proposed that the higher incidence of bacterial transmission via platelets is due to the difference in the storage temperatures. Also important is the duration of storage, which has a direct correlation with the likelihood of bacterial contamination. An important concept in the evaluation of data regarding transfusion-transmitted bacterial infections (TTBIs) is the definition of a case. A widely accepted criterion is based upon separation of the cases into possible, probable, and definite contamination, and they are defined as follows.

1. Possible contamination: The blood culture from a recipient grows a bacterial pathogen, with documentation of no other apparent source, but there is failure to isolate the same bacteria from the donor blood product, either because the culture is negative or it could not be done.

2. Probable contamination: The blood culture from the recipient is negative or could not be done, but there is definite bacterial growth in the donor blood product.

3. Definite contamination: The blood culture from the recipient and the donor blood product grow the same bacteria

Viral infections. Transfusion transmissible viral infections include; human immunodeficiency virus (HIV), hepatitis B virus (HBV), hepatitis C virus (HCV), cytomegalovirus (CMV), hepatitis A virus (HAV), Epstein –Barr virus (EBV), human T-lymphotrophic virus (HTLV) and parvovirus B19. It is mandatory in most countries to test all blood donors HIV, HBV and HCV. However donors in the window phase of these infections (a period of time a person is infectious but has not had time to develop detectable antibodies) may test negative and may potentially cause infection in the recipient. Careful and strict donor selection process and pathogen reduction methods such as leucodepletion of red cells and platelets (reduce risk of CMV which is carried within the leucocyte) and solvent/detergent treatment of plasma fractions can potentially reduce the risk of transmission. HAV and parvovirus infection can be reduced by pooling plasma. A significant number of donors in the pool may have antibodies to these viruses. The development of a nucleic acid test for the HIV-1 RNA has dramatically lowered the rate of donor blood seropositivity to about 1 in 3 million units in countries where this technology is available. The transmission of hepatitis C via transfusion currently stands at about a rate of 1 in 2 million units. Such low rates have mostly been attributed to the ability to screen for both antibody as well as nucleic acid testing for viral RNA in donor blood.

Protozoan infection. Protozoal infections are endemic in mainly tropical low income countries, affecting millions of people. Malaria, trypanosomiasis (Trypanosoma cruzi/Chagas disease) and protozoal tick borne diseases (Babesia), toxoplasmosis and filariasis can be efficiently transmitted by transfusion of cellular blood components. In non-endemic areas like Europe malaria, Chagas disease and Babesia are imported diseases resulting from travelling to endemic areas. Prevention of transfusion-associated protozoal infections in most development and non-endemic countries depends mainly on selection of donors using questionnaires. In most of these countries donors at risk for malaria are often deferred for a period of time.

Trypanosoma cruzi. T cruzi is the causative agent of Chagas disease, which is generally spread by the bite of the reduviid bug. The illness has an acute and a chronic form. The acute form principally affects children in endemic areas that include Central and South America and parts of Mexico and manifests as fever, lymphadenopathy, and hepatosplenomegaly. In severe cases, myocarditis and encephalitis may occur. The disease may take a more indolent course, and after a latency of decades, it can present with serious end-organ damage, causing chagasic cardiomyopathy and megaesophagus. Individuals from endemic areas may become chronic carriers of the T cruzi parasite and are responsible for transmission of T cruzi through blood transfusion. Such cases are well known in high-prevalence areas. Seroprevalence in the US ranges from 0.12 to 0.20%, but only 7 cases have been reported to be transmitted by blood. Serologic testing and deferral of positive donors is a policy in endemic countries, and an enzyme-linked immunosorbent assay (ELISA)–based screening test has been instituted in the US as well.

Babesia microti

B microti is an intraerythrocytic protozoan parasite that produces a malarialike illness and is the principal cause of human babesiosis. The majority of the cases have been reported from the Northeast. The common mode of transmission is via an Ixodes tick bite, but B microti can also be acquired via transfusion of infected blood. The clinical spectrum of B microti infection ranges from asymptomatic individuals to severe disease with massive parasitemias that cause haemolytic anaemia thrombocytopenia, shock, and death. The risk of severe infection is particularly high in patients who have HIV infection, have had a splenectomy, or are immunosuppressed. Leukoreduction does not reduce the transmission risk because B microti is intraerythrocytic.

Leishmania donovani. L donovani belongs to a group of intracellular parasites. The common mode of transmission is a bite by sandflies of the genus Phlebotomus. Cases have been reported in highly endemic areas regarding transmission by transfusion of blood products. For this reason, people returning from war zones in Iraq are being deferred from donations for 1 year in some developed countries.

West Nile virus. A mosquito-borne flavivirus infection causing encephalitis. Recent seasonal epidemics have occurred in North America. West Nile virus can be transmitted by blood donated during the viraemic phase. During the epidemic season, donors may not give blood in the UK for 28 days after returning from an affected area unless a test for viral RNA is negative.

Treponemal infections (syphilis. Through the years, a great controversy had arisen over the need for syphilis testing of blood donors. Although the American Association of Blood Banks (AABB) initially dropped its recommendation that donors be tested for syphilis in 1978, the Food and Drug administration (FDA) of the United States keeps on this requirement. This decision was reinforced by the HIV epidemic. It is now recommended in most countries that surrogate testing including syphilis should be done to prevent those at risk from donating blood.

Creutzfeldt - Jakob disease (CJD). Creutzfeldt - Jakob disease (CJD) is a form of the human transmissible spongiform encephalopathies (TSEs) and is characterized by mental deterioration, cerebellar dysfunctions, involuntary movements, and psychiatric alterations. CJD is a rare disease and occurs at a rate of approximately 1 per million populations annually. The risk of transmission of CJD through blood transfusion has not been established, but it cannot be completely ruled out. The disease has a long incubation period, and studies and surveillance programs have not lasted long enough or included sufficient numbers of cases to conclude that CJD is transmitted through blood transfusion. Many people are concerned that it may be possible to transmit CJD through blood and related blood products such as plasma. Some animal studies suggest that contaminated blood and related products may transmit the disease, although this has never been shown in humans.

13. Investigation of Blood transfusion reactions

Blood transfusion is the process of receiving blood products into one's circulation intravenously. Transfusions are indicated in a variety of medical conditions to replace lost components of the blood. Early transfusions used whole blood, but modern evidenced based medical practice commonly uses only components of the blood, such as red blood cells, white blood cells, platelet, fresh frozen plasma and cryoprecipitate. Transfusion reactions are unintended responses in a patient which are associated with the transfusion of blood or blood component. These reaction may be fatal, life-threatening, incapacitating and result in prolong hospitalization and morbidity. Patients receiving transfusion of blood products must be monitored closely for clinical signs of transfusion reactions. The patient's temperature, pulse, blood pressure and respiratory rate must be determined prior to starting the transfusion and regularly during and after the transfusion (to detect signs of delayed transfusion reaction). It is recommended to retain all used transfusion bags for 24 hours before discard. This is to ensure that the donor red cells are available if a transfusion a reaction needs to be investigated.

Pre-transfusion testing. The pre-transfusion testing is made up of the following procedure aimed at ensuring that blood provided for transfusion is compatible and will accomplish the desired aim of improving patient haemoglobin, improving anaemia and improving the oxygen delivery to tissues. The pre-transfusion testing should include the following procedures:

1. Checking the previous transfusion records of patients (manually or computer) for previous grouping and antibody screening result.
2. Check and ensure that the details of patient on request form and hand labelled sample match and contain the minimum data set.
3. Determination of patient ABO and Rhesus blood group using appropriate reagents that have been quality controlled.
4. Performance of antibody screen of patient or mother in case of neonatal transfusion. Identification of alloantibodies in patient with a positive antibody screen.
5. Selection of appriopriate unit for crossmatching. Unit should be negative for antigen for which patient alloantibody is specific.
6. Crossmatching of patient serum and plasma against the donors red cells (Electronic issue, One tube spin or full IAT crossmatch depending on indication).
7. Prepare a worksheet and record all crossmatching testing results. Label units with compatibility labels. Record the batch numbers of reagents used.

Check that reagents are in date before use. Ensure that equipment have had daily maintenance done before use. Sign and date all worksheet.

8. Has the record and testing result been crosschecked.

ABO grouping. Blood grouping must include both a forward (red cell) group and back (serum grouping) using IgM monoclonal anti A, B and AB (cell or forward group) and A_1, B cells (for serum or back group). A negative control of patient own red cells versus serum or plasma or patient plasma against O cell must be included.

Rh D grouping. The rhesus D blood group of a patient can be performed using two different batches of IgM monoclonal anti-D reagents. Reagents must be appriopriately controlled against D positive (positive control) and D negative red cells (negative control). Observed ABO and Rh D group of patient must be compared with previous group in patient records before appriopriate units are selected. All discripancies must be investigated before units are selected for crossmatch.

Antibody screening. The aim of antibody screening is to detect the presence of alloantibody to enable the selection of units that are negative for the antigen to which the alloantibody is specific. The aim is to detect the presence of clinically significant antibodies in the patient plasma, select antigen negative units and prevent immediate or delayed transfusion reaction as well as ensuring that the transfused red cells survives optimally in the patient circulation. Antibody screening invoves testing a patient's serum/plasma by IAT against 2 or 3 antibody screening cells. If antibody screening result is positive, the specificity of the antibody is carried out using a panel of cells (AHG and enzyme) with known antigen status.

14. Compatibility testing

Before a recipient receives a transfusion, compatibility testing between donor and recipient blood must be done. The first step before a transfusion is given is to type and screen the recipient's blood. Typing of recipient's blood determines the ABO and Rh status. The sample is then screened for any alloantibodies that may react with donor blood. It takes about 45 minutes to complete (depending on the method used). The blood bank labotatory scientist also checks for special requirements of the patient (e.g. need for washed, irradiated or CMV negative blood) and the history of the patient to see if they have a previously identified antibody. A positive screen warrants an antibody panel/investigation to determine if it is clinically significant. An antibody panel consists of commercially prepared group O red cell suspensions from donors that have been phenotyped for commonly encountered and clinically significant alloantibodies. Donor cells may have homozygous (e.g. K+k-), heterozygous (K+ k+) expression or no expression of various antigens (K-k+). The phenotypes of all the donor cells being tested are shown in a chart. The patient's serum is tested against the various donor cells using an enhancement method, e.g. Gel or LISS. Based on the reactions of the patient's serum against the donor cells, a pattern will emerge to confirm the presence of one or more antibodies. Not all antibodies are clinically significant (i.e. cause transfusion reactions, HDN, etc.). Once the patient has developed a clinically significant antibody it is vital that the patient receive antigen negative phenotyped red blood cells to prevent future transfusion reactions. A direct antiglobulin test (Coombs test) is also performed as part of the antibody investigation. If there is no antibody present, an immediate spin crossmatch or computer assisted crossmatch is performed where the recipient serum and donor serum are incubated at room tempearture. In the immediate spin method, two drops of patient serum are tested against a drop of 3-5% suspension of donor cells in a test tube and spun in a serofuge. Agglutination or hemolysis in the test tube is a positive reaction and the unit should not be transfused. If an antibody is suspected, potential donor units must first be screened for the corresponding antigen by phenotyping them. Antigen negative units are then tested against the patient plasma using an antiglobulin/indirect crossmatch technique at 37 degrees Celsius to enhance reactivity and make the test easier to read. In urgent cases where crossmatching cannot be completed, and the risk of dropping hemoglobin outweighs the risk transfusing uncrossmatched blood, O-negative blood (C,D,E negative, Kell negative, high titre negative, HBS and CMV negative unit) is used, followed by crossmatch as soon as possible. O-negative is also used for children and women of childbearing age. It is preferable for the laboratory to obtain a pre-transfusion sample in these cases so a type and screen can be performed to determine the actual blood group of the patient and to check for alloantibodies. Cross-matching blood, in transfusion medicine, refers to the complex testing that is performed prior to a blood transfusion, to determine if the donor's blood is compatible with the blood of an intended recipient, or to identify matches for organ transplants. Cross-matching is usually performed only after other, less complex tests have not excluded compatibility. Blood compatibility has many aspects, and is determined not only by the blood types (O, A, B, AB), but also by blood factors, (Rh, Kell, etc.). Cross-matching is done by a certified laboratory scientist, in a laboratory. It can be done electronically, with a computer database, or serologically. Simpler tests may be used to determine blood type (only), or to screen for antibodies (only). (Indirect Coombs test). Cross-matching involves testing the patient serum or plasma against donors red cells. The aim of the crossmatch is to ensure that there are no antibodies in patient plasma or serum that are directed against antigens on the donors red cells. There are 2 types of crossmatch (immediate spin and IAT crossmatch. Immediate spin is indicated in patients with no previous history of alloantibodies and in whom the pre-transfusion antibody screen is negative. The immediate spin is aimed at detecting ABO blood group incompatibility between donor and recipient. An IAT crrossmatch must be carried out in all patients with a previous history of alloantibodies or patients with a positive antibody screen. IAT crossmatch is carried out at 37°C. Tube or IAT card must be inspected for agglutination or haemolysis before washing the cells and adding AHG reagent. If there is agglutination or haemolysis the unit is not compatible and should not be transfused. The IAT crossmatch detect presence of immune antibodies in patient plasma that are specific to antigens on donor's red cells.

Types of

1. Major Cross-match: Recipient serum is tested against donor packed cells to determine if the recipient has alloantibodies against any antigens on the donor's cells. This is a compulsory requirement prior to release of a unit of packed cells.

2. Minor Cross-match: Recipient red cells are tested against donor serum to detect donor antibodies directed against a patient's antigens. This is no longer required. It is assumed that the small amount of donor serum and antibodies left in a unit of packed cells will be diluted in a recipient's plasma volume.

Crossmatch can also be divided into three groups depending on procedure, One tube spin (Saline at room temperature), Full antiglobulin (IAT) crossmatch and Albumin Techniques

One tube spin (Immediate spin). The one tube spin is a crossmatch between donor red cells and recipient's plasma. Donor's red cells is added to recipient's serum or plasma and centrifuged at room temperature after which the tube is observed for agglutination or haemolysis. The presence of agglutination or haemolysis indicates an incompatitible crossmatch and indicates the presence of IGM or cold antibody It is indicated in patients with a negative antibody screen and no previous history of clinically significant alloantibody including suspected prophylactic anti-D.

Procedure for one tube spin

1. Determine ABO and Rhesus group of recipient

2. Determine the antibody screen on patient serum or plasma.

3. Arrange the units in order of outdate, and enter the unit numbers in the appropriate place on the worksheet, oldest units first.

4. Label a 12 x 75 mm tube for each donor unit.

5. Prepare a 3% suspension of each donor unit.

6. Re-check the ABO and Rh type of each donor unit by performing an ABO test (forward grouping only).

7. Confirm the ABO and Rh type of each donor unit by performing an ABO test (forward grouping only).

8. Record donor and recipient's blood typing results in the appropriate spot on the worksheet.

9. Label a tube for each donor unit, using the last 3 digits of the unit number and the patient's initials.

10. Place two drops of patient serum into each tube.

11. Place one drop of washed 3% donor cells into the appropriate tube and allow to stand for 2-5 minutes at room temperature.

12. Shake to mix, and centrifuge for 30-60 seconds or for the length of time for the saline calibration of the centrifuge.

13. Gently re-suspend and examine macroscopically for agglutination and haemolysis. Record results under the Immediate Spin (IS) column of the worksheet.

14. Presence of agglutination or haemolysis indicates an incompatible cross-match. If no agglutination or haemolysis, unit is compatible and a compatibility label is printed.

Antiglobulin (IAT Crossmatch). If the patient has an antibody or a record of a previous alloantibody, the crossmatch must be carried through the antiglobulin phase, and the donor units typed for the corresponding antigen. Frequently a patient may have developed an antibody in the past, which is recorded in his file, but the titer may have dropped and it is no longer detectable in the antibody screen. If this is the case, it is not necessary to set up any panel cells. Merely carry the crossmatch through the LISS and AHG phase but ensure that the donor units are negative for the corresponding antigen to which the antibody is specific. If no typing serum is available in the transfusion laboratory, and the antibody is clinically significant, notify your Blood Transfusion Center that you need antigen-negative blood for the patient. Antiglobulin phase of the crossmatch adds to patient safety, even when the antibody screening test is negative for the following reasons; antibodies might be missed if the corresponding antigens are not present on the screening cells, antibodies might be missed if the screening cells have only a single dose or weak expression of the corresponding antigen, antibodies might be missed if the biomedical scientist performing the test used a slightly less sensitive technique when performing the antibody screen, or if the antibody was missed due to a technical error or an error in reading the test. Detection of immune IgG alloantibodies that have sensitized donors red cell is detectable by using the antiglobulin test (using the AHG reagents. An indirect antiglobulin test (IAT) is indicated and it involves the incubation of patient's serum and donors red cells, incubation at 37°C, and washing 3 times in saline and adding AHG reagent. Polyspecific antiglobulin reagent will agglutinate red cells sensitized with antibodies and or are coated with complements.

Compatibility testing using the IAT Method

1. Label a small clean glass tube with the donor number

2. Pipette 3 drops of the patient's serum into the tube and add 1 volume of washed 3% donor red cell suspension and mix.
3. Centrifuge lightly at 150g for one minute.
4. Gently tilt the tube back and forth and observe for agglutination or haemolysis. Agglutination or haemolysis indicated incompatibility at the saline at room temperature (one tube spin phase of the crossmatch). Re-check donors blood group as well as ensure that the correct patient sample has been tested. This phase will normally detect ABO blood group incompatibility.
5. If there is no agglutination, mix the content of the tube and incubate at 37°C for 20-30 minutes.
6. Centrifuge at slow speed and observe for agglutination or haemolysis. This phase constitute the saline at 37°C phase of the crossmatch. Agglutination or haemolysis indicated incompatibility at the saline at 37°C.
7. Wash the cells three times in saline. At the end of the third wash decant completely the supernatant.
8. Resuspend the cells at the bottom of the tube and add 2 drops of AHG reagent and mix.
9. Centrifuge slowly at 150g for 1 minute and observe for agglutination or haemolysis. Agglutination reaction indicates incompatibility in the IAT phase of the crossmatch and usually indicates the presence of immune IgG antibody in the serum that is reactive against antigens of the donor red cells which may cause a transfusion reaction if donor red cell is transfused. Such incompatible unit must not be transfused.
10. If there is no agglutination, it means that the unit is compatible. However to check that the AHG reagent has worked, add a drop of AHG control (IgG sensitized red cells.
11. The control cell is prepared by adding equal volume of washed group o positive red cells to IgG anti-D. Incubate at 37°C for 30 minutes. Wash 3-4 times in saline and resuspend the deposit in saline to make a 5% suspension. When added to patient serum, donor red cells and AHG mixture should show a visible agglutination.

Compatibility testing using a saline and albumin technique. An albumin technique can also be used when it is not possible to obtain AHG reagent. The following reagents are often required to carry out this crossmatch technique; Patients serum, washed 3% suspension of donor red cells in saline and 20% bovine serum albumin (BSA) reagent. ABO blood group incompatibility and IgG Alloantibodies can be detected by the albumin technique (Anti-D,, other Rhesus antibodies, occasional anti –Lewis, MNSs, Lutheran and P). Albumin technique is not as sensitive as the AHG technique and will miss weak reacting Kell, Kidd and Duffy antibodies.

Procedure

1. Label two tubes with the donor number. Pipette 1 drop of patient's serum into each tube. Add I drop of 3% red cell suspension of donor red cells into each tube.

2. Incubate one tube at 37°C for 45 minutes.

3. Centrifuge the second tube lightly at 150g for 10-15 seconds. Mix gently back and forth and observe for agglutination or haemolysis. This constitute saline at room temperature phase of the crossmatch (One tube spin). Agglutination or haemolysis indicated incompatibility at the saline at room temperature (one tube spin phase of the crossmatch). Recheck donors blood group as well as ensure that the correct patient sample has been tested.

4. At the end of 45 minutes incubation add 1 drop of BSA to the second tube (allowing the reagent to run down the side of the tube).

5. Do not mix but incubate further for 10-15 minutes at 37°C and observe for agglutination. If there is no agglutination observe microscopically. Agglutination indicates an incompatible crossmatch and is an indication of the presence of immune IgG antibody in the patient's serum reactive against the group specific antigens on the donor's red cells.

Electronic issue (computer crossmatch). Electronic cross-matching is essentially a computer-assisted analysis of the data entered from testing done on the donor unit and blood samples drawn from intended recipient. This includes ABO/Rh typing of the unit and of the recipient, and an antibody screen of the recipient. Electronic cross-matching can only be used if a patient has a negative antibody screen, which means that they do not have any active red blood cell atypical antibodies, or they are below the detectable level of current testing methods. If all of the data entered is compatible, the computer will print a compatibility label stating that the unit is safe to transfuse. Electronic issue is based of the principle that if a patient ABO andRh D group is known and patient antibody screen is negative, it should be possible for patient to receive ABO and Rh D compatible unit issued by a computer programme without a serological crossmatch being carried out. The patient in such cases must have a confirmed ABO and Rh D group (group have been determined on 2 different occasion). For this method to be effective there must be in place a validated automated system for confirmed ABO and D grouping and antibody screening including positive sample identification and electronic data transfer of result (no risk of transcription error in manual imput of result). The computer software must be validated to prevent the issue of ABO incompatible unit. A number of safeguards have been advocated to further improve the safety of the electron procedure.

1. There must be two or more ABO & Rh test results on file for the recipient.

2. The ABO group of the donor units must be retested by the hospital Blood Bank.

3. A bar code scanner must be used to enter blood unit numbers and the computer must be used to print the blood bag labels.

Emergency crossmatching. Sometimes in emergency situations, blood may be required urgently such that there is no enough time for a full crossmatch to be performed. Once the ABO, Rh D group and antibody screen has been completed, there may be no need to carry out a one tube spin or IAT crossmactch if the time required to carry out the crossmatch can negatively affect patient care. In such cases patients can be issued ABO and Rh D compatible uncrossmatched units. The crossmatch can however be carried out in retrospect. In the case of an emergency a physician, physician assistant, or nurse practitioner can request "uncross-matched blood", or donor units of blood that have not been cross-matched. It is thought that this lifesaving measure is of more benefit than any risk of an antibody-mediated transfusion reaction. In addition, the risk of a serious transfusion reaction can be minimized if the donor unit is both ABO-compatible and Rhesus (Rh)-compatible. Type O and Rh negative blood can be given if the recipient's blood group is not known, as may happen in an emergency. In an emergency, blood grouping can be done easily and quickly in 2 or 3 minutes in the laboratory on glass slides with appropriate reagents, by trained technical staff. This method depends on the presence or absence of agglutination, which can usually be visualized directly, although occasionally a light microscope may be needed. Every blood bank must have some units of readily available group O negative red cell that can be used in emergency situation when there is not enough time to wait for a compatible unit. However such units must be Kell negative, negative for high titre A and B haemolysin, CMV negative.

Type and screen. For most surgical patients scheduled for a procedure, it is no longer necessary to have units crossmacted prior to the procedure. What is being done is athe determination of the patient ABO, Rh group and antibody screen (type and screen). In such patients, if blood is need intraoperatively or post operatively, blood can be readily available either by carrying out an immediate spin crossmatch or by electronic issue of ABO and RhD compatible unit based on the assurance that since unit issued is ABO and Rh compatible with patient who is himself negative for alloantibody the chances of incompatibility is extremely rare. However if the antibody screen is positive, the specificity must be determined by doing a panel. If the antibody is clinically significant, all effort must be made to get get appriopriate antigen negative unit crossmatched by both immediate spin and IAT for the patient.

Selection of blood component for transfusion. Hospitals are expected to have their own local policies for the selection and issue of blood or blood components. Hospital should have indication coding tool to ensure that transfusion is appriopriate. All staff involved in the transfusion process from the transfusion laboratory scientist to the prescribing clinician must be trained and competency tested on these policies or guidelines. The policy must also have a guide on the use of certain specialised product for specific patients (neonates and infants).

Such policies must contain information on patients in which specialized products such as CMV negative blood products, irradiated, Kell negative, High titre, HLA matched platelet are indicated as well as criteria to transfuse red cells (Giving O donor red cells to A, B and AB patients or giving A and B donor red cells to an AB patient) and plasma against ABO blood group barrier.

Selection of red cells for patient with clinically significant alloantibody. Clinically significant antibodies are antibodies that are capable of causing a haemolytic transfusion reaction (HTR) and haemolytic disease of the foetus and newborn (HDFN). Not all antibodies can cause red cell destruction invivo. However most warm reacting antibodies (react optimally at 37°C) are mostly clinically significant. Most cold reacting alloantibodies are not clinically significant. The general rule is that all patient with a clinically significant alloantibody (anti-D, C, E, c, e, K, k, Fya, Fyb, Jka, Jkb, M and S) must receive red cell negative for the antigen to which the alloantibody is specific. Such red cells must be crossmatched by both immediate spin and IAT and **must only** be transfused if it is compatible by IAT. If antibody is not clinically significant, it is not necessary to select antigen negative units (anti-Kpa, Le^a, Le^b P, C^w, Lu^a and others). **However for patients with anti C^w, C negative unit should be selected.** In such cases ABO and Rh D compatible Kell negative unit should be crossmatched by immediate spin and IAT and **must only** be transfused if it is compatible by IAT. Kell negative unit is most times selected to prevent the patient from developing anti-K particularly those that are Kell negative (most clinically significant and commonly detected after Rh-antibodies).

Dealing with cold reacting antibodies in selection of blood for transfusion. Cold reacting antibodies are not known to cause the destruction of red cell containing the group specific antigen invivo even in hypothermic patients. Even when cold reacting antibodies (anti-Le^a, Le^b, Lu^a, P_1, N and A_1 and others) are reactive by IAT at warm temperature (37°C), ABO and Rh D compatible unit can be crossmatched using donor red cells and patient plasma pre-warmed at 37°C prior to mixing donor cells and patient plasma. This should normally obviate the problem caused by cold reacting antibodies during crossmatching.

Blood group system	Alloantibody present	Clinical significance	Recommended unit/crossmatch type
ABO	Anti-A1	Rarely	Group A and Rh D matched/ IAT crossmatch at 37°C
Rhesus	Anti-D, C, c, E, e, Cw	Yes and Rarely for anti - Cw	Antigen negative unit/IAT crossmatch at 37°C (C negative unit in case of anti- Cw)
Kell	Anti-K, k	Yes	Antigen negative unit/IAT crossmatch at 37°C

Kidd	Anti- Jka and Jkb	Yes	Antigen negative unit/IAT crossmatch at 37°C
MNS	Anti-M, S,s,U	Yes (rarely for anti-M reactive at 37°C	Antigen negative unit/IAT crossmatch at 37°C
Duffy	Anti-Fya, Fyb	Yes	Antigen negative unit/IAT crossmatch at 37°C

Table: Clinically significant alloantibody and unit recommendation for transfusion

Compatibility Label. A compatibility label or slip must be completed for all red cells crossmatch. The label or slip must contain the following relevant information; recipient's name, recipient's hospital number, ABO and Rh group of recipient, ABO and Rh group of donor, identity number of unit, nature of product, date and time of issue, compatibility status of unit and expiry (use by) date.

Difficulties in crossmatching. The following can pose a significant challenge during crossmatching; rouleaux, cold reacting autoagglutinins and bacterial contamination of donor cells.

Rouleaux. Patients with protein abnormality such as multiple myeloma, patients that have received dextran or other crystalloids or sample that have been contaminated with Wharton's jelly can cause red cells to stalk together like a pile of coins giving an appearance of agglutination (pseudo or false agglutination). Rouleaux can be distinguished from a true agglutination by either by adding a drop of saline to the cell or by examining the red cells microscopically. Rouleaux usually disperse within 1-2 minutes following the addition of saline.

Autoagglutinins. Some patient serum contains autoagglutinins (antibodies that show agglutination with patients own red cells and other red cells (autoagglutination). Autoagglutinins are commonly seen in the serum of patients with lymphoma, leukemia, virus pneumonia, systemic lupus erythaematosus, auto immune diseases and occasional in severe Plasmodium falciparum malaria. This pseudo agglutination is often caused by cold reacting agglutinins. When cold agglutinins are present, the auto control is often positive. The effect of autoagglutination due to cold agglutinin can be obviated by washing the patient red cells in warm saline and the auto control read after incubation at 37°C for 10 minutes. The auto control is usually negative after incubating at 37°C.

15. Red Blood Cells alloimmunisation

Patients experiencing alloantibody formation are asymptomatic. The alloantibody is discovered at the time of pre-transfusion testing. It is compulsory to carry out ABO, Rh group and indirect antihuman Globulin (IAT) alloantibody screening. All patients found positive should have their plasma tested against a panel of cell of known antigen status to identify the alloantibody present. Antibody identification was carried out on serum employing commercial two-cell panel (APAN and EPAN). However when test with the two-cell panel using standardized blood bank methods, a third cell panel (B Panel) may be used to facilitate the identification. Alloimmunization significantly concerns the Rhesus, Kell, Duffy and Kidd system which are clinically significant. They can cause, not invariably haemolytic transfusion reactions and limit the ability of safer transfusion while, others are clinically insignificant. Factors for immunization are complex and involve at least three main contributing elements.

1. RBC antigenic difference between the blood donor and the recipient.
2. The recipient's immune status
3. The immunomodulatory effect of the allogenic blood transfusions on the recipient's immune system.

There is relatively high risk of alloimmunization in transfusion-dependent. Red cell alloimmunization should not be overlooked in transfusion-dependent and multi-transfused patients. Alloimmunization must always be considered in certain patients; those who repeatedly suffer from haemolytic transfusion reaction and those who are not able to maintain haemoglobin at a desired level despite having regular transfusions. Regular screening for red cell alloantibodies testing would add towards the better management of these patients. Antibody identification is used as a follow-up test to a positive indirect antiglobulin test (IAT). The IAT is typically performed on all patients that require red cell transfusion and during each pregnancy to determine whether the patient and mother have developed any red blood cell (RBC) antibodies as part of a "Group and Screen" or "Group and Crossmatch request." The antibody identification test is used to determine the RBC antigen(s) that the antibody or antibodies are specific and to determine their clinically significant (Ability to cause a transfusion reaction and ability to cause hemolytic disease of the foetus newborn (HDFN). Some RBC antibodies are known to cause moderate to severe reactions while other less significant ones may cause a positive IAT but few or no symptoms or complications in the blood transfusion recipient or pregnant woman. If one or more clinically significant RBC antibodies are identified, then donor blood that lacks the corresponding RBC antigens must be used for transfusion. When someone has a disease condition that requires recurrent transfusions, they are exposed to many foreign RBC antigens and are more at risk of developing multiple RBC antibodies over time, making the process of finding compatible blood increasingly challenging. Appropriate antigen negative blood will be supplied. Alloimmunisation to the D and K (Kell) antigens is prevented by the provision of Rh (D) negative and Kell negative blood for Rh (D) negative, Kell negative patients. This is particularly important for females with child-bearing potential as these antibodies can cause severe haemolytic disease of the newborn during pregnancy. Patients with sickle cell disease or major haemoglobinopathy syndromes (thalassaemia) and haematological oncology patients who are chronically transfused are at greatest risk of allo-antibody formation. Prior to commencing transfusion, patients with these condition should have extended red cell phenotyping performed to enable the selection of blood matched for the patient's Rhesus and Kell antigens is supplied for transfusion.

The development of red blood cell (RBC) isoimmunisation with alloantibodies and autoantibodies complicate transfusion therapy particularly in multiply transfused patients. Alloimmunization to red cell antigens is still a current problem in many settings in Saharan Africa for several reasons; alloantibody testing for antenatal women and patients who require red cell transfusion is often lacking, alloantibody testing of transfusion recipients to ensure that they receive red cells negative to alloantibody they may have developed is often lacking, there is absence of universal access to prophylactic immunoglobulin D for the prevention of Rh isoimmunisation in Rh negative women and the absence of cost effective means of estimating Feto Maternal Haemorrhage (FMH) in Rhesus negative mothers delivered of Rhesus positive babies and following sensitizing event during pregnancy. It is obvious that the additional testing of blood donors for clinically significant red cell antigens as well as alloantibody screening of all recipients for which red cell transfusion is indicated should be implemented as a routine to prevent as far as possible the incidence of alloimmunization. It would also be cost-effective, bearing in mind the fact that there are laborious and expensive laboratory testing necessary to provide compatible blood for alloimmunized patients.

Challenges of red cell alloimmunization. Red blood cell (RBC) alloimmunization results from genetic disparity of RBC antigens between donor and recipients. Alloimmunization are significant especially when it involves a clinically significant alloantibody that causes haemolytic transfusion reactions and haemolytic disease of the newborn. It is very important that they be correctly, and some of them routinely, typed in blood donors as well as in patients. The development of red blood cell (RBC) isoimmunization with alloantibodies and autoantibodies complicate transfusion therapy particularly in multiply transfused patients. Alloimmunization to red cell antigens is still a current problem in many settings in SSA. Alloantibody testing of transfusion recipients to ensure that they receive red cells negative to alloantibody they may have developed is often lacking; there is absence of universal access to prophylactic immunoglobulin D for the prevention of Rh isoimmunization in Rh negative women coupled with the absence of cost effective means of estimating Feto Maternal Haemorrhage (FMH) in many settings in sub Saharan Africa. These factors all complicate transfusion practice in this region. It is obvious that the additional testing of blood donors for clinically significant red cell antigens as well as alloantibody screening of all recipients for which red cell transfusion is indicated should be implemented as a routine to prevent as far as possible the incidence of alloimmunization. It would also be cost-effective, bearing in mind the fact that there are laborious and expensive laboratory testing necessary to provide compatible blood for alloimmunized patients. Extended blood typing should be implemented for some categories of polytransfused patients as well. This strategy is another step forward to improving the safety of blood transfusion in Africa.

Providing blood and blood products for patients with clinically significant alloantibodies. Red blood cell (RBC) alloimmunization results from genetic disparity of RBC antigens between donor and recipients. Alloimmunization are significant especially when it involves a clinically significant alloantibody that causes haemolytic transfusion reactions and haemolytic disease of the newborn. It is very important that they be correctly, and some of them routinely, typed in blood donors as well as in patients. The development of red blood cell (RBC) isoimmunization with alloantibody and autoantibodies complicate transfusion therapy particularly in multiply transfused patients. Alloimmunization to red cell antigens is still a current problem in many settings in Saharan Africa. Alloantibody testing of transfusion recipients to ensure that they receive red cells negative to alloantibody they may have developed is often lacking; there is absence of universal access to prophylactic immunoglobulin D for the prevention of Rh isoimmunisation in Rh negative women coupled with the absence of cost effective means of estimating Feto Maternal Haemorrhage (FMH) in many settings in sub Saharan Africa. These factors all complicate transfusion practice in this region. It is obvious that the additional testing of blood donors for clinically significant red cell antigens as well as alloantibody screening of all recipients for which red cell transfusion is indicated should be implemented as a routine to prevent as far as possible the incidence of alloimmunization. It would also be cost-effective, bearing in mind the fact that there are laborious and expensive laboratory testing necessary to provide compatible blood for alloimmunized patients. Extended blood typing should be implemented for some categories of polytransfused patients as well. This strategy is another step forward to improving the safety of blood transfusion in Africa. Antibodies to red blood cells (RBCs) can be produced by the body's immune system in response to being exposed to "foreign" RBC antigens, structures found on the surfaces of RBCs. Apart from antibodies of the ABO blood group system that universally common, those of other blood group system are immune and results in response to stimulation by a foreign antigen introduced via a blood transfusion and as a result of a foreign foetal red cell entering the maternal circulation during pregnancy or during delivery. Antibody stimulation is dependent on a number of factors;

1. The immunogenicity of the antigen
2. The dosage of the antigen to which the body is exposed
3. The frequency of exposure
4. The immune competence of the individuals immune system

Most antibodies that react in-vitro at 37°C by AHG technique are generally clinically significant and can cause HDFN and transfusion reaction. It is important to investigate the alloabtibody status of patient prior transfusion and during pregnancy. The clinical significance of alloantibodies depends on a number of factors;

1. The blood group specificity
2. Medium and temperature of optimum reactivity
3. Ability to activate complement
4. The immunoglobulin class of the antibody

5. The titre of the antibody

Alloantibody stimulation processes

Transfusion. Following exposure of an individual to an antigenic stimulus (primary immune response), antibody is usually detectable within 3 months (IgM). When the individual subsequently encounters the antigen (secondary response or booster dose), there is a more frequent antibody production and a switch of the immunoglobulin class of the antibody to IgG. Transfusion of red cells containing antigens which the recipient lacks can trigger an immune response leading to the development of antibody against the foreign antigen. Subsequent encounter with this foreign antigen can result in a transfusion reaction resulting from the antibody produced destroying the red cells containing the offending antigen. Such reaction may range from severe intravascular haemolysis in the patients circulation to extravascular sequestration of the antibody coated red cell by the reticuloendothelial system (macrophages in liver and spleen). It is vital that all individuals for which a red cell transfusion is intended have an antibody screen before transfusion. A positive antibody screen indicates a risk of a transfusion reaction irrespective of the compatibility status. The specificity of the antibody must be identified and specifically selected antigen negative blood is transfused.

Pregnancy. During pregnancy and especially during delivery, foetal red cells may enter into maternal circulation. If these foetal cells contain antigens inherited from the father and which the mother lacks, these foreign fortal red cells can stimulate the mother to produce antibodies (immune). This test identifies the specificity of red blood cell antibodies in the blood that were produced in response to a previous exposure to someone else's RBCs either through blood transfusion or prior pregnancy. It is often done as a follow up to a positive screening result by an indirect antiglobulin test (IAT) or when an antibody is detected attached to a patient's RBCs by a positive direct antiglobulin test (DAT). The type of RBC antibodies that you may produce depends on the specific combination of surface antigens on your RBCs that you inherited from your parents. Normally your body will only produce antibodies directed against antigens not found on your own cells. The major RBC antigens are A, B and the Rh factor (D antigen). They determine a person's basic blood type (for more on this, see Blood Type and Blood Banking). The Rh factor (D antigen) is a potent stimulus for antibody production. It is estimated that if an Rh negative person is exposed to only one or two drops of Rh positive blood, their immune system can be triggered to begin producing anti-D antibodies. For these reasons, blood that is to be transfused must be compatible with the patient. When a person with a RBC antibody is again exposed to RBCs bearing the "foreign" antigen, whether by another transfusion or pregnancy, the RBC antibodies may attach to the specific antigens on the foreign RBCs and target the RBCs for destruction. Depending on the antigen and antibody involved and the quantity of RBCs affected, this can cause a reaction ranging from mild to severe and potentially life-threatening. It may happen immediately, such as during a blood transfusion, or take longer, from one to several days following a transfusion. When antibodies attach to antigens, the red blood cells can be destroyed, termed hemolysis. This can occur within the blood vessels or in the liver or spleen and cause symptoms and signs such as fever, chills, nausea, flank pain, low blood pressure, bloody urine, and jaundice. Antibody identification tests that detect antibodies directed against the minor RBC blood group antigens are not routinely done but are performed when the presence of an antibody is detected through a positive IAT or DAT. Antibody identification is used as a follow-up test to a positive indirect antiglobulin test (IAT). The IAT is typically performed during each pregnancy to determine whether the mother has developed any red blood cell (RBC) antibodies and before RBC transfusions as part of a "type and screen" or "type and crossmatch." The antibody identification test is used to determine the RBC antigen(s) that the antibody or antibodies are directed against to determine if they are likely to be clinically significant, i.e., if they are likely to cause a transfusion reaction or hemolytic disease of the newborn (HDN). Some RBC antibodies are known to cause moderate to severe reactions while other less significant ones may cause a positive IAT but few to no symptoms or complications in the blood transfusion recipient or baby. If one or more clinically significant RBC antibodies are identified, then donor blood that lacks the corresponding RBC antigens must be used for transfusion. When someone has a condition that requires recurrent transfusions, they are exposed to many foreign RBC antigens and may develop multiple RBC antibodies over time, making the process of finding compatible blood increasingly challenging. An IAT and antibody identification test may be used as part of an investigation if a person has a transfusion reaction. Sometimes an RBC antibody may be present in such a small quantity that it does not cause a positive IAT during pre-transfusion blood compatibility testing. But after the blood is given to the recipient, it can trigger renewed, rapid antibody production and cause a delayed hemolytic transfusion reaction several days later. If RBC antibodies have been identified in a pregnant woman, then the baby's condition will be monitored. Whether or not the antibodies will affect the baby's condition depends upon the antibody present, the RBC antigens that the fetus has, and when the mother's antibodies come into contact with the fetus's blood. Some antibodies can cross the placenta from mother to baby and cause HDN.

Cell	**Rh**	**Rhesus**								**Kell**						**Duffy**		**Kidd**		**Sex linked**	**Lewis**		**MNS**				**P**	**Lutheran**	
		D	C	E	c	e	f	CW	V	K	k	Kpa	Kpb	Jsa	Jsb	Fya	Fyb	Jka	Jkb	Xga	Lea	Leb	S	s	M	N	P1	Lua	Lub
1	R1RI	+	+	0	0	+	0	+	0	0	+	0	+	0	+	+	0	+	0	+	0	+	0	+	+	0	0	0	+
2	R2R2	+	0	+	+	0	0	0	0	0	+	0	+	0	+	+	+	0	+	+	0	+	+	0	+	0	+	0	+
3	Rr	0	0	0	+	+	+	0	0	+	+	0	+	0	+	0	+	+	+	+	0	0	0	+	0	0	+	+	+

Table: Antibody screening cells
Yellow = Indicates those antigens which are destroyed or depressed by enzyme treatment

When is antibody identification test ordered? When a RBC antibody is identified, it means that an antibody that specifically targets an RBC antigen or antigen group is present in the blood. If the antibody is considered clinically significant, then it will need to be taken into account with each transfusion and/or pregnancy. If it is not considered clinically significant, then it is not likely to cause a transfusion reaction in the patient or hemolytic disease of the newborn. The antibody identification test may be ordered whenever an IAT or a DAT is positive and may be repeated, when a person has a transfusion reaction and when a mother has a baby with HDN and DAT is positive.

Cell Number	D	C	E	c	e	f	M	N	S	s	P1	Lea	Leb	K	k	Fya	Fyb	Jka	Jkb	IS	37	AHG
1	0	+	0	+	+	+	+	+	+	+	+	+	0	0	+	+	+	+	0			
2	+	+	0	0	+	0	+	+	0	+	+	0	+	0	+	0	+	+	0			
3	+	+	0	0	+	0	+	0	+	+	+	0	+	+	+	+	+	0	+			
4	+	0	+	+	0	+	+	+	0	+	+	+	0	0	+	0	+	+	+			
5	0	0	+	+	+	+	0	+	+	0	+	0	+	0	+	0	+	+	+			
6	0	0	0	+	+	+	+	0	0	+	+	0	+	0	+	+	0	+	+			
7	0	0	0	+	+	+	+	+	+	+	+	+	0	0	+	0	+	0	+			
8	0	0	0	+	+	+	+	+	0	+	+	0	0	+	+	0	0	+	0			
9	0	0	0	+	+	+	+	0	+	0	0	+	0	0	+	0	+	+	+			
10	0	0	0	+	+	+	+	0	0	+	0	0	+	0	+	+	0	+	0			
11	0	0	0	+	+	+	0	+	0	+	0	0	+	0	+	+	+	+	+			
Patient Typing																						
INTERPRETATION:																						

An example of Panel used for antibody identification

Cell number	D	C	E	C	E	K	Fya	Fyb	Jka	Jkb	Lea	Leb	1/IAT	1/ENZ	2/AIT	2/ENZ	3/IAT	3/ENZ	4/IAT	4/ENZ	5/IAT	5/ENZ
1	+	+	0	0	+	0	0	+	0	+	0	+	2	3	2	3	0	0	0	0	0	0
2	+	+	0	0	+	+	+	0	+	0	0	+	2	3	2	3	0	0	3	3	3	0
3	+	0	+	+	0	0	0	0	0	+	0	0	2	3	0	0	2	3	0	0	0	0
4	+	0	0	+	+	0	0	0	+		0	0	2	3	0	0	0	0	0	0	0	0
5	0	+	0	+	+	0	+	+	+		+	0	0	0	2	3	0	0	0	0	3	0
6	0	0	+	+	+	+	+	+	+	+	0	+	0	0	0	0	2	3	3	3	3	0
7	0	0	0	+	+	+	0	+	+	+	0	0	0	0	0	0	0	0	3	3	0	0
8	0	0	0	+	+	0	+	0	+	+	+	0	0	0	0	0	0	0	0	0	3	0
9	0	0	0	+	+	0	0	0	+	0	0	+	0	0	0	0	0	0	0	0	0	0
10	0	0	0	+	+	0	0	+	0	+	0	+	0	0	0	0	0	0	0	0	0	0
11	+	+	0	0	0	0	0	+	+	+	0	+	2	3	2	3	0	0	0	0	0	0

Interpretation : Sample 1= Anti-D 2 = Anti-C 3 = Anti-E 4 = Anti-K 5 = Anti-Fy^a

Table: Antibody Panel result

Cell number	D	C	E	c	E	K	Fya	Fyb	Jka	Jkb	Lea	Leb	6/IAT	6/ENZ	7/AIT	7/ENZ	8/IAT	8/ENZ	9/IAT	9/ENZ	10/IAT	10/ENZ
1	+	+	0	0	+	0	0	+	0	+	0	+	0	0	2	3	3	0	0	0	2	3
2	+	+	0	0	+	+	+	0	+		0	+	2	3	0	0	0	0	0	0	2	3
3	+	0	+	+	0	0	0	0	0	+	0	0	0	0	2	3	0	0	0	0	0	0
4	+	0	0	+	+	0	0	0	+		0	0	2	3	0	0	0	0	0	0	0	0
5	0	+	0	+	+	0	+	+	+		+	0	2	3	0	0	3	0	2	3	0	0
6	0	0	+	+	+	+	+	+	+	+	0	+	2	3	2	3	3	0	0	0	2	3
7	0	0	0	+	+	+	0	+	+	+	0	0	2	3	2	3	3	0	0	0	0	0
8	0	0	0	+	+	0	+	0	+	+	+	0	2	3	2	3	0	0	2	3	0	0
9	0	0	0	+	+	0	0	0	+	0	0	+	2	3	0	0	0	0	0	0	2	3
10	0	0	0	+	+	0	0	+	0	+	0	+	0	0	2	3	3	0	0	0	2	3
11	+	+	0	0	0	0	0	+	+	+	0	+	2	3	2	3	3	0	0	0	2	3
Interpretation : Sample 6 = Anti- Jka 7 = Anti-Jkb 8 = Anti- Fyb 9 = Anti-Lea 10 = Anti-Leb																						

Table: Antibody Panel result

Cell number	D	C	E	c	E	K	Fya	Fyb	Jka	Jkb	Lea	Leb	6/IAT	6/ENZ	7/AIT	7/ENZ	8/IAT	8/ENZ	9/IAT	9/ENZ	10/IAT	10/ENZ
1	+	+	0	0	+	0	0	+	0	+	0	+	0	0	2	3	3	0	2	3	2	3
2	+	+	0	0	+	+	+	0	+	0	0	+	2	3	2	3	0	0	2	3	2	3
3	+	0	+	+	0	0	0	0	0	+	0	0	2	3	2	3	2	3	0	0	0	0
4	+	0	0	+	+	0	0	0	+	0	0	0	2	3	2	3	2	3	0	0	0	0
5	0	+	0	+	+	0	+	+	+	0	+	0	2	3	0	0	3	3	2	3	3	0
6	0	0	+	+	+	+	+	+	+	+	0	+	2	3	2	3	3	3	0	0	2	3
7	0	0	0	+	+	+	0	+	+	+	0	0	2	3	2	3	3	3	0	0	0	0
8	0	0	0	+	+	0	+	0	+	+	+	0	2	3	2	3	3	3	2	3	3	0
9	0	0	0	+	+	0	0	0	+	0	0	+	2	3	0	0	3	3	0	0	2	3
10	0	0	0	+	+	0	0	+	0	+	0	+	0	0	2	3	3	3	0	0	2	3
11	+	+	0	0	0	0	0	+	+	+	0	+	2	3	2	3	3	0	2	3	2	3

Interpretation : Sample 6 = Anti- E + Jka 7 = Anti-D + Jkb 8 = Anti- c + Fyb 9 = Anti-C + Lea 10 = Anti- Fya + Leb

Table: Antibody Panel result

Characteristics of panel cells used for antibody identification

1. An antibody panel usually includes at least 11 panel cells.
2. Group O red cells are often used for the preparation of panel cells since group O red cells lack ABO blood group antigens.
3. Each of the panel cells has been antigen typed shown on antigram as either (+) to indicate the presence of the antigen and (-) to indicate absence.
4. Cells homozygous for the corresponding antibodies are often used to enhance agglutination reaction.
5. Antibodies vary in their optimum temperature of reactivity (saline at room temperature and at 37°C and AHG at 37°C). Most antibodies detectable in AHG at 37°C (warm reacting IgG) are clinically sgnificant).
6. The activity of certain antigens are destroyed or depressed by enzyme (ficin, papain and bromeline) treatment (Duffy, MNS and Xga) while others are enhanced (Rhesus, Kidd, Lewis, I and P antigens).
7. Some antigens exhibits a dosage effect. Their reaction with the corresponding antibody is stronger if the patient is homozygous for the corresponding antigen.
8. The key in antibody identification is that an antibody will only react with cells that have the corresponding antigen; antibodies will not react with cells that do not have the antigen

There are a few basic steps to follow when interpreting panels for alloantibody identification. They include:

1. "Ruling out" means crossing out antigens that did not react (Cross out antigens that show no reaction in any phase. Do **NOT** cross out heterozygous antigens that show dosage.
2. Circle the antigens that are not crossed out. Circle the entire antigen that you could not eliminate during the crossing out process.
3. Consider antibody's usual reactivity pattern such as temperature and medium of optimum reactivity. The Lewis antibody (anti-Le^a) for example is normally a cold-reacting antibody (IgM), so it makes sense that we see the reaction in the saline phase of testing; The E antigen will usually react at warmer temperatures (37°C).
4. Look for a matching pattern to enable you conclusively identify the antibody. Single antibodies usually shows a pattern that matches one of the. Multiple antibodies are more difficult to match because they often show mixed reaction strengths.

5. Again, it's important to look at the a**uto control result.** A negative auto control is an indication that the antibody detected is an alloantibody rather than an autoantibody. A positive control indicates the presence of an autoantibody.
6. **The strength** of the reaction also plays a key role in the determination of the presence of a single or multiple antibodies. Consistent strength usually indicates the presence of one antibody. Different reaction strengths may indicate the presence of multiple antibodies or dosage. Strength of reaction may also be due to "dosage" effect. If panel cells are homozygous, a strong reaction may be seen while If panel cells are heterozygous, reaction may be weak or even non-reactive
7. Panel cells that are heterozygous should not be crossed out because antibody may be too weak to react.

To identify an antibody, the rule of three must be met to confirm the presence of the antibody. Patient serum **must;** show a positive reaction with at least 3 cells with the antigen on the panel cell and show a negative reaction with 3 cells without the antigen on the panel cell. If there are not enough cells in the panel to fulfill the rule, then additional cells from another panel could be used. Example is the B panel cells. Most labs also carry different lot numbers of panel cells. In addition to the rule of three, **antigen typing** the patient red cells can also play a role in the **confirmation of the identity of an antibody. You must however o**nly perform this if the patient has NOT been recently transfused (donor cells could react). The principle of antigen testing is based on the fact that a patient can only produce antibody against a red cell antigen that he lacks. If reagent antisera (of the suspected antibody) are added to the patient RBCs, a **negative** reaction should result. Antigen testing of patients with an alloantibody (phenotyping) is based on the principle that an individual will only produce antibody to a blood group antigen that he himself lacks. Identification of multiple antibodies may be quite challenging. Several procedures can be performed to identify multiple antibodies. These include:

Use of selected Cells. Selected cells are chosen from other panel or screening cells to confirm or eliminate the antibody. The cells are "selected" from other panels because of their characteristics. The number of selected cells needed depends on how may antibodies are identified. Every cell should be positive for each of the antibodies and negative for the remaining antibodies. For example if you ran a panel and identified 3 different antibodies: anti-S, anti-Jk^a, and anti-P_1. Selected cells 1 positive for S and negative for Jka and P1 while cell 2 should be positive for Jka but negative for S and P1 and cell3 should be positive for P1 and negative for S and Jka.

Neutralization. Some antibodies may be neutralized by certain commercial substances and can play a role in alloantibody confirmation. Certain commercial "substances" bind to the antibodies in the patient serum (neutralize), causing them to show no reaction when tested with red cells containing the corresponding antigen. Manufacturer's instruction should be followed and a dilutional control should always be used. The control should contain saline and serum (with no neutralizing substance) and should give a positive reaction. A control shows that a loss of reactivity in the test (serum treated with the neutralizing substance) is due to the neutralization and not to the dilution of the antibody strength when the substance is added. Many of these neutralizing substances neutralize COLD antibodies. Cold antibodies can sometimes **mask** more clinically significant antibodies (IgG). This is an important reason to use neutralization techniques.

Examples of common neutralizing substances are:

1. P_1 substance (sometimes derived from hydatid cyst fluid)
2. Le^a and Le^b substance (soluble antigen found in plasma and saliva)
3. I substance can be found in breast milk
4. Sd^a substance derived from human or guinea pig urine
5. Chemical treatment

Proteolytic enzymes. Proteolytic enzymes can also be used to enhance or destroy certain blood group antigens. Enzymes remove the **sialic acid** from the RBC membrane, thus "destroying" it and allowing other antigens to be "enhanced". Some antigens are destroyed by enzyme treatment while the activities of others are enhanced. Examples of antigens that are positive, negative or show variable reactions with enzyme treatment is shown in the table below. In addition, enzyme procedures may be either one-step or Two-step. If there is no agglutination after treatment, then it is assumed the enzymes destroyed the antigen. In the One-stage test, enzyme is added directly to the serum/cell mixture while in the Two-stage test, panel cells are pre-treated with enzyme, incubated and washed and patient serum is added to panel cells and tested.

Enzyme utility in antibodies identification

<table>
<tr><th>Antigens destroyed enzyme treatment</th><th>Antigens enhanced by Ficin/ Papain treatment</th><th>Antigen with variable reaction with enzyme treatment</th></tr>
<tr><td>M, N,S,s</td><td>Rhesus, A, B, H</td><td rowspan="4">Cartwright (Yt)</td></tr>
<tr><td>Sex linked Xga, Hagen (JMH), Gerbich (Ge2 and Ge4)</td><td>Kidd, Dombrock (Do), Landsteiner-Weiner (LW)</td></tr>
<tr><td>Duffy (Fya, Fyb)</td><td>Lewis, Scianna (Sc), Colton (Co), Kx, Ok</td></tr>
<tr><td>Indian (In), Chido (Ch), Rodgers (Rg), John Milton</td><td>I, P, Cromer, Lutheran, Diego(Di), Knops (Kn)</td></tr>
</table>

Several enzymes exist:
Ficin (figs)
Bromelin (pineapple)
Papain (papaya)

Sulfhydryl reagents. Ability of sulfhydryl reagents to cleave the disulfide bonds of IgM molecules can help in the differentiation between IgM and IgG antibodies. It is good to use these agents when you have a mixture of both IgG and IgM antibodies (warm/cold). Examples of Sulfhydryl reagents include; Dithiothreitol (DTT) is a thiol and will denature Kell antigens and 2-mercaptoethanol (2-ME)

ZZAP. Sometimes, patients with autoantiobodies require red cell transfusion. The most important technical issue faced by the transfusion laboratory is determining if the patient's serum contains alloantibodies in addition to the autoantibody. Between 15 and 40% of patients with autoimmune haemolytic anaemia have alloantibodies. The most common alloantibodies detected in the sera of patients with AIHA in descending order are: anti-E, K, C, Fy^a, Jk^a, and c. The most frequently used method for detecting alloantibodies in the presence of a broadly reactive autoantibody is the warm auto adsorption procedure. Autoantibody is removed by treating the autologous red cells with ZZAP, which is a combinination of dithiothreitol and papain. Autoantibody is then adsorbed from plasma with these treated autologous red cells. Several adsorptions may be necessary to remove all of the autoantibody. If no antibody is detected, the adsorbed plasma can be used for crossmatching donor units. If alloantibody is present, it must be identified and antigen negative units selected for crossmatching. A combination of proteolytic enzymes papain and DTT help denatures **Kell, M, N, S, Duffy** and other less frequent blood group antigens but does not denature the Kx antigen. ZZAP is good for adsorption techniques. It "frees" autoantibody off patient's cell, so that the clinically significant antibody which it is masking can be identified. It may also help in the possible identification and study of the autoantibody.

Autoantibodies

The recipient's immune system may also react to someone else's white blood cells, platelets, and may sometimes form autoantibodies that target their own red blood cells. Rarely, antibodies in the plasma of the blood donor may target the RBCs of the transfusion recipient. Some RBC antibodies may not target a specific RBC antigen but may react with a broad range of different red blood cell antigen types, including the patient's own. These types of antibodies can occur in association with autoimmune disorders, lymphomas and chronic lymphocytic leukaemia, certain viral or mycoplasma infections, and some medications. Autoantibodies can be cold or warm reacting. Auto-antibodies can sometimes "mask" clinically significant allo-antibodies, so it's important to differentiate between auto- and allo-antibodies. React at room temperature with most (if not all) of the panel cells and give a positive auto control. The DAT is usually positive with anti-C3 AHG (detects complement). A positive DAT may be indicative of the following:

1. Could be due to Mycoplasma pneumoniae, infectious mononucleosis, or cold haemagglutinin disease (CHAD).
2. A positive auto control or DAT may indicate that an auto-antibody is present
3. Sometimes the auto control may be positive, but the antibody screening may be negative, meaning something is coating the RBC. DAT in such

cases are usually positive indication that the patients red cells are coated with possibly an autoantibody.

4. The direct antiglobulin test (DAT) is a tests for the determination of in vivo coating of RBCs with antibody (in the body)

5. AHG serum is added to wash patient red cells to determine the presence of antibody coating on the surface of the patient red cells.

Although not always performed in routine pre-transfusion testing, a positive DAT can offer valuable information; If the patient has been transfused, the patient may have an alloantibody coating the transfused cells and if the patient has NOT been transfused, the patient may have an autoantibody coating their own cells. Mini-cold panels can be used to help identify cold auto antibodies. Since anti-I is one of the commonest autoantibody, cord blood cells which contain no I antigen are usually included in the mini cold panel. Cold auto antibodies can be a nuisance at times. There are a few ways to avoid the effect of their reactions:

1. Use anti-IgG AHG instead of polyspecific reagent. Most cold antibodies react with polyspecific AHG and anti-C AHG because they fix complement.

2. Skipping the Saline at room temperature phase avoids the attachment of cold auto antibodies to the red cells.

3. Use 22% Bovine Serum Albumin (BSA) which is a potentiating medium and facilitates the detection of clinically significant warm reacting IgG antibodies instead of LISS.

4. If the antibodies remain, then **pre-warmed techniques** can be performed. Red cells, serum, and saline are incubated at 37° before being combined.

5. Auto adsorption is another technique in which the autoantibody is removed from the patient's serum using their own red cells. The serum can be used to identify any underlying alloantibodies.

6. More common than cold autoantibodies, positive DAT can also be due to IgG antibodies coating the red cell. In such cases the majority of panel or screening cells will be positive. The Rh system (e antigen) seems to be the main target amongst others.

7. IgG antibodies coating the red cell cause warm autoimmune hemolytic anemia (WAIHA). These warm autoantibody can either be: Idiopathic occurring either as a result of known disorder; Systemic Lupus Erythematosis (SLE), Rheumatoid Arthritis (RA), Leukemia, pregnancy, infectious diseases and lymphoma) or as a result of long term use of certain medications.

Several techniques are used when warm autoantibodies are suspected. They include;

Elution techniques. Elution techniques "free" antibodies from the sensitized red cells so that the antibodies can be identified. The **eluate** is a term used for the removed antibodies. Testing the eluate is useful in investigations of positive DATs. The red cells can also be used after elution for RBC phenotyping if needed. When tested with panel cells, the eluate usually remains reactive with all cells if a warm autoantibody is present. Warm autoantibody may be present in the following condition; HDN, transfusion reactions and autoimmune disease. The most common elution techniques

1. Acid elutions (glycine acid). This method lowers pH, causing antibody to dissociate

2. Organic solvents (ether, chloroform). This help to dissolve the lipid bi-layer of RBC

3. Heat (conformational change)

4. Freeze-Thaw technique (this lyses cells and releases the antibody coating on the red cells)

5. Adsorption procedures can be used to investigate underlying alloantibodies

6. **ZZAP or chloroquine diphosphate** can be used to dissociate IgG antibodies from the RBC. After the patient RBCs are incubated, the adsorbed serum is tested with panel cells to ID the alloantibody (if present)

Clinically Significant	Sometimes Clinically Significant	Usually not Significant	Not Considered Significant
Rh (C, E, c, e)	MNS (U, Vw, Mur)	Lutheran (Lua, Lub)	Chido/Rodgers (Cha, Rga)
Kell (K, k, Ku)	Vel	Lewis (Lea, Leb)	JMH
Duffy (Fya, Fyb, Fy3)	Ge	MNS (M, N)	Bg
Kidd (Jka, Jkb, Jk3)	Hy	A1	Csa
Diego (Dia, Dib, Wra)	Yta	P1	Xga
MNS (S, s)			

Table: RBC antibodies and their clinical significance.

There are two types of adsorption techniques:

Autoadsorption. Carried out in those patients who have not had a recent transfusion. Autoantibodies are removed using patient RBCs, so alloantibodies can be identified and patient red cell can be phenotyped.

Allogenic (Differential) adsorption. This method is used in patients who have recently been transfused. It uses other cells (allogenic) with the patient's serum. The figure below shows the 2 different types of autoadsorption principles. Many of elution tests can damage the antigens on the RBC. **Choroquine diphosphate** (CDP) and glycine acid EDTA reagents can dissociate IgG from the RBC without damaging the antigens. This technique is very useful if the RBC needs to be antigen typed. Quinilone derivative often used as an antimalarial can also be used. It may however not remove autoantibody completely from DAT positive cells. Partial removal may be enough to antigen type the cells or to be used for autoadsorption of warm autoantibodies.

16. HDFN and management of Rh negative pregnancies

The human red blood cell (RBC) membrane is complex and contains a variety of blood group antigens, the most clinically significant being the ABO system and the Rh system. The Rh system consists of two related proteins, RhD and RhCE, which express the D and CE antigens, respectively. People who have the D antigen on their RBCs are said to be RhD-positive, whereas those who do not are said to be RhD-negative. If the mother is RhD-negative and the fetus RhD-positive, the mother may react to fetal blood cells in her circulation by developing anti-D antibodies, a process known as RhD sensitization. Sensitization is unlikely to affect the current foetus but may result in haemolytic disease of the foetus and newborn (HDFN) during a second RhD-positive pregnancy. In its mildest form the infant has sensitized RBCs, which are detectable only in laboratory tests; however, HDFN may result in jaundice, anaemia, developmental problems, or intrauterine death.1 The frequency of RhD-negative phenotype in previous studies in Nigeria 4.44%, 3.9% in Kenya, 4.06% in Guinea and 2.4% in Cameroon. These findings are much lower than the ≥14% prevalence of Rh-negative phenotype observed in studies among Caucasians. In most Sub-Saharan African countries, there are challenges associated with Rh pregnancies. A previous report indicated the effectiveness of anti-D prophylaxis in the prevention of HDFN despite poor access. The utilization rate of anti-Rh antiserum in South African population groups for the years 1983–1985 was investigated. The crude utilization rate of anti-Rh antiserum was 41%–44% for all population groups combined. The rate for Blacks, Whites, Indians, and Coloreds was 14%–20%, 89%–94%, 59%–64%, and 45%–51%, respectively. The potential risk of rhesus alloimmunization and the ensuing risk of fetal death with increasing parity were investigated in two groups of parturients: primiparous and grand multiparous Mozambican parturients. The difference did not reach statistical significance. Anti-D immunoglobulin remains the most important alloantibody causing HDN, regardless of the availability of anti-D immunoglobulin for prophylaxis in resource-limited settings and suggests that all patients at booking should have an antibody screen. Care management with anti-D prophylaxis in patients presenting with severe alloimmunization is difficult to access in Sub-Saharan Africa. Beyond the challenge of access to anti-D prophylaxis, there is lack of alloimmunization prevention during illegal abortions and poor documentation of adequate information in patients' medical notes. These factors are highly responsible for the difficult management of Rh-negative patients. To prevent HDFN in most developed countries, RhD-negative women are given anti-D immununoglobulin (IgG) after delivery and often also between 28 and 34 weeks of gestation.

At delivery, Rh D phenotype of the newborn is determined even if RhD fetal genotype is known. Maternal blood is drawn for quantification of fetomaternal transfusion within 72 hours of delivery of an Rh-positive baby and the optimum amount of anti-D immunoglobulin administered. Anti-D prophylaxis has significantly reduced the incidence of erythroblastosis fetalis caused by sensitization to the D-antigen and perinatal deaths from alloimmunization have fallen 100-fold in the developed world.

The anti-D immununoglobulin is prepared from the plasma of immunized human donors and therefore exists in limited supply. Monoclonal anti-D antibodies have been developed to replace polyclonal anti-D and in vivo assays for these have been predominantly based on their ability to clear erythrocytes from the maternal circulation. Although the implementation of a program of routine antenatal anti-D prophylaxis (RAADP) has led to a significant decline in the residual numbers of women becoming sensitized in most developed countries, a significant number of women are not fortunate enough to have access in Sub-Saharan Africa and thus continue to be affected. This is an ethical issue of utmost public health importance. The aim of this study is thus to highlight the challenges associated with the effective management and prevention of Rh alloimmunization among Rh-negative women in Sub-Saharan Africa.

Anti-D immunoglobulin. Anti-D immunoglobulin is produced by the pooling and fractionation of plasma from large numbers of donors who themselves are RhD-negative and have been exposed to RhD-positive RBCs to stimulate the production of RhD antibodies. The future of anti-D immunoglobulin might involve monoclonal or recombinant products, thus eliminating the risks associated with human blood products. Costs would probably increase if recombinant products were used. Anti-D, a polyclonal IgG product is routinely and effectively used to prevent HDFN. The mechanism of anti-D has not been fully elucidated. However, a correlation has frequently been observed between anti-D-mediated RBC clearance and prevention of the antibody response, suggesting that anti-D may be able to destroy RBCs without triggering the adaptive immune response. Anti-D opsonized RBCs may also elicit inhibitory FcgammaRIIB signaling in B cells and prevent B cell activation. The ability of antigen-specific IgG to inhibit antibody responses has also been observed in a variety of animal models immunized with a vast array of different antigens, such as sheep RBCs. This effect has been referred to as antibody-mediated immune suppression.

Antenatal antibody screening. It is recommended that all women in most developed countries should have a blood group and antibody screening at first antenatal visit. It has been reported that 1.5%–2% of pregnant women show atypical blood group sensitization. Opinion is divided as to the clinical importance of a repeat anti-D antibody screen at 28 weeks' gestation. Those in support of 28 weeks' testing argue that there is the potential advantage to identify about 0.18% or fewer women particularly Rh-negative who become alloimmunized after their first antenatal screen possibly as a result of potential sensitizing event occurring after the first antenatal visit. The American Society of Clinical Pathology recommends that testing for unexpected antibody be carried out before antenatal anti-D is given to Rh-negative pregnant women and that repeat Rh testing be omitted if two documented test results confirming the Rh-negative status of the woman are on her record. Prior to 1970, HDFN due to anti-D was a significant cause of morbidity and mortality. By 1990, a reduction in mortality from 1.2 per 1000 births to 0.02 per 1000 births had been achieved in response to the introduction of immunoprophylaxis with anti-D immunoglobulin. At that time the sensitization rate dropped to about 1.2%. A further reduction to between 0.17% and 0.28% was achieved by introducing universal prophylaxis during the third trimester of pregnancy. These findings contributed to the National Institute for Clinical Excellence (NICE) in the UK for example recommend that all D-negative pregnant women who do not have immune anti-D should be offered anti-D immunoglobulin routinely during the third trimester of pregnancy. Some developed countries have also endorsed studies into the feasibility of mass fetal blood group by analysis of fetal DNA in maternal plasma. The benefits of this testing would be twofold. Firstly, there would be a substantial reduction in the use of anti-RhD immunoglobulin, an expensive blood product in short supply. Secondly, women with an RhD-negative fetus would be spared unnecessary exposure to this pooled human blood product with its associated discomfort and perceived risk from viral or prion contamination. Paternal testing of a baby's father may be offered to all Rh-negative pregnant women to eliminate unnecessary blood product administration. It is recommended that partners of Rh-negative pregnant women should be routinely tested. It is being suggested that the most important application of blood group genotyping by molecular genetics is the prediction of fetal RhD phenotype in pregnant women who are Rh-negative and in pregnant women with immune anti-D, in order to assess the risk of HDFN. This diagnostic test performed on cell-free fetal DNA in the maternal plasma is now available in some laboratories. High-throughput RhD genotyping of fetuses in all RhD-negative women is feasible only in developed countries and would substantially reduce unnecessary administration of anti-RhD immunoglobulin to RhD-negative pregnant women with an RhD-negative fetus.

Routine Anenatal Anti-D Prophylaxis (RAADP). Organized preventive screening programs for antenatal care were first introduced in Western Europe in the twentieth century with the hope that routine antenatal care would contribute to a reduction in maternal and infant mortality rates. Figures on maternal mortality in the developed world show that the risk of death as a result of pregnancy and child birth is approximately 1 in 7000 compared with 1 in 23 for women living in parts of Africa where antenatal care is poor or sometimes nonexistent. It is part of modern antenatal care to give all RhD-negative pregnant women an anti-RhD immunoglobulin IgG injection at about 28 weeks' gestation with or without a booster at 34 weeks' gestation. This reduces the effect of the vast majority of sensitizing events which mostly occur after 28 weeks' gestation. Anti-RhD immunoglobulin is also given to non-sensitized Rh-negative women immediately within 72 hours after potentially sensitizing events that occur during pregnancy. All these advances in antenatal management of Rh-negative pregnant women in developed countries are beyond the reach of a vast majority of women in Sub-Saharan Africa. In most Sub-Saharan African countries, the recommendation is that:

1. Women should have an ABO and Rh blood group test done at the time of antenatal booking.

2. Women found to be Rh-negative and who are married to Rh-positive men and run the risk of carrying an Rh-positive fetus and who can afford

treatment are offered prophylactic D immunoglobulin of 500 -1500 IU at 28 weeks' gestation.

3. Tests to determine the presence of clinically significant alloantibodies in antenatal care patients should be carried out.

4. At delivery the blood group of the baby should be determined and if the baby is found to be Rh-positive, 500 -1500 IU of D immunoglobulin is administered.

5. Facilities for determination of FMH should be available in developing countries.

6. There should be provision of prophylactic D immunoglobulin following potential sensitizing events during pregnancy.

In most developing countries including Nigeria, these requirements are not met. The result effect of this failure in management is that anti-D remains the most important alloantibody causing HDFN in Sub-Saharan Africa despite the availability of anti-D immunoglobulin for prophylaxis. Only in an insignificant number of centers do Rh D-negative women have an antibody screen at booking and repeat antibody screens during the rest of their pregnancy. Rh-negative women should be given an injection of human anti-D immunoglobulin after the termination of pregnancy procedure to prevent blood incompatibility complications in future pregnancies. There are many challenges to meeting this requirement in most countries in sub Saharan Africa:

1. Unsafe abortion, defined by the World Health Organization as a procedure for terminating an unwanted pregnancy either by persons lacking the necessary skills or in an environment lacking the minimal medical standards, or both, is prevalent and continues to put Rh-negative women who cannot afford anti-D immunoglobulin at risk of Rh isoimmunization.

2. A broad array of personnel performs unsafe termination of pregnancy in Africa. Aside from the woman herself, others include physicians working at clandestine sites or in hospital operating theaters after normal working hours.

3. Others with medical experience include midwives, traditional birth attendants, pharmacists and nurses needs training on anti-D prophylaxis in Rh negative pregnancy.

4. Most worrisome are 'untrained quacks' whose motives may be financial and their skills negligible.

Women who are Rh-negative should be given an injection of human anti-D immunoglobulin after the termination of pregnancy procedure unless the father of the fetus is also Rh-negative. This prevents blood incompatibility complications in future pregnancies. The costs associated with providing routine antenatal anti-D prophylaxis are the cost of the anti-D immunoglobulin IgG and the cost of treatment administration. The price of anti-D Immunoglobulin differs according to its manufacturers: Bio Products Laboratory (BPL; Elstree, UK) offers anti-D IgG at a unit prize of £27 (US$41) for 500 IU vial while Baxter Healthcare (Deerfield, IL) anti-D IgG is offered at a unit prize of £23.90 (US$36) for a 1250 IU vial. Offering antenatal anti-D prophylaxis will cost an Rh-negative woman £47.80 (US$72) to £54 (US$82) per pregnancy depending on whether she is administered the BPL or Baxter product at 28 and 34 weeks. Cost-effectiveness analysis indicates that offering routine antenatal anti-D prophylaxis to RhD-negative women is economical and results in a marked impact upon the death rate associated with hemolytic disease of the newborn.

Way forward to universal access to anti-D prophylaxis in developing countries

1. Drug manufacturers need to be more humane by reducing the cost of providing anti-D prophylaxis particularly in low-income countries in Sub-Saharan Africa. Cost constraints have remained a limiting factor preventing people from access to best possible treatment and care in Sub-Saharan African countries like their counterparts in most developed countries.
2. There is also the urgent need for African leaders to take up the bold challenge to provide universal access to anti-D prophylaxis for Rh-negative women. Per capita income in most settings is Sub-Saharan Africa is low and continues to affect affordability to prophylactic anti-D treatment.
3. In the absence of anti-D prophylaxis to prevent incidence of HDFN, options such as exchange blood transfusion and intrauterine transfusion (IUT) can significantly reduce mortality and prevent stillbirths. However, safety of blood and blood products remains a great concern. One of the biggest challenges to blood safety particularly in Sub-Saharan Africa is accessing safe and adequate quantities of blood and blood products. Government and societies in Africa need to address several enduring challenges; universal access to anti- D, provision of appropriate infrastructure, trained personnel, and financial resources to support the effective management of Rh negative pregnancies and provision of ultrasonographically guided IUT. This has improved the ability to treat severely anemic fetuses earlier in gestation and has increased the chances of survival of more severely affected foetuses. Around 10%–12% of fetuses affected by HDN will require IUT and a relatively high proportion of IUT survivors may suffer neurodevelopmental problems such as cerebral palsy, deafness, and motor and speech delay that will require specialist input and, in some cases, special education while others will suffer some degree of developmental delay requiring physiotherapy or speech therapy.

Antepartum and postpartum prophylaxis. Current guidelines in most countries recommend that a minimum of 500 IU anti-D IgG be offered to all non-sensitized RhD-negative women at 28 and 34 weeks gestation in order to prevent the risk of RhD sensitization in pregnancy. It is recommended that a minimum anti-D immunoglobulin of 500 -1500 IU be administered:

1. After miscarriage or threatened abortion or induced abortion
2. Ectopic pregnancy
3. Following chorionic villous sampling
4. Amniocentesis
5. Cordocentesis
6. Placental abruption
7. Blunt trauma to the abdomen
8. Placenta previa with bleeding, external cephalic version and any other potentially sensitizing events at less than 20 weeks gestation in non-sensitized D-negative women.

However in the event of any sensitizing event after 20 weeks' gestation, a minimum of 500 IU of anti D is administered and blood must tested for FMH and if the estimated fetal bleed is greater than 4 mL, additional anti-D is administered (125 IU per 1 mL bleed). Before termination of pregnancy, blood type and antibody screen is done and if lady or mother is a confirmed RhD-negative a minimum of 500 IU of anti D is given. Anti- D should ideally be administered with 72 hours of a potentially sensitising event. However if anti-D immunoglobulin is not given within 72 hours of delivery or other potentially sensitizing event; anti-D immunoglobulin should be given as soon as the need is recognized, for up to 28 days after delivery or other potentially sensitizing events. Anti-D immunoglobulin of a minimum of 500IU should be given routinely to all Rh-negative non-sensitized women at 28 weeks' gestation when fetal blood type is unknown or known to be Rh-positive. All pregnant women (D-negative or D-positive) should be typed and screened for alloantibodies with an indirect antiglobulin test at the first prenatal visit and again at 28 weeks. When paternity is certain, Rh testing of the baby's father may be offered to all Rh-negative pregnant women to eliminate unnecessary blood product administration. Non-sensitized D-negative women are given a minimum anti-D of a minimum of 500 IU after:

1. Miscarriage or threatened abortion
2. Induced abortion during the first 12 weeks of gestation
3. Ectopic pregnancy at less than 12 weeks' gestation
4. Molar pregnancy
5. Following chorionic villous sampling at less than 12 weeks.

At therapeutic termination of pregnancy, blood type and antibody screen is done unless results of blood type and antibody screen during the pregnancy are available, in which case antibody screening need not be repeated. Anti-D of 500IU should be given to all non-sensitized D-negative women, following conditions; amniocentesis, placental abruption, blunt trauma to the abdomen, cordocentesis, placenta previa with bleeding, external cephalic version and placenta previa with bleeding. There is a substantial risk of FMH over 30 mL with above events, especially with blunt trauma to the abdomen. If FMH is in excess of the amount covered by the dose given additional anti-D should be given for every additional fetal RBC by ensuring that patients receive 125IU for every 1ml FMH. Failures of anti-D immunoglobulin prophylaxis can occur when there is increased FMH and/or insufficient anti-D immunoglobulin administration was observed. The causes of prophylaxis failure in developing countries include; facilities for the determination of FMH to allow for optimum dosing of anti-D immunoglobulin are often lacking in most settings in Africa. Countries in Sub-Saharan Africa could learn from good practices in developed countries to help reduce the incidence of Rh isoimmunisation and hemolytic disease of the newborn. The proposal to use human Anti-D immunoglobulin prophylactically in pregnancy should not detract from the most expedient approach to further the reduction of Rh disease; ensure that every eligible woman is given Anti-D immunoglobulin after delivery, abortion, and other potentially sensitizing events like their counterparts in the developed world, ensure that Rh-negative women at risk are offered family planning with the potential to limit the number of pregnancies in these women who are already immunized. This is likely to be an effective way to reduce the current incidence of hemolytic disease in Sub-Saharan Africa. Present evidence shows that blanket antepartum Anti-D immunoglobulin prophylactic treatment may be very costly but beneficial to a significant number of women who may not be fortunate enough to have access as a result of unaffordability. There is need for sensitive and practical laboratory testing for FMH to be clinically available to provide new data on FMH. It is suggested that the KB testing should become the minimal cost-effective alternative to flow cytometric testing of FMH in low-income countries in Sub-Saharan Africa because of the cost implication of procuring flow cytometric equipment and lack of trained personnel. There is the urgent need for pregnant women truly at risk for Rh isoimmunization to be identified by analysis of their blood during first antenatal visit and that this should become the rational basis for antepartum Anti-D immunoglobulin treatment. There are compelling advantages in cost, risks, and benefits for an approach of selective antepartum Anti-D immunoglobulin therapy as opposed to routine prophylaxis for all Rh-negative gravid women. The knowledge of anti-D prophylaxis among obstetricians can be improved. A continual system of education to raise awareness of evidence-based practices as well as clinical audit can be implemented to address this. Rh-negative women in Sub-Saharan Africa will benefit immensely from programs such as the RAADP, but costs remains a major hindrance.

Potentially sensitising events in Rh (D) negative pregnancy after 20 weeks gestation

1. Amniocentesis and cordocentesis
2. Antepartum haemorrhage and per vaginal bleed

3. External cephalic version
4. Fall and other abdominal trauma
5. Intrauterine death (IUD and still birth)
6. Intrauterine therapeutic interventions like amniocentesis, intrauterine transfusion and surgery
7. Miscarriage
8. Therapeutic termination of pregnancy (TOP)

Managing intermittent bleeds in Rh (D) negative pregnancy

1. If recurrent bleed occur after 20 weeks gestation, anti D will be required in 6 weekly intervals.
2. FMH should be performed every 2 weeks.
3. If FMH is detected, additional anti-D should be administered irrespective of whether passive anti-D is present or not.
4. Follow up sample should be repeated after 72 of initial intervention to confirm clearance of fetal red cells from maternal circulation.
5. If repeat is positive, flow cytometric test for FMH may be required to confirm that the circulating fetal cells is D positive cells.

Testing for Feto Maternal Haemorrhage (FMH). Rh immunization in pregnancy most commonly results from the fact that at delivery a variable amount of fetal blood enters the maternal circulation when the placenta separates from the uterine wall. The KB test (acid elution) is a blood test used to quantify FMH. It measures the amount of fetal haemoglobin transferred from a fetus to a mother's bloodstream. It is based on the differential properties of haemoglobin F containing foetal red cell to withstand elution by an acid stain. It is usually performed on Rh-negative mothers to identify women with a large fetomaternal haemorrhage (>4 mL of packed fetal RBCs) who may need additional anti-D immunoglobulin to ensure complete clearance of all fetal RBCs from maternal circulation and thus prevent them from being sensitized to produce immune antibodies against D- antigen on the surface of the fetal RBCs. A standard dose of 125 IU is the required dose of Anti-D immunoglobulin required to inhibit 1 mL bleed of fetal RBCs and thus prevent the formation of Rh- antibodies in the mother and prevent Rh- disease in future Rh-positive children. The KB test is the standard method of detecting FMH. It takes advantage of the differential resistance of fetal haemoglobin to acid elution. A standard blood smear is prepared from the mother's blood, and exposed to an acid bath. This removes adult haemoglobin, but not fetal haemoglobin, from the RBCs. Subsequent staining with eosin makes fetal cells (containing fetal haemoglobin) appear rose-pink in color, while adult RBCs are only seen as 'ghosts'. A large number of cells (>5000) are counted under the microscope and a ratio of fetal to maternal cells generated. In those with positive tests, follow-up testing as a postpartum check should be done to rule out the possibility of a false positive. This could be caused by:

1. A process in the mother which causes persistent elevation of fetal haemoglobin
2. Sickle cell trait
3. Hereditary persistence of fetal haemoglobin (HPFH).

Comparison with other more expensive or technologically advanced methods such as flow cytometry has shown that the KB test, like the more advanced methods, is sensitive for the detection of FMH. Testing at the time of birth and postpartum is indicated if baby is Rh-positive. A cord sample is collected from all babies born of Rh-negative mothers. Where the cord sample is Rh positive, a KB or flow cytometric determination of FMH is carried out and anti-D immunoglobulin optimal to clear the volume of FMH is administered preferably within 72 hours of delivery.

Procedure for KB. Since fetal and maternal blood cells have the same life expectancy in the maternal bloodstream, it is possible to obtain informative results from a KB stain for a fair period of time after a stillbirth. However, if the mother and fetus are ABO incompatible, it is more crucial to quickly perform the KB stain following a stillbirth, as the fetal RBCs will be eliminated from the maternal bloodstream very quickly, causing the KB stain to underestimate the degree of FMH, if any. The KB technique, based on acid elution of maternal RBCs, is the mostly widely used technique in the developed world for estimating the volume of FMH and for determining the need for additional doses of anti-D immunoglobulin to prevent maternal alloimmunization. Finally, anything that causes persistence of fetal haemoglobin in maternal blood cells will make interpretation much trickier. Certain hemoglobinopathies, the most common of which is sickle cell trait and HPFH do this. The KB test has been used worldwide since the 1950s to quantify the FMH and to ensure that an appropriate dose of anti-D immunoglobulin is administered both antenatally and postnatally to RhD-negative women to prevent Rh alloimmunization. Although apparently a simple test to perform, recent reports have suggested that unless meticulous attention is paid to both technique and interpretation, the accuracy of the test cannot be guaranteed and that it should be replaced with a flow cytometric test which would give more relevant and accurate results. Flow cytometers are not, however, available to all laboratories performing estimations of FMH. The comparability of results was assessed using a standardized KB technique with flow cytometry suggest that if careful attention is paid to performing a standardized KB test, then it is of value in estimating the size of FMH, and that flow cytometry may be of additional value for cases in which the Kleihauer result is equivocal or indicates that a large FMH has occurred which requires the administration of additional anti-D immunoglobulin. Patient samples identified by KB testing as having FMH >4 mL were sent for flow cytometric analysis. The report indicated that flow cytometry is helpful for the accurate quantification and management of patients with large FMH, and in cases where the presence of maternal haemoglobin F-containing cells renders the KB technique inaccurate, worthwhile reductions in the use of anti-D immunoglobulin can be achieved.

Principle. Foetal haemoglobin containing red cells are resistant to both alkali denaturation and acid elution. Dry blood films fixed in 80% ethanol and immersed in acid buffer solution, red cells containing adult haemoglobin A are eluted leaving red cell ghost while red cells containing foetal haemoglobin F are resistant and the haemoglobin can be stained. In preparing the slides, the sample must be properly mixed and samples must be taken within 72 hours of the sensitising event. Film should not be too thick. Thin film is made by diluting maternal sample 1:2 with phosphate buffered saline. Positive and negative samples should be run along with the test sample.

How to prepare positive and negative control samples. To prepare positive control sample add 9 drops of any female patient EDTA anticoagulated sample into 2 tubes. To the first tube add 1 drop of a foetal sample of the same ABO group. Mix very well and add a1 drop from the first tube into the second tube. Add 5 drops of phosphate buffered saline. To prepare a negative control sample, add 15 drop of well mixed adult male EDTA anticoagulated sample into a tube and add 5 drops of phosphate buffered saline

Shephards stain preparation. Shephards stain is made up of 3 components; Solution 1, solution 2 and 80% ethanol. To prepare 40 mls of working solution of Shepards stain for staining Kleihauer;

1. Measure 2 parts (20mls) of solution one into a staining jar
2. Add 1 part (10mls) of solution 2
3. Add 1 part (10mls) of 80% ethanol
4. Mix the components

Staining

1. Fix thin film in 80% alcohol for 5 minutes and allow to air dry
2. Place slide in shepherd stain for 20 seconds
3. Rinse in running tap water and allow to dry and stain with eosin for 3 minutes. Rinse thoroughly in running water
4. Air dry and examine at least 25 fields under the microscope at low power(x10 objective). Examine the positive and negative controls slides.
5. If any foetal cells are seen in the test film, the foetal cell count must be counted to determine the size of the bleed.

Foetal cell counting

1. Replace one of the objective of the microscope with a graticule (Miller square)

2. Focus the microscope making sure the graticule is on the top left hand corner.

3. Select the x 40 lens and count at least 50 fields of the area of the film where the red cells are just touching each other.

4. For each field count all the foetal cells in the large and small square.

5. Count all the maternal cells in the small square. Count fields with at least 25-30 maternal cells.

6. To calculate the total number of maternal cells, add the total number of maternal cells together and multiply by 9. Also add the total number of foetal cells from the 50 fields.

7. The calculation of FMH is done using mollison's rule.

$$\text{Mollison Rule} = \frac{\textit{Number of foetal cells}}{\textit{Number of maternal cells}} \text{x } 2400$$

8. For example if the number of foetal red cells is 9 and the maternal cells is 2000, the FMH = 9/2000 x 2400 =10.8 mls bleed.

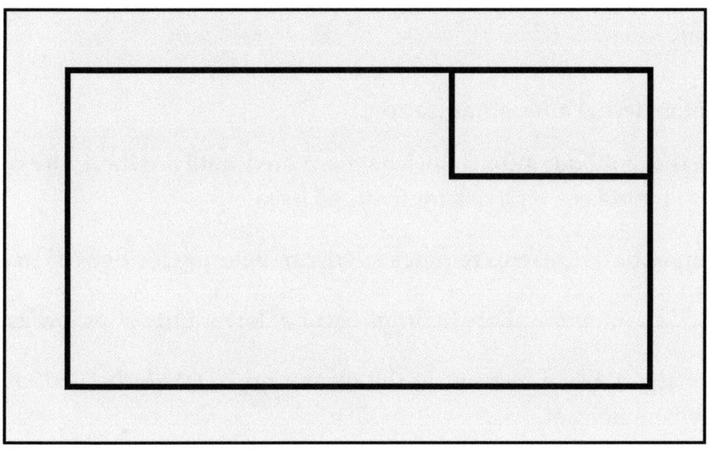

Figure: Diagram of Miller square (graticule)

Calculation of dose of anti-D. Anti-D administered is calculated by giving 125 IU per ml of FMH. For a 10.8 ml bleed you will have to administer 10.8 x 125 IU = 1350 IU of anti-D. For films where there is no foetal cells you assume that bleed is < 4mls and administer a minimum of 500 IU. Samples with raised FMH may need to be referred to the reference laboratory for flow cytometric estimation of bleed. If flow cytometric result is higher, you will need to administer more anti-D using the 125 IU per 1 ml bleed rule. A repeat sample is re-tested 72 hours post anti-D administration to see if there are any residual foetal red cells. If any, count and administer more anti-D.

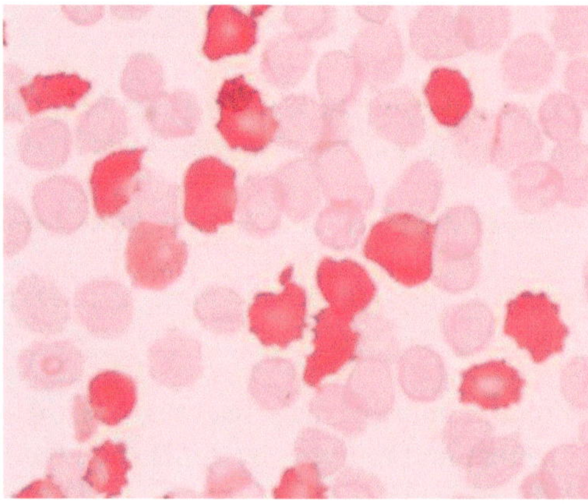

Figure: Show positive FMH with the eluted maternal cells and the elution resistant intensely stained foetal cells.

Testing for FMH is not indicated in the following cases

1. Rh (D) negative women who have immune anti-D
2. Women delivered of a Rhesus negative baby
3. If sensitizing event occur less than 20 weeks gestation (you give 500-1500 iμ only)

Management of maternal alloimmunization

1. Maternal antibody titre should be monitored until a critical titre of 1:32 which indicates a high risk for hydrops foetalis
2. At this critical titre fetus requires intense monitoring for signs of anaemia
3. In Kell alloimmunization, hydrops occur at lower titres of as low as 1:8
4. Generally a 4-fold increase in the titre of an HDN –associated alloantibody is significant.
5. At such critical title amniocentesis can be performed as early as 15 weeks gestation.
6. It may be necessary to do a foetal genotype on maternal plasma at 16 weeks gestation if mum has anti-D and partner is Rh (D) positive. If anti-D level is 4-15 iu (moderate risk) and if > 15iu (high risk for HDN)

7. If maternal antibody is anti K, confirm partner Kell phenotype. If positive do foetal genotype at 20 weeks gestation and monitor antibody level and monitor baby for signs of anaemia. A titre of 1:32 or greater is indicative of HDN risk.

8. If mum is anti-c positive and partner is heterozygous for c and maternal anti-c is >7.5 iu, there is a high risk of HDN.

9. If amniocentesis indicates high risk and there are signs of anaemia, intrauterine transfusion may become necessary.

Management of a sensitized neonate (HDN)

1. Direct anti-human Globulin (DAT) test is positive
2. Neonate may be anaemic (HB<14)
3. Minimal haemolyis with associated neonatal bilirubin level of <4mg/dL may be observed in 50% of such neonate
4. Phototherapy may be indicated and neonate should be monitored for signs of anaemia (3-6 months)
5. In cases of moderate haemolytic disease of the newborn (25%) there is moderate anaemia and elevated neonatal bilirubin levels. Baby may not be jaundiced at birth but hyperbiluribinaemia may occur 24 hours post delivery. Peripheral blood picture may indicates numerours nucleated red cells, immature neutrophils (band forms) and decreased platelet count
6. There may be hepatosplenomegaly and increased risk of developing bilirubin encephalopathy without urgent exchange blood transfusion with O Rh (D) negative fresh red cells or a unit compatible with mum and baby.
7. In severe haemolytic disease child may either be still birth (Blue baby) or hydropic at birth.

Challenges of Rh isoimmunisation in Africa

Despite the fact that the prevalence of Rh-negative phenotype is significantly lower among Africans than in Caucasians, alloimmunization to RhD remains a major factor in perinatal morbidity and continues to compromise women's obstetric care in Nigeria and the African continent due to the following reasons:

1. Unaffordability of anti-D immunoglobulin. A preliminary study of 67 RhD-negative women over a 2-year period in Nigeria has shown that isoimmunization due to Rh incompatibility is poorly studied among Nigerian women, with many questions unanswered.
2. Absence of a management protocol for this condition, which will include both the clinicians and the laboratory biomedical scientist.

3. Lack of alloimmunization prevention during illegal abortions and the lack of information about patients' medical files are highly responsible for the difficult management of Rh-negative patients.
4. Cost of procuring anti-D immunoglobulin; absence of a universal access program for all Rh-negative women.
5. Failure to recognize potential sensitizing events in pregnancy as such and to treat them appropriately.
6. Failure and absence of facilities to assess the extent of FMH; poor and sometimes absence of alloimmunization prevention during illegal termination of pregnancy in Rh-negative women
7. Dearth of information about previous pregnancies and termination in patients' medical files due to poor data management
8. Failure to comply with postpartum prophylaxis guidelines to offer further anti-D immunoglobulin to all Rh-negative women delivered of Rh-positive babies with 72 hours of delivery depending on the extent of FMH; failure to offer Rh-negative pregnant women anti-D immunoglobulin following any potentially sensitizing event during pregnancy; and failure of obstetrician to offer these Rh-negative women the maximum standard of antenatal and postnatal care.
9. Suboptimal antenatal management of Rh-negative pregnant women due to several health system challenges: socioeconomic realities, lack of adequate qualified staff, inadequate referral services, shortage of supplies, and shortages of midwives, counselors, laboratory, and obstetrics and gynecology personnel.
10. Lack of innovative low-cost devices and diagnostic methods such as the use of the KB test for determination of FMH could improve the quality of care offered these women. Improving the uptake of quality antenatal, intrapartum, and postpartum care as well as innovative community-based strategies, combined with health systems strengthening and the development of an evidenced-based protocol for the management of Rh isoimmunization, are critical for evidence-based interventions required to deliver interventions to improve screening and treatment for risk factors and reduce the risks of Rh isoimmunization.

17. Transfusion alternatives and exemplary stewardship in the management of blood and blood product

As a resource, allogenic blood has never been more in demand than it is today. Escalating elective surgery, shortages arising from a fall in supply, lack of a national blood transfusion service, policies, appropriate infrastructure, trained personnel and financial resources to support the running of a voluntary non-remunerated donor transfusion service, old and emerging threat of transfusion –transmissible infections (TTIs) have all conspired to ensure that allogenic blood remains very much a vital but limited asset to healthcare delivery particularly in sub Saharan Africa. Concerns about adverse effects of allogenic blood transfusion have prompted the review of transfusion practices and justify the need to search for transfusion alternatives to decrease or avoid the use of allogenic blood. Some of the complications associated with allogenic blood are immunological, and are thought to be responsible for the increase in tumour recurrence after surgical resection, increased postoperative infection rates, increased progression of HIV infection and multi-organ failure.

Use of Erythropoietin. The availability and use of haemopoietic growth factors on a large scale for in vivo and in vitro management of anaemia has opened a new era in transfusion medicine. Erythropoietin (EPO) was the first haemopoietic growth factor identified. Many anaemic patients being managed with erythropoietin alone or with some combined strategy of erythropoietin plus red cell replacement has shown that the red cell transfusion requirement is substantially reduced. Anaemia is frequently diagnosed in patients with cancer. A systematic literature review (1996–2003) to produce evidence-based guidelines on the use of erythropoietin in anaemic patients with cancer shows that red blood cell (RBC) transfusion requirements are significantly reduced with erythropoietic protein therapy in patients with chemotherapy-induced anaemia or when used to prevent cancer anaemia. Level I and III evidence indicates that patients with chemotherapy-induced anaemia or anaemia of chronic disease initially classified as non-responders to standard doses proceed to respond to treatment following a dose increase. Similarly report on treatment with epoetin alfa as a single weekly dose significantly increased Hb levels in patients with cancer who were undergoing radiotherapy. The response was greater in patients treated with radiotherapy alone than in those receiving combined therapy. The duration of EPO treatment was shorter in the group treated with radiotherapy alone than in the combined treatment group. Experience with preoperative single weekly dose of 150 ug/kg of EPO, in Ghanaian patients has shown that it is effective in raising the pre-operative haemoglobin. Previous report to assess the effectiveness and safety of early initiation of EPO (initiated before eight days after birth) in reducing red blood cell transfusions in preterm and/or low birth weight infants indicates that early administration of EPO reduces the use one or more red blood cell transfusions, the volume of red blood cells transfused, and the number of donors and transfusions the infant is exposed. Cost and availability of EPO is a major challenge in SSA. Previous report has indicated that poor use of EPO is more likely in countries that had lower annual per capita health care expenditures, lower proportions of privately funded health care, and a national health service. Financial considerations and a haemoglobin level <10 g/dL appear to influence erythropoietin use in the United States, whereas financial considerations alone determine erythropoietin use abroad particularly in SSA.

Use of oral and intravenous iron. A previous report has estimated that most pre-school children and pregnant women in developing countries and at least 30-40% in developed countries are iron deficient. The high prevalence in Africa is due to multiple and complex factors related to several underlying mechanisms which include:

1. Inadequate diet.
2. Poor iron absorption in the alimentary canal.
3. Increased iron requirements owing to low birth weight, growth, pregnancy or lactation.
4. Chronic blood loss resulting from parasitic infection including hookworm.

Intravenous iron treatment is a readily available option in treating women with postnatal anaemia. Several studies have evaluated the therapeutic effectiveness, safety, and cost of intravenous iron and oral iron therapy over red cell transfusion and have found iron therapy more cost effective particularly because;

1. Crossmatching is not required
2. Absence of risk of iso-immunisation to foreign protein
3. Fear of transfusion transmissible disease can be ignored.

The incidence of repeated red blood cell (RBC) transfusion in anaemic gynaecologic cancer patients receiving platinum-based chemotherapy iron has shown that Intravenous iron is an alternative treatment for anaemic gynaecologic cancer patients receiving platinum-based chemotherapy and reduces the incidence of RBC transfusion without serious adverse events. Although the cost of intravenous iron sucrose therapy may seem high compared to oral, a lack of adherence to therapy and side effects including gastrointestinal irritation during oral iron therapy were not experienced during intravenous therapy. However, advocacy exist that concurrent blood transfusion and iron supplementation should be avoided.

Antifibrinolytics. Concerns regarding the safety of transfused blood have led to the development of a range of interventions to minimise blood loss during major surgery. Although use of antifibrinolytics may not seem cost effective in most African settings, studies have shown that antifibrinolytic (aprotinin, tranexamic acid, epsilon-aminocaproic acid) reduce blood loss in orthopedic surgery, scoliosis and coronary bypass surgery. Aprotinin and tranexamic acid reduced significantly the proportion of patients requiring allogeneic erythrocyte transfusion according to a transfusion protocol. Recently, questions have been raised regarding the comparative performance of the drugs and the safety of the most popular agent, aprotinin. Report indicates that anti-fibrinolytic drugs provide worthwhile reductions in blood loss and the need for allogeneic red cell transfusion. Post partum haemorrhage is a leading cause of maternal death particularly in SSA. It also contributes to maternal morbidity as women may require a hysterectomy to control bleeding, or may require a blood transfusion, which can transmit viral infections. Anti-fibrinolytic agents have been proposed as a treatment for post partum haemorrhage. The administration of tranexamic acid was associated with a reduction in blood loss of 92 millilitres (95%CI 76 to 109). A review of the use of aprotinin as prophylaxis to prevent bleeding indicates that it reduces the need for red cell transfusion, and the need for re-operation due to bleeding, without serious adverse effects.

Factor V11a. Prothrombin complex concentrate (PCC) is presented as a powder and solvent for solution for injection containing human prothrombin complex. It nominally contains; human factor 11, V11, IX X, Protein S and C. It is indicated for the treatment of bleeding and perioperative prophylaxis of bleeding in acquired deficiency of the prothrombin complex coagulation factors, such as deficiency caused by treatment with vitamin K antagonists, or in case of overdose of vitamin K antagonists, when rapid correction of the deficiency is required. There are an increasing number of anecdotal reports and trials of recombinant activated factor VII (rFVIIa) for bleeding during surgery. Major blood loss can often be life-threatening and is most commonly encountered in the settings of surgery and trauma. Patients receiving anticoagulant therapy are also at increased risk of bleeding. There is a potential role for PCC in controlling bleeding in patients undergoing cardiac surgery and other surgical procedures and reduce, and sometimes abolish, the need for allogenic blood in surgical and non surgical patients. Although some of these may remain unavailable to patients particularly in SSA because of financial constraints on the health care system. Nonetheless, physicians in Africa must always keep in mind that the first and foremost strategy to avoid transfusion of allogenic blood is their thorough understanding of the pathophysiologic mechanisms involved in anaemia and coagulopathy, and their thoughtful adherence to evidence based good practices in the developed world can potentially reduce the likelihood of allogenic blood transfusion in many patients groups.

Use of restrictive red cell transfusion practices and transfusion Triggers. Most clinical practice guidelines recommend restrictive red cell transfusion practices, with the goal of minimising exposure to allogeneic blood. The current evidence supports the use of restrictive transfusion triggers in patients who are free of serious cardiac disease and suggests that critically ill patients tolerate anaemia well and that blood transfusions may increase the risk of adverse outcomes. However, data from randomized controlled trials suggest that overall morbidity (including cardiac) and mortality, hemodynamic, pulmonary and oxygen transport variables are not different between restrictive (transfusion threshold between 70 and 80 g/l) and liberal transfusion strategies and that a restrictive transfusion strategy is not associated with increased adverse outcomes. In fact, a restrictive strategy may be associated with decreased adverse outcomes in younger and less sick critical care patients. The majority of existing guidelines conclude that transfusion is rarely indicated when the haemoglobin concentration is greater than 100 g/l and is almost always indicated when it falls below a threshold of 60 g/l in healthy, stable patients or more in older, sicker patients. A retrospective audit over a 1-year period in two Dutch hospitals has shown that a proportion of red blood cell (RBC) transfusions seem unnecessary and advocated that evaluation of the indications for and the appropriateness of RBC transfusions in the postpartum patient is vital.

Use of artificial Oxygen carriers. The expected cost-explosion in transfusion medicine resulting from an increasing imbalance between donors and recipients, treatment of transfusion-associated complications has increased the socio-economic significance of the development of safe and effective synthetic oxygen carriers as an alternative to the transfusion of allogeneic red blood cells. However, a recent review of artificial oxygen carriers (AOC) indicates that despite decades of preclinical and clinical research on AOC, the results were disappointing. In

Russia, a perflourocarbons (PFC) called Perftoran is available locally and the only approved hemoglobin-based oxygen carrier (HBOC) called Hemopure in South Africa is not being used much. Other products, just prior to filing for FDA approval, did not achieve convincing study results and research and production was stopped. Adverse reactions such as hypotension and pulmonary complication have significantly affected their widespread use despite its potential role in the reduction of preoperative allogeneic blood transfusion. In the light of these challenges, it seems that the global clinical establishment of artificial oxygen carriers is not to be expected in the near future. Fluid resuscitation after massive hemorrhage in major surgery and trauma may result in extensive hemodilution and coagulopathy. After extensive hemodilution, fibrin clots are more prone to fibrinolysis because major antifibrinolytic proteins are decreased. Cryoprecipitate are considered the mainstay hemostatic therapies in such situation. Purified factor concentrates (fibrinogen) of plasma origin and from recombinant synthesis are increasingly used in the management of bleeding associated with dilutional coagulopathy to rapidly restore targeted factors. Purified fibrinogen concentrate has been used extensively in the management of major obstetric haemorrhage.

Avoidance of wastage of blood components. Blood is becoming an increasingly scarce and valuable resource. Shortages occur periodically because of a fall in supply. There is the need to avoid unnecessary wastage. A successful and sustainable future demands exemplary stewardship from all players in the careful management of both blood supply and demand issues. Wastage of this precious gift is an unacceptable failure in the stewardship of our products. It is not something to be discarded casually because it was left out of a fridge for too long. Information from the national blood stocks management project reported wastage of 2.25% in 40 NHS hospitals in the UK. In the United States, an estimated 9.7% of available allogeneic red cell units were wasted. Red blood cell (RBC) product wastage in hospitals is reported to range from 0.1% to 6.7%. Data indicated that approximately 87% of wasted RBC units were either individual unit that were out of blood bank for more than 30 minutes. Factors identified as contributors to RBC wastage most amenable to improvement are; lack of awareness and training of staff ordering and handling RBC products, poor management of temperature-validated containers and inconsistent interpretation of RBC temperature indicators.

Monitoring requests for blood components using transfusion indication criteria, monitoring categories of health care workers responsible for blood wastage, not accepting short-dated units from blood distribution centres, and if short-dated units were accepted, being allowed to return those units to the blood distribution centre can help optimize the use of blood products. Data has shown that three factors can significantly affect RBC outdating; Distance from the blood supplier, mean monthly transfusion activity and month of the year. There may be the need to transport near-outdate RBC units to a high-usage hospital site, which would reduce overall discard rates, thereby increasing overall stock levels available in the blood system and that such redistribution systems can be an effective way to reduce RBC unit discard rates. Even simple transportation systems have many factors affecting the RBC unit temperature. Novel temperature stabilizing materials may make future transportation of RBC units more reliable. Outdating rate varieS among different blood groups (group 0 less than A = B less than AB). Blood product production planning can bring about a significant reduction in outdating and substantial economic savings for a regional blood supplier. Home transfusion practices are becoming very popular in most developed countries particularly for transfusion dependent patients. There is however increasing concern about effective cold chain monitoring of blood products intended for home transfusion. Home care nurses face many challenges in transporting and storing medications and blood products in their vehicles and in patients' homes. Unlike climate-controlled institutions, products subject to the cold of winter and the heat of summer can easily be damaged, which can be harmful to the patient. Additionally, several regulations and protocols demand that products be cared for in a certain manner, stored in the proper container, and labelled appropriately to reduce the incidence of blood product wastage. Despite considerable advances in the safety of blood components, transfusion associated bacterial infection (TABI) remains an unresolved problem. Bacterial contamination of blood product also plays a significant role in blood product wastage.

18. Blood components therapy

Whole blood is a living tissue that circulates through the heart, arteries, veins, and capillaries carrying nourishment, electrolytes, hormones, vitamins, antibodies, heat, and oxygen to the body's tissues. It contains red blood cells, white blood cells, and platelets suspended in fluid called plasma. If blood treated with anticoagulant which prevent it from clotting is centrifuged the denser red blood cells, settle to the bottom leaving the plasma on top; and the white blood cells and platelets will remain suspended in the buffy coat between the plasma and the red blood cells. The platelet-rich plasma is then removed and placed into a sterile bag, and it can be used to prepare platelets, fresh frozen plasma or cryoprecipitate. Platelets can be produced by a further centrifugation of the platelet-rich plasma. This process allows the platelets to settle at the bottom of the blood bag. Plasma and platelets are then separated and made available for transfusion. The supernatant plasma can be pooled with plasma from other donors fractionated, to provide purified plasma proteins such as albumin, immunoglobulin (IVIG), and clotting factors. As a resource, allogenic blood has never been more in demand than it is today. Factors responsible for an increasing demand for blood and blood products include:

1. Escalating elective surgeries
2. An ageing population
3. Malaria associated anaemia in children and pregnant women
4. Poor management of intraoperative and intra and post partum bleeding

Periodic shortages arising from a fall in supply, old and emerging threat of transfusion – transmissible infections and spiralling costs due to various safety interventions introduced in developed countries, the risk of transfusion transmitted infections has become exceedingly small in these countries. However, emerging pathogens still represent a serious challenge, as demonstrated by West Nile virus in the US and more recently by Chikungunya virus in the Indian Ocean. In addition bacterial contamination, particularly in platelets, and protozoa transmitted by blood components still represent sizeable risks in developed countries. In developing countries the risk of all transfusion transmitted infections is still high due to insufficient funding and poor organization of the health service. Safety introductions have all conspired to ensure that allogenic blood remains very much a vital but limited asset in healthcare delivery warranting the optimum utilization of whole blood separated into various components to meet the specific clinical need of multiple patients. Medical treatments are becoming more complex and sophisticated, with patient receiving the specific component indicated for the management of their condition. This constitutes a justification for the implementation of component therapy particularly in developing countries to ensure optimum utilization of donated whole blood.

Whole blood transfusion. Widespread use of whole blood has continued particularly in resource poor developing countries despite a general move to blood component therapy in the developed world in recent years particularly because leukocytes present in allogeneic cellular blood components, intended for transfusion, are associated with adverse effects; development of febrile transfusion reactions, graft-versus-host disease, alloimmunization to leukocyte antigens, and the immunomodulatory effects that might influence the prognosis of patients with a malignancy coupled with findings that leukocytes may be the vector of infectious agents such as CMV, HTLV-I/II, and EBV as well as other viruses. A previous study involving Haematologists in charge of blood banks in England and North Wales to ascertain how much and for which indications whole blood was being requested. More than 90% of hospitals that responded had not requested whole blood during the last 12 months. The evidence for the use of whole blood in preference to component therapy in the massive transfusion setting was reviewed, and no compelling evidence was found for its routine use for this indication. However, US military physicians have used FWB in every combat operation since the practice was introduced in World War I and continues to do so during current military operations. Indications for the use of whole blood include;

1. Neonatal exchange transfusion or paediatric surgery

2. Infrequent use in adult practice was for major bleeding particularly when whole blood was available, and in cardiac surgery, when post-operative bleeding was unresponsive to standard replacement therapy.

Red blood cells transfusion. Red cells are perhaps the most recognizable component of whole blood. Red blood cells contain haemoglobin, a complex iron-containing protein that carries oxygen throughout the body. Patients who benefit most from transfusions of red blood cells include those with chronic anaemia resulting from disorders such as malignancy, acute blood loss resulting from trauma, surgery, obstetrics haemorrhages, chemotherapy –induced anaemia. The red blood cell (PRBC) transfusion has been shown to impact survival in trauma patients with massive hemorrhage. Red blood cells contains an insignificant amount of plasma and thus is indicated for the treatment of anaemia in patients with congestive heart failure and elderly patients with cardiovascular risk who might not tolerate the increased volume in whole blood. Massive obstetric haemorrhage is a major cause of maternal death and morbidity; abruptio placentae, placenta praevia and postpartum haemorrhage being the main causes. Postpartum hemorrhage (PPH) is an obstetric emergency that can occur following vaginal or cesarean delivery. Traditional blood components, including packed red blood cells should be used in patients with significant bleeding. Upper gastrointestinal haemorrhage affects 50 to 150 per 100,000 adults per year and has a high mortality. Red blood cell transfusions are frequently given. Improvements in cell preservative solutions over the last decade have increased the shelf life of red blood cells from 21 to 42 days. Red blood cells (RBC) can be frozen in glycerol solutions and stored for many years. Thawed RBC must have the glycerol removed, but the recovered cells have normal survival in humans. Freezing has been used to store RBC of rare phenotypes for more than 40 years.

White blood cells. White blood cells play a role in protecting the body from invasion by foreign substances. Several types of white blood cells exist; granulocytes and macrophages protect against infection and destroying invading bacteria and viruses while lymphocytes play a key role in host defence mechanism. Granulocytes can be collected by aphaeresis or by centrifugation of whole blood. Leukocytes have ability to distinguish between self cells (body own cells) and foreign (allogenic) cells on the basis of human leukocyte antigen (HLA) proteins that are present on the cell membrane and are effectively unique to a person. During allogenic whole blood transfusion a person receives large number of allogenic donor leukocytes and these are recognized as foreign cells by the recipient immune system which leads to several adverse reactions. To avoid such leukocyte-mediated adverse reactions leukodepleted blood transfusion is required. The effectiveness of white blood cell transfusion has been an issue of intense debate among scientists. The presence of leukocytes in cellular blood components is thought to be associated with a number of significant adverse effects in recipients. Leukocyte reduction reduces the:

1. Frequency of human leukocyte antigen alloimmunization
2. Cytomegalovirus virus and human T-cell leukemia virus infections
3. *Reduction* in the occurrence of febrile non-hemolytic transfusion reactions
4. Reduction in the risk transfusion –transmissible variant Creutzfeldt-Jakob disease (vCJD).
5. Leukoreduction by filtration may reduce the incidence of post-operative infections and adverse outcomes in patients undergoing elective major aortic surgery as well as in patients undergoing abdominal Aortic surgery.

Plasma. Plasma is the liquid portion of the blood and a protein-salt solution in which red and white blood cells and platelets are suspended. Plasma, which is 90 percent water, constitutes about 55 percent of blood volume. Plasma serves a variety of functions, from maintaining a satisfactory blood pressure and volume to supplying critical proteins for blood clotting and immunity. Fresh frozen plasma is plasma frozen within hours after donation in order to preserve clotting factors, stored for one to seven years, and thawed before it is transfused. It is most often used to treat certain bleeding disorders, when a clotting factor or multiple factors are deficient and no factor-specific concentrate is available. It also can be used for plasma replacement via a process called plasma exchange. Definite indications for the use of FFP include replacement of single factor deficiencies, acute disseminated intravascular coagulation, thrombotic and thrombocytopenic purpura and inherited deficiencies of inhibitors of coagulation. There is no justification for the use of FFP in cases of hypovolaemia, plasma exchange procedures, nutritional support, protein-losing states and treatment of immunodeficiency states. FFP must be used with 24 hours of thawing. The earlier it is used after thawing, the better. A higher FFP: PRBC ratio is an independent predictor of survival in massively transfused patients and that aggressive early use of FFP may improve outcome in massively transfused trauma patients. Education on indications of FFP transfusion and improved identification of bleeding may reduce transfusion rates. FFP can partially correct abnormal coagulation. Although the overall risks of FFP are low, they are the least safe blood components, due to the following factors; Immunologic reactions such as allergy/anaphylaxis, Transfusion-related acute lung injury (TRALI) and Haemolysis due to high titre anti-A or anti-B haemolysin which may be present in the plasma of donors.

Information on use of FFP

1. FFP is not indicated in disseminated intravascular coagulation without bleeding, is only recommended as a plasma exchange medium for thrombotic thrombocytopenic purpura (for which cryosupernatant is a possible alternative).

2. FFP should never be used to reverse warfarin anticoagulation in the absence of severe bleeding, and has only a very limited place in prophylaxis prior to liver biopsy. Octaplex (prothrombin complex concentrate) is indicated for the reversal of warfarin effect.

3. When used for surgical or traumatic bleeding, FFP and cryoprecipitate doses should be guided by coagulation studies, which may include near-patient testing.

4. FFP is not indicated to reverse vitamin K deficiency for neonates or patients in intensive care units.

5. In the UK, methylene blue treated FFP from countries with a low bovine spongiform encephalopathy incidence is recommended by the Departments of Health for children born after 1 January 1996 or children less than 16 years on the date of transfusion.

Cryoprecipitate. Cryoprecipitate is the portion of plasma that is rich in certain clotting factors, including Factor VIII, fibrinogen, von Willebrand factor, and Factor XIII. Cryoprecipitate is removed from plasma by freezing and then slowly thawing the plasma. It is used to prevent or control bleeding in individuals with hemophilia and von Willebrand's disease, which are common, inherited major coagulation abnormalities. Afibrinogenaemia is a rare bleeding disorder with an estimated prevalence of 1:1,000,000. It is an autosomal recessive disease resulting from mutations in any of the 3 genes that encode the 3 polypeptide chains of fibrinogen and are located on the long arm of chromosomes 4. Replacement therapy is the mainstay of treatment of bleeding episodes in these patients and plasma-derived fibrinogen concentrate is the agent of choice. Cryoprecipitate and fresh frozen plasma are alternative treatments that should be used only when fibrinogen concentrate is not available. Until the mid-80s, cryoprecipitate has been the mainstay of treatment of patients with von Willebrand disease who were unresponsive to desmopressin. The advent of virally-inactivated factor VIII (FVIII) concentrates containing von Willebrand factor (VWF), originally devoted to hemophiliacs, provided a better therapeutic approach to von Willebrand disease. The International Society for Thrombosis and Haemostasis (ISTH) Disseminated Intravascular Coagulation (DIC) scoring system provides objective measurement of DIC. Where DIC is present the scoring system correlates with key clinical observations and outcomes. In DIC there is a global deficiency of coagulation factors. Severe hypofibrinogenaemia (<1 g/l) that persists despite FFP replacement may be treated with fibrinogen concentrate or cryoprecipitate. Predetermined transfusion guidelines, pretransfusion approval, and transfusion audits are useful tools in the education of those ordering blood components, potentially resulting in the reduction of inappropriate use of blood components. Cryoprecipitate should be used within 4 hours after thawing.

Platelets. Platelets (or thrombocytes) are very small cellular components of blood that help the clotting process by sticking to the lining of blood vessels. The platelet is vital to life, because it helps prevent massive blood loss resulting from trauma. Transfused platelets are either pooled random-donor platelet concentrates or single-donor aphaeresis platelets. When stored for 5 days, all of these products are equally efficacious. A 10,000/microL prophylactic platelet transfusion trigger has been documented to be both hemostatically efficacious and cost effective in reducing platelets transfusion. Units of platelets are prepared by using a centrifuge to separate the platelet-rich plasma from the donated unit of whole blood. The platelet-rich plasma is then centrifuged again to concentrate the platelets further. Platelets also may be obtained from a donor by a process known as apheresis, or plateletpheresis. Apheresis instrument, which, using centrifugation, separates the blood into its components, retains the platelets, and returns the remainder of the blood to the donor. The resulting component contains about six times as many platelets as a unit of platelets obtained from whole blood. The advantages of aphresis platelet over pooled platelets include; the reduction in donor exposures and reduction in the risk of transfusion-transmitted infections and the incidence of platelets alloimmunization. Platelets are used to treat a condition called thrombocytopenia, in which there is a shortage of platelets, and in patients with abnormal platelet function. It is stored at room temperature for up to five days. Leukoreduction and ABO matching of platelet transfusions also have been associated in preliminary observational studies with reduced morbidity and mortality in surgical patients and reduced infections in patients with leukemia. There are clear indications for providing leukoreduced platelet products; reduction of platelet alloimmunization rates, prevention of cytomegalovirus (CMV) transmission by transfusion and reduction in febrile transfusion reactions. In addition, there are studies that suggest that white cells that contaminate platelet and red-cell transfusions may contribute to possible immunomodulatory effects of transfusion, such as an increased incidence of postoperative infections and metastasis formation in cancer patients. Gamma irradiation of platelet is indicated to prevent transfusion-related graft-versus-host disease (GVHD), which is uniformly fatal. Proven situations where -irradiation should be performed are for patients receiving allogeneic stem cell transplants, for patients receiving blood products from related donors, and for patients who are severely immunocompromised, usually because of their disease or its treatment for example patients with Hodgkin disease or other lymphomas. Three aspects of prophylactic platelet transfusions can be controlled by the physician; whether to provide prophylactic platelet transfusions to patients with chronic thrombocytopenia, what platelet count should initiate a platelet transfusion (appropriate platelet transfusion trigger) and what dose of platelets should be used. Previously, a platelet count of 20,000/μL was considered to be an indication for a prophylactic platelet transfusion. Generally accepted WHO bleeding grades are:

1. Grade 0: No bleeding or bleeding-related risk.
2. Grade 1: Presence of petechiae, ecchymosis, occult blood in body secretions, and mild vaginal spotting.
3. Grade 2: Evidence of gross hemorrhage not requiring red cell transfusions over routine transfusion needs (epistaxis, hematuria and hematemesis).
4. Grade 3: Haemorrhage requiring transfusion of 1 or more units of red cells/day.
5. Grade 4: Life-threatening hemorrhage, defined as massive bleeding causing hemodynamic compromise or bleeding into a vital organ (intracranial, pericardial, or pulmonary hemorrhage.

In spite of prophylactic platelet transfusions given at transfusion triggers of 10,000 to 20,000 platelets/μL, several clinical trials have demonstrated that bleeding still occurs. The risk of bleeding varies substantially among studies; depending on the study, WHO grade 1 bleeding was observed in 46% of patients, WHO grade 2 in 12% or 58% of patients, and WHO grades 3 and 4 in 5%, 11%, 20%, or 36% of patients. Refractoriness to platelet transfusions can be separated into immune- and non-immunemediated mechanisms. Because isolated poor responses to an individual platelet transfusion are not uncommon, a determination of platelet refractoriness requires two serial platelet transfusions with poor responses. A and B red cell antigens are expressed on platelets and ABO-incompatible platelets have reduced post-transfusion platelet recoveries but normal survivals. ABO compatible means the donor has no A or B antigens incompatible with the recipient's A or B antibodies. Therefore, providing ABO-compatible platelets is important both to achieve the best post-transfusion platelet increments but also to reduce the incidence of alloimmune platelet refractoriness. Several prospective randomized platelet transfusion trials have clearly documented the effectiveness of transfusing leukoreduced platelet and red cells compared with standard blood products (control) in preventing the development of HLA antibodies. There are basically three strategies for managing allo-immunized platelet refractory patients:

1. Select HLA-compatible donors from an HLA-typed registry of apheresis donors
2. Identify HLA-antibody specificities.
3. Select antigen-compatible apheresis donors; and perform platelet cross-match tests to select compatible platelets.

Childhood idiopathic thrombocytopenic purpura (ITP). Childhood idiopathic thrombocytopenic purpura (ITP) is a common disorder. However, single-institution, long-term, natural history data are limited. ITP is a common paediatric disease presenting at any age with low morbidity and mortality. Most cases can be managed by paediatricians without Haematology referral. Several equally successful therapeutic options exist. Chronic cases present at an older age with higher platelet counts. Up to 50% of cases of chronic ITP will resolve with ongoing follow-up. The overall prognosis in childhood ITP is excellent. Thrombopoietin receptor agonists are currently under clinical investigation for the treatment of ITP and may represent an alternative treatment option in the future. Treatment of immune thrombocytopenic purpura (ITP), the most common bleeding disorder of childhood, is a controversial subject for most practitioners. To address the controversies, the American Society of Hematology (ASH) and the British Society for Hematology (BSH) have developed ITP practice guidelines. These guidelines, based on expert opinion. The ASH guidelines favour therapy based on a low platelet count, and the more current BSH guidelines recommend a more conservative 'wait and watch' approach. In addition to treating children with severe bleeding symptoms, there is a tendency (not evidence based) to treat early in order to prevent a life-threatening bleeding episode, including intracerebral haemorrhage. Treatment for immune thrombocytopenic purpura includes:

1. Corticosteroids are a highly effective therapy, inexpensive, and can usually increase the platelet count within hours to days. However, chronic or prolonged use is associated with toxicity.
2. Intravenous Rh immunoglobulin (IV RhIG), Inravenous Immunoglobulin (IVIG), are preferred by many paediatricians prefer to treat with IVIG and IV RhIG, reserving corticosteroid treatment for serious bleeding or refractory disease. However, in the UK, for the most part, corticosteroids are used as first-line therapy in children with ITP.
3. Splenectomy is rarely indicated in children except for those with life-threatening bleeding and chronic, severe ITP with impairment of quality of life.

Plasma derivatives. Plasma derivatives are concentrates of specific plasma proteins that are prepared from pools of plasma. Plasma derivatives are obtained through a process, known as fractionation. They are heat-treated and/or solvent detergent-treated to kill certain viruses, including HIV and hepatitis B and C. Plasma derivatives include:

Factor VIII Concentrate

Antihemophilic factor that is part of the factor VIII/von Willebrand factor complex. It is produced in the liver and acts in the intrinsic pathway of blood coagulation. It serves as a cofactor in factor X activation and this action is markedly enhanced by small amounts of thrombin. Haemophilia is a rare genetic bleeding disorder that almost always occurs in males. A person has haemophilia when he or she inherits problems with certain blood clotting making them unable to work properly. Blood-clotting factors are needed to help stop bleeding after a cut or injury and to prevent spontaneous bleeding. The haemophilia gene can contain many different errors, leading to different degrees of abnormality in the amount of clotting factor produced. There are two major types of haemophilia; Haemophilia A is caused by a deficiency of active clotting factor VIII. Approximately 1 out of every 5,000 male babies is born with haemophilia and Haemophilia B (Christmas disease) is caused by a lack of active clotting factor IX. It is less common, occurring in 1 out of every 30,000 male babies. von Willebrand's disease (VWD) is an inherited bleeding disorder characterized by deficient levels of or dysfunctional von Willebrand factor (VWF). Plasma-derived concentrates containing von Willebrand factor and factor VIII (VWF/FVIII concentrates) are the mainstay of treatment of patients with inherited von Willebrand's disease (VWD) who are unresponsive or have a contraindication to desmopressin (DDAVP) therapy. A previous study evaluated the efficacy and safety of BIOSTATE(R), a high purity plasma-derived double-virus inactivated FVIII/VWF concentrate, when used in non-surgical bleeds, surgical procedures and prophylactic therapy in VWD patients for whom desmopressin treatment was deemed ineffective, inadequate or contraindicated. Report indicates that BIOSTATE was shown to be efficacious and well tolerated when treating patients with VWD. Similarly previous reports recommended that acute and prophylactic treatment of bleeding in von Willebrand disease (VWD) patients with von Willebrand factor (VWF)/factor VIII (FVIII) concentrates.

Factor IX Concentrate. Factor IX is one of the proteins of the coagulation system. Deficiency of this protein causes haemophilia B. Haemophilia B is an inherited bleeding disorder associated with a deficiency of coagulation factor IX. The hallmark of the severe phenotype is recurrent and spontaneous bleeding into joints, which can lead to joint deformity and arthritis at an early age. Recombinant factor IX is now increasingly regarded as the treatment of choice because it does not transmit human pathogens. All patients in the UK now receive this product exclusively. Conventional treatment now consists of the administration of recombinant factor IX concentrate on a prophylactic basis to prevent bleeds and, hence, minimise disability in the long -term. A prospective clinical study of recombinant factor IX (BeneFIX (R); rFIX), designed to allow investigator prescribed prophylaxis according to customary practices, was conducted in children <6 years old with severe haemophilia B. Routine prophylaxis with 1 or 2 rFIX infusions per week over an average of greater than 6 months of therapy resulted in near complete prevention of spontaneous breakthrough haemorrhages (<1 per year), with most children (77%) having none, including seven patients (32%) who had no bleeding episodes at all. Haemorrhages in joints were less common than those outside joints (27% vs. 73%) of haemorrhages. Factor IX Grifols (R) is a new high-purity plasma derived FIX concentrate with two specific pathogen elimination steps. Efficacy and safety study of a plasma-derived factor IX concentrate Mononine has shown that infusion therapy is safe and effective in the treatment of haemophilia B patients undergoing surgery, exposed to trauma, or experiencing severe spontaneous haemorrhage.

FACTOR V11a. Octaplex is presented as a powder and solvent for solution for injection containing human prothrombin complex. It nominally contains; human factor 11, V11, IX X, Protein S and C. It is indicated for the treatment of bleeding and perioperative prophylaxis of bleeding in acquired deficiency of the prothrombin complex coagulation factors, such as deficiency caused by treatment with vitamin K antagonists, or in case of overdose of vitamin K antagonists, when rapid correction of the deficiency is required. There are an increasing number of anecdotal reports and trials of recombinant activated factor VII (rFVIIa) for bleeding during surgery. Factor V11a use for the management of bleeding following complex cardiac surgery has shown that use of rFVIIa in cardiac surgery may be effective, but definitive clinical trials are needed to clarify its role in clinical practice and safety. Following immediate measures to control bleeding, the broad principles for managing massive blood loss have been summarized as follows: restore volume (administer colloids or crystalloids), perform laboratory investigations (full blood count, blood group and cross-match, coagulation screening and biochemistry), administer blood component therapy (red blood cells, platelets, fresh frozen plasma [FFP] or cryoprecipitate), and administer appropriate pharmacological agents (for instance, antifibrinolytic drugs or recombinant activated factor VII. Major blood loss can often be life-threatening and is most commonly encountered in the settings of surgery and trauma. Patients receiving anticoagulant therapy are also at increased risk of bleeding. There is a potential role for PCC in controlling bleeding in patients undergoing cardiac surgery and other surgical procedures. Major bleeding among patients receiving oral anticoagulant therapy (OAT) is common, affecting some 6.5% of patients per year.

Anti-Inhibitor Coagulation Complex (AICC). Strategies for the management of perioperative bleeding in patients with haemophilia and inhibitors have evolved rapidly as a result of the development of the bypassing agents; Factor Eight Inhibitor Bypassing Activity, Anti-inhibitor Coagulant Complex (FEIBA) and activated recombinant factor VII (rFVIIa). There are currently no established guidelines for perioperative use of bypassing agents, and few controlled clinical studies have been carried out. The experiences in a recent case review demonstrate that both major and minor surgical procedures can be safely performed in patients with haemophilia and high-titre inhibitors under the cover of bypassing agents, with a high expectation of success. Safety and efficacy study of combined rFVIIa and FEIBA therapy in patients with haemophilia A and inhibitors during bleeding episodes indicates that concomitant infusion of low-dose rFVIIa and low-dose FEIBA, seems to be safe, efficacious and economical in patients refractory to rFVIIa and probably other haemophilia A patients with an inhibitor.

Albumin. The major protein in plasma is albumin. Albumin helps keep fluid from leaking out of blood vessels and into tissues, and albumin binds to and carries substances such as hormones and certain drugs. Evidence-based guidelines for severe traumatic brain injury (TBI) do not include strategies for fluid administration. A previous study investigated the use of albumin administration in traumatic brain injury to maintain normal colloid osmotic pressure and advocates a neutral to slightly negative fluid balance. Findings indicated that albumin administration in combination with a neutral to a slightly negative fluid balance was associated with low mortality in patients with severe TBI. In children with severe malaria, resuscitation with albumin infusion results in a lower mortality than resuscitation with saline infusion. In patients with cirrhosis and spontaneous bacterial peritonitis, renal function frequently becomes impaired. This impairment is probably related to a reduction in effective arterial blood volume and is associated with a high mortality rate. In patients with cirrhosis and spontaneous bacterial peritonitis, treatment with intravenous albumin in addition to an antibiotic reduces the incidence of renal impairment and death in comparison with treatment with an antibiotic alone. Albumin is a large molecule which plays an essential role in generating colloido-osmotic pressure which facilitates fluid retention in the intravascular space. Human Albumin is quiet useful in burnt patients. Licensed indications are the emergency treatment of shock and other conditions where restoration of blood volume is urgent, burns, and hypoproteinaemia.

Immune Globulins, including Rh Immune Globulin. The administration of Rh immune globulin (RhIG) to D–negative women after parturition is a remarkably successful therapy and has prevented many thousands of D+ infants worldwide suffering from hemolytic disease of the fetus and newborn (HDFN) since its introduction nearly 40 years ago. The mechanism of action is due to the role for immunomodulatory cytokines and foetal red cell clearance. Rh (D)-negative women with a large fetomaternal haemorrhage (FMH) from an Rh (D) positive fetus are at risk for anti-D alloimmunization if they do not receive adequate Rh immune globulin (RhIG). Determination of the adequate RhIG dose for these women is a critical laboratory procedure for protecting their future Rh (D)+positive children. Laboratories performing quantification of FMH should review their procedures and training for calculating RhIG dosage. Intravenous immunoglobulin and intravenous anti-D are common therapies in the management of patients with immune thrombocytopenia (ITP). Despite immediate increases in the platelet count, the duration of response is limited, with platelet increments lasting between 2 and 4 weeks. Infusion reactions are common but adverse events are rare.

Anti-Inhibitor Coagulant Complex (AICC). Anti-Inhibitor Coagulant Complex is a freeze-dried sterile human plasma fraction with Factor VIII inhibitor bypassing activity. In vitro, it shortens the activated partial thromboplastin time (APTT) of plasma containing Factor VIII inhibitor. Factor VIII inhibitor bypassing activity is expressed in arbitrary units. It is indicated for the control of spontaneous bleeding episodes or to cover surgical interventions in hemophilia A and hemophilia B patients with inhibitors. Prophylactic infusion of factor concentrates is a safe, effective intervention for preventing arthropathy in patients with haemophilia; on demand treatment is insufficient to prevent the orthopaedic complications and subsequent haemophilic arthropathy that stem from recurrent joint haemorrhages. Patients with haemophilia and inhibitors with bleeding episodes treated with bypassing agents showed that when APCC was administered regularly, most patients exhibited a reduction in the numbers of haemorrhages, an improvement in orthopaedic status, and an improvement in quality of life.

Alpha 1-Proteinase Inhibitor Concentrate. Alpha-antitrypsin (AAT) is a serine protease inhibitor, which inhibits the proteolytic enzyme elastase. Alpha (1)-Antitrypsin (AAT) deficiency is a common but underrecognised condition. Since its first description by Laurell and Eriksson in 1963, significant advances have been made in understanding the genetics, physiology and pathophysiology of this condition. The intravenous administration of purified AAT to AAT-deficient individuals has been shown to confer biochemical efficacy by raising the serum AAT level above an epidemiologically established 'protective threshold' while preserving the biochemical properties and functional capacity of the protease inhibitor. Individuals with a deficiency of AAT may develop clinical manifestations that include a decline in lung function. Deficiency of AAT can lead to many clinical manifestations, most commonly chronic obstructive pulmonary disease in the form of emphysema. Severe forms of alpha (1)-antitrypsin (AAT) deficiency require augmentation therapy by intravenous administration of purified preparations of AAT concentrate. Aralast is one of three approved human plasma-derived treatment options used to prevent the progression of emphysema associated with AAT deficiency disorder.

19. Management of major haemorrhage

Haemorrage is a leading cause of early death following traumatic injury, intra and post surgical and ante and post partum. In most severely injured patient with injury severity score > 25 the mortality rate is between 60-70%. Patient who suffer from uncontrolled haemorrage do so within the first 6 hours following injury. Haemorrhage accounts for 40% of deaths from trauma and is the most common cause of preventatable mortality in developing countries due to:

1. Chronic blood shortages, high prevalence of transfusion-transmissible infection
2. Reliance on whole blood transfusion and lack of other component required to manage coagulopathy
3. Absence of national blood transfusion service and reliance on family replacement and commercial blood donation
4. Inadequate use of pharmacologic and non pharmacologic alternatives to allogenic blood.

What is a major haemorrhage? Major haemorrhage is the replace of patient's blood volume or transfusion of > 10 units of packed red cells with a 24 hours period. It can also be defined as the loss of 50% of blood volume within a 3 hours period or a loss of 150ml per minute. The aim of blood volume replacement with concentrated red cells and other plasma products following massive haemorrhage are:

1. To rapidly and effectively restore adequate blood volume and prevent hypovolaemic shock and to allow for adequate haemostasis, oxygen carrying capacity and blood biochemistry.
2. To allow for an early and aggressive correction of coagulopathy
3. Allow for optimal resuscitation.
4. Reduce potentially preventable deaths.

Haemorrhage control measures

1. Direct pressure /tourniquet if appriopriate
2. Stabilization of fractures
3. Surgical interventions such as: Damage control surgery, Interventional radiology and use of endoscopic and obstetrics techniques

Use of haemostatic drugs such as:

1. Use of antifibrinolytic (aprotinin, tranexamic acid, epsilon-aminocaproic acid) to reduce blood loss. Aprotinin and tranexamic acid reduced significantly the proportion of patients requiring allogeneic erythrocyte transfusion according to a transfusion protocol. Tranexamic acid (1g bolus followed by 1g over 8 hours).
2. Vitamin K and prothrombin complex concentrate (PCC) particularly for warfarinised patients. Prothrombin Complex Concentrate PCCs are a human blood product and both pasteurisation and nanofiltration are used for viral inactivation. Prothrombin Complex Concentrate PCCs contain the clotting factors II, VII, IX, X and Protein C. Warfarin and other coumarin derivatives exert their anticoagulant affect by preventing the production of biologically active Vitamin K dependent co-factors (II, VII IX and X). These effects can be reversed by the administration of Vitamin K but the onset of action is delayed by 4-6 hours. Therefore, in situations where more rapid reversal of anticoagulation is required and where the thrombotic risks of complete reversal are less than the risks of continued bleeding, the use of a Prothrombin Complex Concentrate.
3. Novo 7: Nova 7 is a vitamin K-dependent recombinant human coagulation Factor VIIa (rFVIIa), intended for promoting hemostasis by activating the extrinsic pathway of the coagulation cascade. It is a glycoprotein. It is an important factor in the clotting of blood that forms a complex with

tissue thromboplastin and calcium to activate the prothrombinase, thus acting to accelerate the conversion of prothrombin to thrombin.

Cell salvage. Intraoperative blood salvage, also known as autologous blood salvage, is a medical procedure involving recovering blood lost during surgery and trauma-related blood and re-infusing it into the patient. Several processes have been developed to assist in salvaging the patient's own whole blood in the perioperative setting. These can be categorized into three general types of salvage procedures: Cell processors and salvage devices that wash and save red blood cells (cell washers or RBC-savers). Cell processors are red cell washing devices that collect anticoagulated shed or recovered blood, wash and separate the red blood cells (RBCs) by centrifugation, and reinfuse the RBCs. RBC washing devices can help remove byproducts in salvaged blood such as activated cytokines, anaphylatoxins, and other waste substances that may have been collected in the reservoir suctioned from the surgical field. Direct transfusion is a blood salvaging method that are used in surgery such as coronary artery bypass grafts (CABG), valve replacement, or surgical repair of the great vessels. Ultrafiltration devices filter the patient's anticoagulated whole blood. The filter process removes unwanted excess non-cellular plasma water, low molecular weight solutes, platelet inhibitors and some particulate matter through hemoconcentration, including activated cytokines, anaphylatoxins, and other waste substances making concentrated whole blood available for reinfusion.

Management plan in case of massive haemorrhage

1. Patient bleeding/collapses (loss of 150 mls/minute or in clinical shock)
2. Emergency group O (2 units) located in the nearest transfusion fridge can be used immediately in dare emergency. The managing clinical team must remember to inform the transfusion laboratory that emergency units have been taken to enable immediate replenishment.
3. Resuscitate (Ensure airway is clear, breathing and circulation)
4. Identify location of patient and call for help and allocate roles (team lead, communicator, samples, documenter and transporter).
5. Alert emergency response team as well as blood transfusion laboratory.
6. Take blood and send to laboratory for crossmatch, Full blood counts (FBC), Coagulation test (PT, APTT and Fibrinogen), Urea and creatinine, calcium and Blood gases).
7. Ask the managing clinician if major haemorrage pack 1 (MHP 1) required or tailored therapy. If major haemorrhage pack 1 required, prepare 8 units of red cells, 8 units of FFP and 2 doses of platelet. If tailored therapy ask how many units of red cells, FFP and palatelets required.
8. Depending on urgency with which the product is required, emergency group O positive, group specific blood or fully crossmatched blood may be made available.

- Emergency O positive blood (male, women >60, not known to have allo anti-D). Unlimited issue until a suitably identified sample is received and a secure group is obtained.
- Group specific (ABO/D matched) – suitable sample/secure group obtained. Not fully crossmatched.
- Full crossmatch (ABO/D matched, antibody screen performed, specifically 'crossmatched' patient's plasma versus donor's red cells).

1. Give the ordered blood products and reassess patient for suspected continuing haemorrhage requiring further transfusion. Take and send post transfusion blood samples to the laboratory for repeat FBC, PT, APTT, Fibrinogen, Urea and creatinine, Calcium and Blood gas.
2. The aim of any further intervention is to maintain the following:
    - Haemoglobin between 8-10g/dl
    - Platelet count above 75 x 10^9/l
    - International normalized ratio below 1.5
    - APTT ratio below 1.5
    - Fibrinogen above 1g/l. If not met; consider giving 2 units of cryoprecipitate.
    - Calcium above 1mmol/l. If not met, consider giving 10 mls of calcium chloride (10%) over 10 minutes period.
    - Temerature above 36°C. If not met, use warm fluid device or use forced air warming blanket.
    - Ph above 7.35
3. If the above aim is not achieved and patient continue to bleed, order MHP 2 (4 red cells, 4 FFP, 1 platelet and 2 units of cryoprecipitate if fibrinogen is <1g/l or <2g/l in case of obstetric haemorrhage.
4. Give blood products in MHP 2/tailored therapy and reassess patient for suspected continuing haemorrhage. Take and send post transfusion blood samples to the laboratory for repeat FBC, PT, APTT, Fibrinogen, Urea and creatinine, Calcium and Blood gas.
5. If further blood product is required inform the transfusion laboratory. At this point if patient continue to bleed you can seek the advice of the Haematologist to consider the use of Novo 7. If bleeding ceases send a stand down call to transfusion, return all unused blood component to the transfusion laboratory, complete all transfusion-related documentation. Com-

plete an audit of the management and identify any non-conformances, determine root causes, identify the preventive and corrective action as well as lessions learnt that can potentially improve subsequent management of massive haemorrhage in the hospital.

Acute Traumatic coagulopathy. Most (25%) severe trauma patients seen in emergency department often present with a triad of; Hypotherma, Acidosis and Acute traumatic coagulapathy (ATC). Acute traumatic coagulapathy is assocaited with a four-fold increase in trauma-related mortality. Damage control suscitation is immediately required to effectively and urgently address this triad. This involves the silmutaneous replacement of plasma component and red blood cells. The FFP: RBC OF 1:1, 1:2 and 1:3 has been suggested. Evidenced based findings however show that ratio of > 1:1 does not seem to offer any additional advantage. There is growing advocacy for the application of thromboelastometry. Thromboelastometry (TEM) is an established viscoelastic method for haemostatis testing in whole blood. TEM investigates the interaction of coagulation factors, their inhibitors, anticoagulant drugs, blood cells, specifically platelets, during clotting and subsequent fibrinolysis. It can serve as a guide with regards to componet usage in traumatic massive haemorrhage. There is also growing advocacy for the increased use of alternatives to conventional blood component particularly fibrinogen concentrate for fibrinogen replacement.

20. Storage conditions, shelf life indication and mode of transfusion

Red blood cells

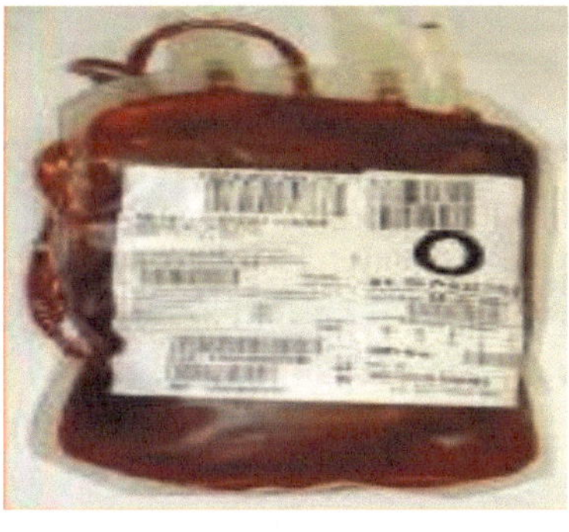

Red cell optimum storage temperature is 4°C ± 2°c. Time out of storage should not exceed 30 minutes at any material time (or must be discarded). Transfuse over 2-3 hours per unit. Used to treat acute blood loss to maintain HB above 7g/dl in otherwise fit patients and above 8g/dl in elderly patient or in peri operative situation when HB is < 7g/dl or <8g/dl in patients with known cardiovascular disease (elderly patients, those with hypertension, diabetes mellitus and other vascular diseases), in critical care to maintain HB >7 g/dl, in post chemotherapy to maintain HB > 8g/dl and in post radiotherapy to maintain HB > 10g/dl and in patients with chronic symptomatic anaemia with the hope of maintaining HB >8g/dl.

Fresh frozen plasma

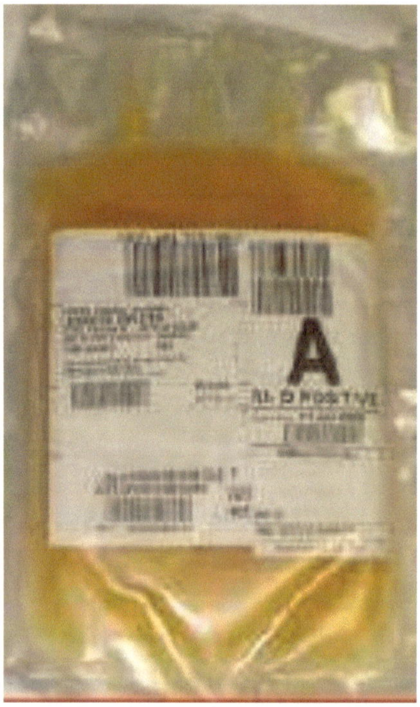

The optimum storage temperature for FFP is < - 30°C. Takes about 20-30 minutes to thaw. Once thawed, it should be used within 4 hours for optimum benefit or for up to 24 hours if stored at 4°C. Adult therapeutic dose is 4 units. Transfuse at rate of 12-15 ml/kg body weight. Transfuse over 30 mins per unit. FFP is indicated in the following situations; for the replacement of single coagulation factor deficiencies where the specific or combined factors is not available for example factor V with INR > 1.5, in liver disease patients with a pt >4 seconds of the control value (>1.5), in massive transfusion and surgery-related bleeding with INR > 1.5, in thrombotic thrombocytopenic purpura (TTP) in conjunction with plasma exchange with INR >1.5, in cases of Disseminated Intravascular Coagulation (DIC) in the presence of bleeding and abnormal coagulation results and for the immediate reversal of warfarin effect in the presence of life threatening bleeding. However prothrombin complex concentrate (PCC) is the optimal preferred treatment since FFP only has a partial effect.

Cryoprecipitate

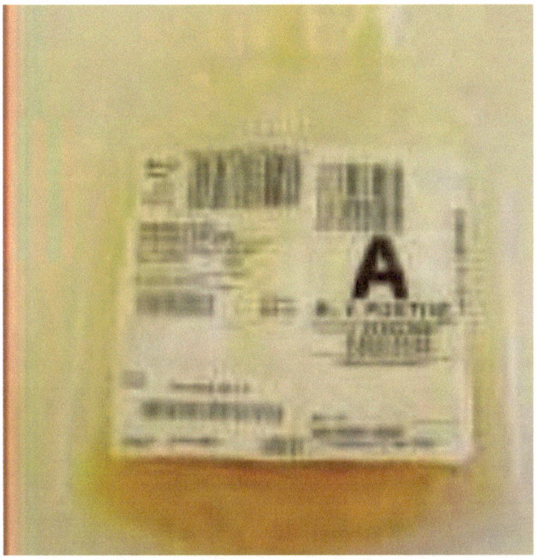

t

The optimum storage temperature for cryoprecipitate is < - 30 0c. Takes about 20-30 minutes to thaw. Once thawed, it should be used immediately within 4 hours. Adult therapeutic dose is 2 units. Transfuse at rate of 12-15 ml/kg body weight. Transfuse over 30 mins per unit. Cryoprecipitate is indicated in the following conditions; in cases of Disseminated Intravascular Coagulation (DIC) in the presence of bleeding and a fibrinogen level of < 1g/L, in cases of renal failure with bleeding and fibrinogem level of <1 g/L, in cases of hypofibrinogenaemia secondary to massive blood transfusion with fibrinogem level of <1 g/L, in cases of bleeding associated with thrombolytic therapy and associated hypofibrinogenaemia and in advanced renal disease to correct bleeding or as a prophylaxis in surgery in patients with fibrinogem level of <1 g/L.

Receipient group	**O**	**A**	**B**	**AB**
1st choice	O*	A	B	AB***
2nd choice	A	AB***	AB***	A**
3rd choice	B	B**	A**	B**
4th choice	AB***	-	-	-

Table: Selection of FFP for transfusion

Key

* = Group O FFP must be reserved only for O recipients

** = All FFP for use against ABO blood group barrier must be test for high titre haemolysins and found negative

***= AB FFP are often in short supply

Platelet

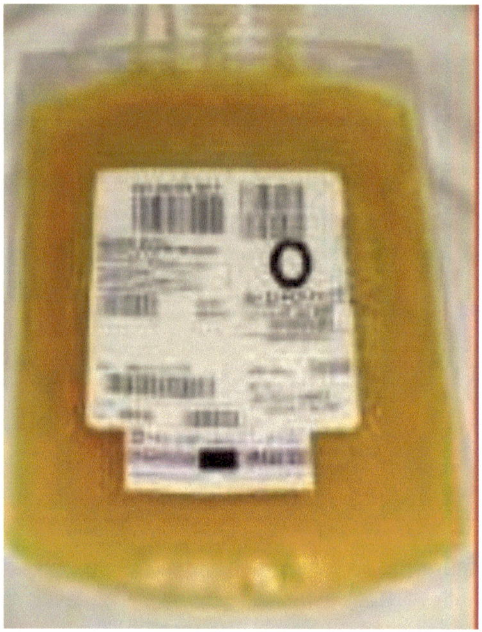

The optimum storage temperature in the platelet agitator is 22 0C. Maximum shelf life is 5 days. Transfuse at rate of 15 ml/kg body weight. Transfuse over 30 mins per unit. Platelet concentrate is indicated in the following conditions; When thrombocytopenic patients do not achieve the expected post-transfusion platelet count increment they are said to be refractory. This usually occurs in patients receiving frequent platelet transfusions. There are clinical and immunological causes of platelet refractoriness. Clinical causes include; sepsis, DIC, bleeding, fever, some drugs, and enlarged spleen. Immunological causes include the development of antibodies to human leucocyte antigens (HLA) or human platelet antigens (HPA). Immunological refractoriness can be managed by the provision of HLA or HPA matched platelets. Leucocyte reduction of blood products to levels less than 10^6/unit reduces the likelihood of alloimmunisation. This can be achieved through the use of pre storage or bedside leucocyte reduced blood products. Platelet concentrate is indicated; to prevent spontaneous bleeding in patients with a platelet count <10 x 10^9/l, in cases of autoimmune thrombocytopenia in the presence of major bleeding, in cases of acute Disseminated Intravascular Coagulation (DIC) in the presence of bleeding and thrombocytopenia, in cases of neonatal alloimmune thrombocytopenia to treat haemorrhage or as a prophylaxis prior to surgery, in cases of post transfusion purpura in the presence of life threatening haemorrhage and in patients with an inherited platelet dysfunction such as Glanzman, s thrombosthenia associated with haemorrhage or as a prophylaxis prior to surgery, in patients with haemorrhage that is not surgically corrected (post-cardiopulmonary bypass surgery) and associated with acquired platelet dysfunction and in patients on anti-platelet drugs like Clopidogriel, in a massively transfused patient (1.5-2 times the blood volume replacement) who are bleeding with a platelet count < 50 x 109/l. The aim is to maintain platelet count above 50 x 109/l, to prevent spontaneous bleeding in patients with platelet count of <20 x 109/l in the presence of other bleeding risk factors such as sepsis and other coagulopathies, to prevent bleeding associated with invasive procedures (lumbar puncture, insertion of intravascular lines, epidural anaesthesia, trans-bronchial and liver biopsy and laparotomy) in thrombocytopenic subjects. The platelet count should be raised to 50 x 109/l. In cases of surgery of critical sites such as the brain and eyes, the aim is to maintain platelet count >100 x 109/l.

21. Use of indication coding system to ensure the appriopriate use of blood components

In a bid to protect the national blood inventory and optimally maximize the use of our blood stock, there is need to develop a conservative approach in deciding whether transfusion is required in the managements of patients. Transfusion of the right unit of blood to the right patient at the right time, and in the right condition and according to appropriate guidelines. A chain of integrated events that begins with a correct decision that the patient needs blood and ends with an assessment of the clinical outcome of the transfusion. Its goal is to achieve optimal use of blood. Optimal use of blood ensures:

- Transfusion are safe (No adverse reactions or infections)
- Clinically effective (Benefits the patient)
- Efficient use of donated human blood (No unnecessary transfusions and that transfusion should only be given at the time the patient needs it).

Apprioprite use of blood component has become very important in the last few years for the following reasons; The cost of providing blood components has increased as a result of new safety requirements and other technical developments, the safety of hospital treatment and the effectiveness of care have become major concerns in healthcare systems. Blood transfusion has been the subject of legal proceedings and investigations in most countries. Hospitals should are now expected to be in a position to show that their practice of blood transfusion is safe, clinically effective and efficient, blood is a human tissue and is a precious and scarce resource. Many countries have difficulties matching supplywith demand. There is increasing challenge with supply of blood components (recruitment and retention issues) in most countries coupled with the fact that population in most countries are ageing. As well as the obligation for hospitals and blood collection services to demonstrate to blood donors that each gift of human tissue is carefully, wisely and effectively used and that it can be fully accounted for, legal actions, public inquiries, investigations or adverse media attention stimulated by transfusion-related harm to patientsare gainimg serious management attention and are helping to define the application of blood resource ensure effective use and to avoid future problems. The indications for transfusion provided below are taken from UK national guidelines for the use of blood components. Clinical judgement plays an essential part in the decision to transfuse or not to transfuse and help clinicians decide when blood transfusion is appropriate, and to minimise unnecessary exposure to transfusion. Each indication has been assigned a number, which may be used by clinicians when requesting blood or for purposes of audit.

Red cell concentrates. Red cell concentrate are indicated to treat anaemia in the following clinical situations.

R1. Acute blood loss:-In acute blood loss the objective is to maintain circulating blood volume and haemoglobin (Hb) concentration > 7 g/dl in otherwise fit patients, and > 8g/dl in elderly patients and those with known cardiovascular disease. If there is 15-30% loss of blood volume (800-1500ml in an adult) you can transfuse crystalloids or synthetic colloids. Red cell transfusion is unlikely to be necessary. 30-40% loss of blood volume (1500-2000ml in an adult): rapid volume replacement is required with crystalloids or synthetic colloids. Red cell transfusion will probably be required to maintain recommended Hb levels. >40% loss of blood volume (>2000ml in an adult): rapid volume replacement including red cell transfusion is required. For Peri-operative transfusion, many patients undergoing elective surgical operations should not require transfusion support if their Haemoglobin (Hb) concentration is normal before surgery. Assuming normovolaemia has been maintained, the Hb can be used to guide the use of red cell transfusion.

R2. Patient Hb concentration below 7g/dl. Anaemia with haemoglobin concentration of <70g/l in otherwise healthy/critical care patients may require red cell transfusion.

R3. Hb concentration below 8g/dl in a patient with known cardiovascular disease, or those with significant risk factors for cardiovascular disease (for example elderly patients, and those with hypertension, diabetes mellitus, peripheral vascular disease).

R4. Critical Care. Transfuse to maintain the Hb >7g/dl.

R5. Post-chemotherapy. There is no evidence-base to guide practice. Most hospitals use a transfusion threshold of a Hb of 8 or 9g/dl.

R6. Radiotherapy. Transfuse to maintain Hb above 10g/dl.

R7. Chronic anaemia. Transfuse to maintain the haemoglobin just above the lowest concentration which is not associated with symptoms of anaemia. Many patients with chronic anaemia may be asymptomatic with a haemoglobin concentration >8g/dl.

Fresh frozen plasma (FFP). The normal adult dose of FFP is 12-15 ml/kg body weight equivalent to 4 units for an adult. FFP are indicated in the following clinical situations.

F1. Replacement of single coagulation factor deficiencies, where a specific or combined factor concentrate is unavailable for example factor V.

F2. Immediate reversal of warfarin effect, in the presence of life-threatening bleeding. FFP only has a partial effect and is not the optimal treatment; prothrombin complex concentrates are preferred.

F3. Acute disseminated intravascular coagulation (DIC) in the presence of bleeding and abnormal coagulation results.

F4. Thrombotic thrombocytopenic purpura (TTP), usually in conjunction with plasma exchange.

F5. Massive transfusion and surgical bleeding; the use of FFP should be guided by timely tests of coagulation including near patient testing.

F6. Liver disease; patients with a prothrombin time (PT) within 4 seconds of the control value are unlikely to benefit from the use of FFP.

Cryoprecipitate. The optimum dose for cryoprecipitate is 1 unit/5kg body weight equivalent to 10 units for an adult. Cryoprecipitate is indicated in the following clinical situations.

C1. Acute disseminated intravascular coagulation (DIC), where there is bleeding and a fibrinogen level < 1g/l.

C2. Advanced liver disease, to correct bleeding or as prophylaxis before surgery, when the fibrinogen level <1g/l.

C3. Bleeding associated with thrombolytic therapy causing hypofibrinogenaemia.

C4. Hypofibrinogenaemia (fibrinogen level <1g/l) secondary to massive transfusion

C5. Renal failure or liver failure associated with abnormal bleeding where DDAVP is contraindicated or ineffective

Platelet concentrates. The optimum dose of platelet concentrate is 15 ml/kg body weight for children <20kg; 1 adult therapeutic dose for adults and older children. Platelet concentrateare indicated in the following clinical situations.

P1. Bone marrow failure: To prevent spontaneous bleeding when the platelet count <10 x 10^9/l.

P2. To prevent spontaneous bleeding when the platelet count <20 x 10^9/l in the presence of additional risk factors for bleeding such as sepsis or haemostatic abnormalities.

P3. To prevent bleeding associated with invasive procedures. The platelet count should be raised to >50 x 10^9/l before lumbar puncture, epidural anaesthesia, insertion of intravascular lines, transbronchial and liver biopsy, and laparotomy, and to >100 x 10^9/L before surgery in critical sites such as the brain or the eyes.

P4. Critical care/surgery: Massive blood transfusion. The platelet count can be anticipated to be <50 x 10^9/l after 1.5-2 x blood volume replacement. The aim in massively transfused patient is to maintain platelet count >50 x 10^9/l.

P5. In cases of bleeding, not surgically correctable and associated acquired platelet dysfunction e.g. postcardiopulmonary bypass, possibly combined with the use of potent anti-platelet agents such as clopidigrel.

P6. In acute disseminated intravascular coagulation (DIC) in the presence of bleeding and severe thrombocytopenia.

P7. In inherited platelet dysfunction for example Glanzmanns thrombasthenia with bleeding or as prophylaxis before surgery.

P8. Immune thrombocytopenia. Autoimmune thrombocytopenia, in the presence of major haemorrhage.

P9. Post-transfusion purpura, in the presence of major haemorrhage.

P10. Neonatal alloimmune thrombocytopenia, to treat bleeding or as prophylaxis to maintain the platelet count >50 x 109 /l.

Blood component	Shelf life	Optimum storage temperature	Monitoring Equipment
Red cells	35 days in CPDA	4°C ± 2°C	Temperture recorder and alarm system when temperature is sub-optimal.
Platelets	5 Days	22°C ± 2°C	Temperture recorder and alarm system when temperature is sub-optimal.
Fresh frozen plasma	2 years	< -30°C	Temperture recorder and alarm system when temperature is sub-optimal.
Cryoprecipitate	2 years	< -30°C	Temperture recorder and alarm system when temperature is sub-optimal.

Table: Storage condition of blood components

Special transfusion requirements

Irradiated Blood Component. Graft versus host disease is a serious and often fatal disease that occurs as a result of histocompatibility differences between donor and recipients. It often results from recipient receiving immunocompetent donors' cells or marrow. It often occurs in immunocompromised patients (congenital immunodeficiency, marrow transplant patient and patients on myeloablative therapy such as chemotherapy and radiotherapy) and seldom in immunocompetent subjects. The viable lymphocytes contained in the blood components can cause fatal GVHD in susceptible subjects. GVHD is thought to occur when the donor is HLA homozygous and haploidentical with the recipient. In such a situation, even though the patient is immunocompetent, it is unable to identify the donor's cells as foreign thus allowing for its proliferation and eventual GVHD. To prevent transfusion-associated GVHD, blood components are subjected to radiation (gamma radiation or x-ray) which damages the DNA and interfere with the ability of the lymphocyte to proliferate by forming electrically charged particles or ions. Commonly used isotopes for irradiation is Cs or Co at a minimum dose of 3,000 rads. It is essential to put a quality control measure in place for blood irradiators to ensure that, irradiation was performed as intended and daily check to ensure that timer is working optimally and periodic surveys to prevent leakages of isotope.

Disease conditions	When to prescribe/provide
Acute leukaemia in the absence of bone marrow transplantation	All HLA matched platelets and donations from 1st and 2nd degree relatives
Patients who has received autologous bone marrow and peripheral blood stem cell transplant	Irradiated product required from initiation of chemotherapy until 3-6 months post transplant. It may be safer to continue with lifelong irradiated products
Patients who have received allogeneic haemopoietic cell transplant	From initiation of chemotherapy until 6 months post transplant and if patient continues to be on immunosuppressive drugs
Patients having allogeneic haemopoietic cell donation and peripheral stem cell donation for possible use in future autologous infusion	A week before, during and until harvest is completed.
Hodgkin's disease, T cell Lymphoma &	Indefinitely from time of diagnosis &
Aplastic Anaemia	In transplant patients treated with (ATG)/Alemtuzamab.
Transplant patients and patients with CLL and lymphoma on purine analogues (Fludarabine, Cladribine, Eshap and others)	Irradiated products are indicated indefinitely from diagnosis/treatment
Patients with cellular immunodeficiency syndromes (Di George syndrome, Wiskott –Aldrich syndrome and others.	Irradiated products are indicated indefinitely from diagnosis.
Exchange and intrauterine (IUT) transfusion	Red cells and platelets must be irradiated for IUT and for exchange and top up transfusion provided delay of irradiation does not put patient at risk.
Granulocytes transfusions and transfusions from 1st or 2nd degree relatives.	Red cells and platelets must be irradiated

Indication for Gamma/X-irradiated red cells and platelets

Indications for CMV negative blood components. Cytomegalovirus (CMV) can be transmitted by blood transfusion and sometimes be fatal. Although most previously infected CMV donors may no longer be infectious despite being CMV antibody positive, providing susceptible CMV negative patient with CMV negative blood is a viable way to prevent transfusion-transmitted CMV disease. Providing CMV negative blood products is sometimes difficult because a significant number of blood donors are CMV positive. Since leucocytes are reservoirs of CMV in asymptomatic blood donors, leucodepletion can potentially reduce the risk of transfusion-transmitted CMV infection

Condition	When to prescribe
Pregnancy	All components must be CMV negative prior to delivery.
Intrauterine transfusion	All components transfused in utero
Infants and neonates < 1 year	All blood for IUT, exchange and top up red cell for neonatal use must be CMV negative.
Patients who have received bone marrow/peripheral blood progenitor cell transplants	Continue until CMV status of patient is known and indefinitely if patient is CMV negative.
Patients who has received allogeneic bone marrow/ peripheral blood stem cell transplant/kidney transplant	Continue until CMV status of patient is known and indefinitely if patient is CMV negative.
HIV/AIDS infected and Congenital immune deficient Patients as well as patients receiving extensive chemotherapy	If patients are CMV negative, they should receive CMV negative blood products.

Table: Indication for CMV negative blood products

Condition	When to prescribe
Emergency O Negative red cells	Select rr, Kell Negative, High titre Negative and CMV negative units for emergency use
Rhesus Negative women < 60 years old	Select Rh (D) Negative and Kell negative except in life threatening haemorrhage when Rh (D) Negative and Kell negative is unavailable.
Patients with clinically significant alloantibodies	Select red cells that are antigen negative for antibody patient has.
Autoimmune haemolytic anaemia	Check for presence of any alloantibodies and give units that are negative for antibody patient has as well as ABO and Rh (D) matched, Kell negative.

Sickle cell patients with alloantibodies	Select units that are rr, Hb S negative and negative for antigen to which patient antibody is specific. Sometimes it may be more effective to do an exchange transfusion to reduce the burden of haemoglobin S.
Transfusion –dependent patients	Provide ABO, Rh (D) matched Kell negative unit.
Recipients of allogeneic haematopoietic stem cells transplant	In these patient, if there will be ABO mismatch, transfuse patient with own ABO group until their ABO blood group antibody disappear and DAT is negative and donor group takes over. If minor ABO mismatch, transfuse donor ABO group that is plasma depleted until patient original group are no longer detected. For Rh positive patient that receives an Rh negative graft, transfuse them with Rh(D) red cells.

Summary of indications for antigen/phenotyped Red cells

Condition	**When to prescribe**
HLA or HPA matched platelets	
Platelet refractoriness	Patients that show a poor increment in platelet count after 2 or more platelet transfusion should be tested for refractoriness. Patient may have antibodies to HLA class A and B antigens and should receive HLA-matched platelets. If patient is negative for HLA antibodies then test patients for HPA antibody. If positive give HPA matched platelets
Neonates and neonatal alloimmune thrombocytopenia	Patients should receive ABO/Rh (D) matched HPA-1A-5b that is compatible with maternal alloantibody.
IgA Deficient Blood products	
Condition	When to prescribe
Patients with IgA deficiency or with anti-IgA antibody	Patients should receive IgA deficient units that is saline washed.

Table: Indications for HLA or HPA matched platelets and IgA deficient blood products

Methelene Blue treated plasma products. Methelene blue is an important nuclear stain commonly used in cytology. It is useful in the inactivation of pathogens. Methyelene blue inactivation property is bourne of its ability to attach to the base pairs in the nucleic acid double helix. Exposure of methylene blue treated plasma products to light (yellow spectrum at wavelength of 590nm) activates the methylene blue with attendant destruction of the genetic material of the infective agent including vCJD and prevention of replicaion and infectivity. Methelene blue treatment must only be done after leucodepletion of the product. Methylene blue plasma products are **indicated in neonate and children below 16 years on the day of transfusion.** Method of red cell and platelet inactivation are being developed. Red cells photo- inactivation agent using psolalens (amotosalen) and platelet inactivation agent (riboflavin) are in the validation phases of possible use.

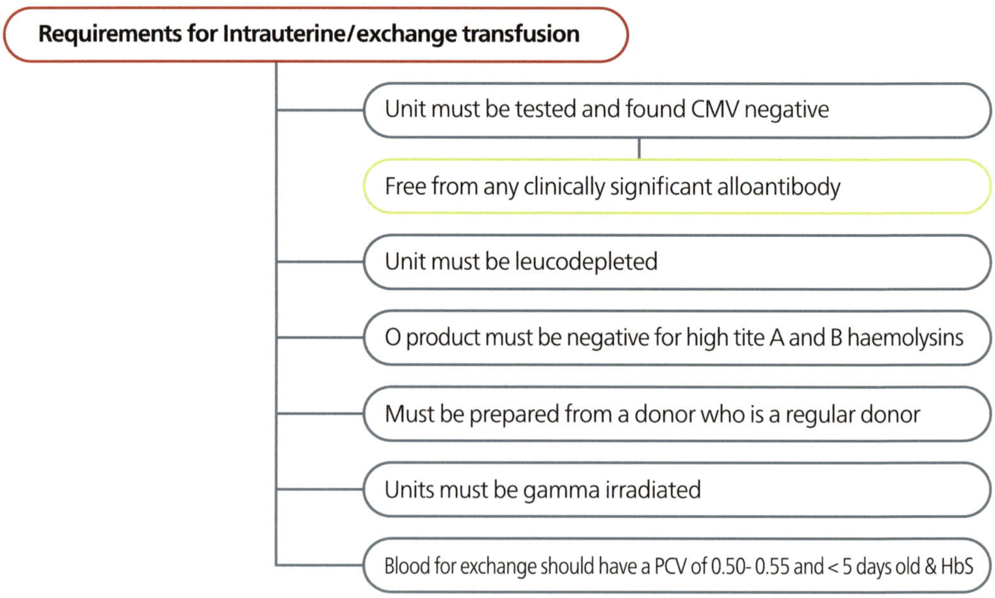

22. Fractionated plasma products

Plasma fractionation involves the use of selective precipitation and extraction of plasma proteins using cold alcohol. A large volume of pooled and microbiologically tested plasma is often used. Use of different alcohol concentration, PH and temperature precipitates different plasma proteins. Fractionated products includes; albumin, immunoglobulins and coagulations products. The fractionation process involves thawing the frozen plasma first to produce cryoprecipitate which is a raw material for production of coagulation factors. Secondly the reminant crosupernatant is treated at cold temperature with various concentration of ethanol and buffers to precipitate fractions containing different plasma proteinsThe purified fractions are then either freeze dried or in stabilized ready to use solutions.

Examples of fractionated plasma products

Albumin. Human albumin solution (HAS) is prepared as 5% (50g/l) or 20% (200g/l) solution. The final product is sterilized by filtration and heat treatment (60°C) for ten hours. The shelf life and optimum storage temperature are 3 years and 20°C respectively. Albumin is commonly used to restore plasma volume and plasma colloid osmotic pressure after trauma, surgery and shock. Albumin **must not** be used as a supplemental source of protein calories in patients requiring nutritional intervention. Indications for albumin includes;

1. Albumin is quiet useful for the management of extensive burns. Large volumes of crystalloids can be infused following extensive burns within the first 24 hours to restore depleted extracellular fluid. However post 24 hours albumin must be used to maintain plasma colloid osmotic pressure.
2. Albumin should not be administered in conjunction with phototherapy in exchange blood transfusion.
3. Albumin may be a useful adjuvant to exchange transfusions when administered concurrently with blood transfusion but it should not be used before transfusion.
4. Using albumin alone to treat ascites without large-volume paracentesis or to treat patients with noncirrhotic postsinusoidal portal hypertension should be avoided. Albumin and nonprotein colloids may be useful for postoperative liver transplant patients to control ascites and severe pulmonary and peripheral edema. Albumin may be used if the following conditions are met; serum albumin less than 2.5 g/dL, pulmonary capillary wedge pressure less than 12 mm Hg and haematocrit greater than 30 percent.
5. The use of albumin in conjunction with large volume plasma exchange (greater than 20 mL/kg in one session, or greater than 20 mL/kg/week in repeated sessions) is appropriate.
6. If cerebral edema is a concern, albumin should be used in concentrated form (25 percent) as a colloid to maintain Cerebral Perfusion Pressure.
7. Using albumin to maintain effective circulation volume following major hepatic resection (greater than 40 percent) is appropriate.
8. Albumin is indicated when clinically important edema develops secondary to crystalloid administration.

Immunoglobulin products. Human immunoglobulin is derived from fractionation of pooled normal plasma. The immunoglobulin content of product is a reflection of the immune status of the donor population. Human immunoglobulin are used in the treatment of several disorders as well as usage prophylactically to prevent several diseases. It can also be used to treat a variety of autoimmune disorders and patient with immunodeficiency. Immunoglobulins can also be used to provide passive immunization against a number of infections such as rabies. Immunoglobulin D is prepared from pooled plasma donation that contains a high titre anti-D and is used to prevent haemolytic disease of the foetus and newborn. Nearly 70 percent of primary immune deficient patients use intravenous immune globulin (IVIG) to maintain their health. IVIG is a pooled plasma derivative administered intravenously every three or four weeks that replaces antibodies in patients who are unable to adequately produce these protective proteins themselves. Examples of immunoglobulin products includes; Anti-D immunoglobulin (250 IU, 500 IU, 1500 IU and 2500 IU), anti-Tetanus (250 IU), Anti-Hepatitis B (200IU and 500IU), Anti-Varicella Zoster (250mg), Anti –Rabies (250IU) and Anti-Hepatitis A. These products are typically given as an intramuscular injection. Antibody replacement therapy, the use of IgG concentrates administered intravenously, is an important therapeutic option for patients who are unable to produce adequate amounts of antibodies. The IgG product, prepared from large pools of human plasma to assure a broad spectrum of antibodies, is known as immunoglobulin, gammaglobulin, or immune serum globulin. The intravenous preparations are known as IVIG (intravenous immunoglobulin) or immunoglobulin intravenous (IGIV).

Coagulation factors. Coagulation products (freeze dried concentrate) powders of known potency and purity can be produced by fractionating pooled plasma. Typical products includes;

Factor V111. Factor VIII (FVIII) is an essential blood clotting factor also known as anti-hemophilic factor (AHF). Antibody formation to Factor VIII can also be a major concern for patients receiving therapy against bleeding; the incidence of these inhibitors is dependent of various factors, including the Factor VIII product itself Factor VIII participates in blood coagulation; it is a cofactor for factor IXa which, in the presence of Ca+2 and phospholipids forms a complex that converts factor X to the activated form Xa. FVIII concentrated from donated blood plasma or alternatively recombinant FVIII can be given to hemophiliacs to restore hemostasis.

High purity factor V111. Commercial virus-inactivated high-purity factor VIII concentrate contains native von Willebrand factor. High-purity factor VIII concentrate is efficacious and safe product for use in cases of von Willebrand's disease when pharmacological correction of the hemostatic defect is not possible. In the surgical patients, the bleeding time can be corrected and clinical hemostasis can be achieved with use of high-purity factor VIII concentrate in patients in whom they are indicated.

High purity factor 1X. Patients with factor IX deficiency may be treated with a factor IX complex to manage an acute hemorrhage. Factor IX high purity (Factor 9 high purity) is a fractionated plasma product which is used in a number of thromboembolic diseases. Factor IX high purity (Factor 9 high purity) is used in haemophilia B and people who need additional factor IX for proper blood clotting. Factor IX high purity (Factor 9 high purity) is a medicine which is used in haemophilia, haemophilia B, haemophilia A, acquired haemophilia and haemophilia with inhibitors.

Anti-thrombin 111. Antithrombin III (ATIII) is a potent inhibitor of the coagulation cascade. It is a nonvitamin K-dependent protease that inhibits coagulation by lysing thrombin and factor Xa. Antithrombin III activity is markedly potentiated by heparin; potentiation of its activity is the principle mechanism by which both heparin and low molecular weight heparin result in anticoagulation. Congenital antithrombin III deficiency is an autosomal dominant disorder in which can individual inherits one copy of a defective gene. This condition leads to increased risk of venous and arterial thrombosis, with an onset of clinical manifestations typically appearing in young adulthood. Acquired antithrombin III deficiency is a deficiency of antithrombin primarily due to consumption. It is observed in situations in which activation of the coagulation system is inappropriate. Antithrombin (AT) concentrates can be therapeutically useful in cases of primary and acquired AT deficiency. Common conditions that result in acquired antithrombin III deficiency include;reduced production, acute and chronic liver disorders, premature neonates, treatment with L-asparaginase, increased excretion/loss, protein-losing enteropathy, nephrotic syndrome, burns, dilutional coagulopathy associated with; massive transfusion, plasma exchange, extracorporeal circulation, increased consumption associated with disseminated intravascular coagulation (DIC), major surgery, heparin infusion, multiple trauma, severe sepsis/septic shock, severe thromboembolism, haemolytic-uraemic syndrome and pre-eclampsia.

Factor V11 concentrate. Factor-VII-rich concentrate may be the treatment of choice in patients with liver disease who require temporary correction of their coagulation defect. Use of the concentrate was associated with uncomplicated delivery and minimal postpartum bleeding in pregnant patient with hereditary factor V11 deficiency. The aim of prophylactic administration of factor VIII to patients with haemophilia A is to reduce their number of bleeds. Factor VIII concentrate can be used in children and adults with severe haemophilia A. Factor VII concentrate appears to be effective in patients with refractory coagulopathy undergoing high-risk cardiovascular surgery. Prophylaxis results in a reduction in the frequency of haemarthroses which has been demonstrated to protect joints from the development and progression of arthropathy.

Factor X1. Factor XI or plasma thromboplastin antecedent is the zymogen form of factor XIa, one of the enzymes of the coagulation cascade. Deficiency of factor XI causes the rare Haemophilia C; this mainly occurs in Ashkenazi Jews and is believed to affect approximately 8% of that population, of both sexes. Individuals with factor X1 deficiency are not likely to bleed spontaneously, and hemorrhage normally occurs after trauma or surgery. Certain procedures carry an increased risk of bleeding such as, dental extractions, tonsillectomies, surgery in the urinary and genital tracts and nasal surgery. Joint bleeds are uncommon. Patients are more prone to bruising, nosebleeds, or blood in the urine. Woman may experience menorrhagia and prolonged bleeding after childbirth. Factor XI (FXI) deficiency is an autosomal disorder that may be associated with bleeding. Currently there are two factor XI concentrates produced in Europe for use in patient with factor X1 defieicency.

Factor V11a. Octaplex is presented as a powder and solvent for solution for injection containing human prothrombin complex. It nominally contains; human factor 11, V11, IX X, Protein S and C. It is indicated for the treatment of bleeding and perioperative prophylaxis of bleeding in acquired deficiency of the prothrombin complex coagulation factors, such as deficiency caused by treatment with vitamin K antagonists, or in case of overdose of vitamin K antagonists, when rapid correction of the deficiency is required. There are an increasing number of anecdotal reports and trials of recombinant activated factor VII (rFVIIa) for bleeding during surgery. Major blood loss can often be life-threatening and is most commonly encountered in the settings of surgery and trauma. Patients receiving anticoagulant therapy are also at increased risk of bleeding. PCC can potentially play a role in controlling bleeding in patients undergoing cardiac surgery and other surgical procedures and reduce, and sometimes abolish, the need for allogenic blood in surgical and non surgical patients. Although some of these may remain unavailable to patients particularly in sub Saharan Africa because of financial constraints on the health care system. Nonetheless, physicians in sub Saharan Africa must always keep in mind that the first and foremost strategy to avoid transfusion of allogenic blood is:

1. Their thorough understanding of the pathophysiologic mechanisms involved in anaemia and coagulopathy
2. Their thoughtful adherence to evidence based good practices in the developed world may potentially reduce the likelihood of allogenic blood transfusion in many patients groups.

23. Rhesus Blood Group System

The Rhesus (Rh) blood group system is one of the most clinically significant blood group systems after the ABO blood group system. The Rh blood group system currently consists of about 50 defined blood-group antigens. The five most significant antigens includes; D, C, c, E, and e. Of these, the D antigen is very important in transfusion and is a most common cause of the hemolytic disease of the foetus and newborn (HDFN) or erythroblastosis fetalis. Based on the presence or absence of D antigen on the surface of an individual's red cells, they are classed as Rh positive and Rh negative respectively. However other antigens of this Rh blood group system are also clinically relevant. In contrast to the ABO blood group, immunization against Rh can generally only occur through blood transfusion or placental exposure during pregnancy. The Rh blood group system was first described in 1939 by Dr Philip Levine and Dr Rufus Stetson when they observed that the serum of a woman who had had a still birth caused a severe haemolytic transfusion reaction to red cells of the same ABO blood group donated by her husband. This serum was also observed to agglutinate the red blood cells of about 80% of the general population despite being of the same ABO blood group. This antibody was faound to have been produced in response to the stimulus of an antigen on the surface of the foetus red cell which he inherited from the father and which the mother lacked. A year later in 1940, Dr Karl Landsteiner and Dr Alexander S. Wiener reported a serum sample obtained by immunizing rabbits with red blood cells from Rhesus macaque which reacted with about 85% of human red blood cells. The antigen responsible for this immunization was termed Rh factor. Based on the serologic similarities between the anibody described by Levine and colleages and those described Landsteiner and Wiener the Rh factor was maintained for antigens, and anti-Rh for antibodies, found in humans. However it was shown in 1942 and clearly demonstrated in 1963 that the clinically described human antibodies were different from the ones related to the Rhesus monkey. This real factor found in Rhesus Macaque was named as Landsteiner-Wiener antigen system. Between 1943-45 the other common antigens of the Rh system were identified. For many years the exact inheritance pattern of the Rh factors were debated. While Weiner promoted the Rh and hr terminology, Fisher-Race utilizing DCcEe for the various Rh antigens. However in 1993 Tippett discovered true mode of Rh inheritance using molecular diagnostics. Although the exact role of the Rh polypeptides are unknown, they are are thought to play a role in cation transport across the red cell membrane. Absence of red cells antigens on the red cell membrane has been associated with stomatocytes (red cells that have a characteristic slit or mouth shaped pallor rather than a central pallor) which have been associated with a mild type haemolytic anaemia. There is a considerable variation in the distribution of Rh (D) antigen in various population groups.

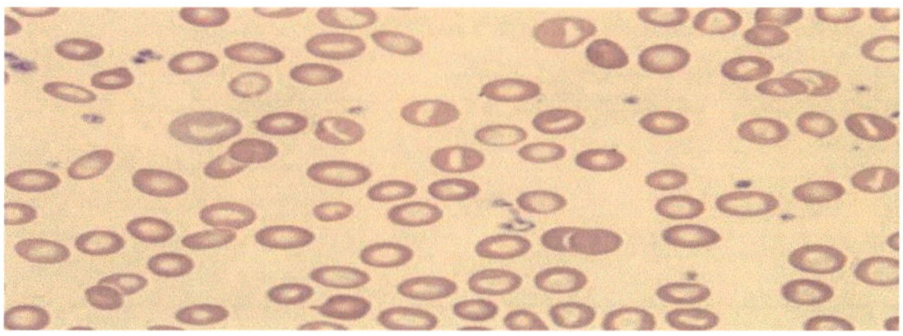

Figure: Stomatocytes in Peripheral blood

Population Groups	Rhesus (D) Antigen	
	Rh (D) Positive (%)	Rh (D) Negative (%)
West Africa	97	3
India	90	10
Europe	83	17
China	93	7
Japan	99.7	0.3

Distribution of the Dantigen in various population groups

Rh Genes and Antigens The Rh gene is located on chromosome 1. There are 2 Rh gene on the locus of chromosome 1 (D and CE). While the D gene control the production of the protein molecule that carry the D antigen, the CE gene control the molecule that carry the other Rh antigen combinations (ce, Ce, cE, and CE). Individuals who are Rh (D) negative lack the D protein are are susceptible to anti-D antibody when exposed to red cells containing the D protein. Although both the D and CE locus produces different protins, they are closely linked on the red cell membrane as a complex of antigens. The combination of the presence or absence of the D protein along with the 4 possible combination of the CE gene products produces 8 gene halotypes. Each of these 8 halotypes have their own shorthand notations. An individual will produce various combinations of these antigens depending upon which halotype is inherited from both parents. The absence of the D antigen is often conventionally expressed as d even though it is not a gene product. The presence of the D antigen is identified with the shorthand nomenclature R while the absence of D is identified with r.

D Gene	CE Gene	Halotype Gene Product (Fisher and Race Nomenclature)	Shorthand nomenclature (Wiener notation)
D	Ce	CDe	R_1
D	cE	cDE	R_2
D	Ce	cDe	R_0
D	CE	DCE	R_Z
D	Ce	Cde	r'
D	Ce	cdE	r"
D	Ce	Cde	R
D	CE	CdE	r^y

Fisher and Weiner model of the Rh gene halotypes

Rh Halotype combination	Rh short-hand notation	Phenptype reaction with anti-sera					Rhesus Group
		Anti-D	Anti –C	Anti-c	Anti-E	Anti-e	
CDe/CDe	R1R1	4	4	0	0	4	RhD+
cDE/cDE	R2R2	4	0	4	4	0	RhD+
CDe/cDE	R1R2	4	4	4	4	4	RhD+
CDE/cde	RZr	4	4	4	4	4	RhD+
CDe/cde	R1r	4	4	4	0	4	RhD+
cDE/cde	R2r	4	0	4	4	4	RhD+
cDe/cDe	R0	4	0	4	0	4	RhD+
Dce/dCE	R0rY	4	4	4	4	4	RhD+

Dce/DCE	RORZ	4	4	4	4	4	RhD+
cde/cde	Rr	0	0	4	0	4	RhD-
Cde/cde	r'r	0	4	4	0	4	RhD-
cdE/cde	r''r	0	0	4	4	4	RhD-
Cde/Cde	r'r'	0	4	0	0	4	RhD-
cdE/cdE	r''r''	0	0	4	4	0	RhD-
CdE/cde	ryr	0	4	4	4	4	RhD-

Phenotype reaction with Rhesus anti-sera

The Rh genotype of an individual is made up of a composition of two of the 8 halotypes inherited from both parents. The genotype of an individual can be expressed as either the halotype combinations (cde/cde), (CDe/cde) and (cDE/cdE) or in shorthand notation (rr), (R1r) and (R2r"). There are at over 50 Rh antigens that have been identified including those that are either combinations of these antigens or weak expressions of the above antigens, but most transfusion and HDFN Rh-related problems are caused by; D, C, E, c or e antigens. There are 5 principle antigens that may be found in most individuals. They are:

1. D found in 85% of the population
2. C found in 70% of the population
3. E found in 30% of the population
4. c found in 80% of the population
5. e found in 98% of the population
6. (d) which has never been identified but refers to the 15% of the population who lack the D antigen

The common alleles are Rh blood group system:

1. C and c are alleles with Cw occasionally seen as a weaker expression of C.
2. E and e are alleles although E is seen only a third as often as e. The e antigen is referred to as a high incidence antigen since it is found in 98% of the population.
3. D and the lack of D (or d) are alleles.

Characteristics of Rh antigens. The Rh antigens are made up of a total of 417 amino acids. These proteins cross the red cell membrane 12 times. The Rh antigens are not as available to react with their specific antibodies and there are fewer antigen determinants than ABO. Unlike the ABO system the Rh antigens are not soluble and are not expressed on the tissues. They are well developed at birth and have been identified in early foetal life (as early as 38 days) as well as immunogenic (ability to stimulate antibody production) and therefore can easily cause hemolytic disease of the foetus and newborn if the baby has a Rh antigen that the mother lacks. Molecular genetic foetal D genotyping can detect small quantity of D genomic DNA and thus allow for the D antigen status of the foetus from small quantity of foetal cells obtaind from a chorionic villus or amniocentesis sample. This is very vital particularly in Rh negative mother with high titre of anti-D (>15 iu) and whose partner is D positive (Dd). The test help to determine the D genotype of the foetus and its predisposition to HDFN. Approximately 60% of Rh negative transfused with Rh positive red cells will produce immune anti-D. After the D antigen, Kell antigen is next most immunogenic. Approximately 10% of kell negative persons develop anti-K when transfused with Kell positice red cells. One third of non-anti-D are anti-K. Unlike the ABO antibodies that are mainly IgM, the Rh antibodies are commonly IgG and formed by immune stimulus due to transfusions or baby's red blood cells entering maternal circulation during pregnancy. Since Rh antibodies are IgG they react optimally at 37°C and their reactions will be observed with the indirect antiglobulin technique. Agglutination reactions are enhanced by high protein (albumin), low-ionic strength saline (LISS), proteolytic enzymes (ficin) and polytheylene glycol (PEG). Rh antibodies exhibit dosage effect and will always react more strongly with homozygous cells than with heterozygous cells. For example, an anti-E will react with strongly with E+E+ cells and more weakly with E+e+ cells. The number of D antigenic determinant on the red cell membrane varies depending of the Rh phenotype/genotype of the individual. These number of antigen sites can be determined by radio-labelled anti-D. T he strongest D reacting red cell an highest antigen sites are the –D-/-D- (CE deletion) followed by R_2R_2 (cDE /cDE).

Rh Genotype	Shorthand notation	Number of D antigenic sites
CDe/cde	R_1r	10,000- 15,000
CDe/CDe	R_1R_1	15,000- 20,000
cDE/ cDE	R_2R_2	16,000 – 33,000
-D-/-D-	CE deletion	111,000 – 202,000

Table: Variation of number of D antigen sites on different Rh genotypes

Both Hemolytic Disease of the Foetus and Newborn and Hemolytic Transfusion Reactions can occur due the various Rh antibodies. To prevent sensitization of a patient the following step must be taken; transfuse Rh-negative individuals Rh-negative red blood cells and platelets and administer prophylactic immunoglobulin –D to all Rh-negative mothers following any potentially sensitizing events during pregnancy to prevent them from producing immune anti-D. The incidence of Rh antibodies

1. Anti-D most common antibody seen in Rh(D) negative people
2. Anti-E most common antibody seen in Rh pos people since only 30% of the population have the antigen
3. Anti-C or Anti-c less common - most people have the antigen

4. Anti-e often seen as autoantibody and will make it difficult to find compatible blood since 98% of the population have the e antigen
5. Anti-C, e or Anti-c, E often seen in combination. If a patient lacks both a C and e and has made an anti-C, then enhancement techniques should be done to make sure that an anti-e is not also present.

Rh System Inheritance. From the 1940's to the 1990's the mechanism for inheritance of the Rh Blood Group System was in question. The terminology that is part of the Fisher-Race Theory is most commonly used even today.

Fisher-Race Theory. The Fisher-Race theory involved the presence of 3 pairs of closely linked genes D, C, and E and their alleles c and e and the absence of D since an anti-d has never been found. These three genes are closely linked on the same chromosome and are inherited as a group of 3. The most common group of 3 genes inherited is CDe and ce (D negative) is the second most common.

Weiner Theory. Weiner believed there was one gene complex with a number of alleles resulting in the presence of various Rh antigens. According to Weiner there were 8 alleles; R^o, R^1, R^2, R^z, r, r', r'', r^y, which ended up with different antigens on the red cells that he called Rh_o, rh', rh'', hr', hr''. Weiner terminology is not use as often today, but you will often see Rh_0 (D) when a person considered to be Rh-positive. At times the gene terms are easier to use than Fisher-Race. If a person has the Fisher-Race genotype of DCe/DCe, it is easier to refer to that type as R^1R^1.

Tippett Theory. In 1986, Tippett predicted that there are two closely-linked genes - RHD and RHCE. The RHD gene determines whether the D antigen that spans the membrane is present. Caucasians who are D negative have no gene at those gene loci. In the Japanese, Chinese, and Blacks of African descent have an inactive or partial gene at this site. The RHCE gene determines C, c, E, e antigens produced from the alleles; RHCe, RHCE, RHcE and RHce.

Rh Halotypes	Gene present	Antigen present	Phenotype	Percentage among Caucasian
R^1	RHD RHCe	D,C,e	R_1	42%
R	RHce	dce	R	37%
R^2	RHD RHcE	DcE	R_2	14%
R^o	RHD RHce (more common in Blacks)	Dce	R_o	4%
r'	RHCe	dCe	r'	2%
r''	RHcE	dcE	r''	1%
R^z	RHD RHCE	DCE	R_z	<1%
r^y	RHCE	Dce	r^y	<1%

Translating From Wiener to Fisher-Race

There are times when you will need to convert Weiner to Fisher-Race or vice versa. It will be easier to do these conversions if you remember the following:

1. R always refers to D whether it is R^o, R^1, R^2, or the very rare R^z.
2. r always refers to the lack of D
3. o refers to having no C or E
4. 1 or ′ always refers to C
5. 2 or ″ always refers to E
6. The very rare haplotypes that have both a C and E are given letters from the end of the alphabet z and y.

Determining genotypes from phenotypes. The following steps will be helpful in determining an individual's phenotype. These rules are based on probability so the least likely genotypes will involve R^z or r^y. Type patient for the five Rh antigens: D, C, c, E, e and start with D: is it positive or negative? If negative, the individual will be homozygous d. If positive for D, you can't tell yet whether the individual is homozygous or heterozygous for D. Therefore, put D on just one chromosome. Look at C: is it positive or negative. If negative, put c on each chromosome. If positive, look at c result to determine if the C is homozygous or heterozygous. If there is no c present, there would be two C and it would be homozygous. If a c is present as well as C, they are heterozygous. If homozygous, and then put C on each chromosome. If heterozygous, put C on same chromosome as D; put c on other. Look at E: is it positive or negative. If negative, put e on each chromosome. If positive, look at e result to determine if homozygous or heterozygous. If homozygous, put E on each chromosome. If heterozygous, put E on same chromosome as the D unless the D already has a C; put e on other chromosome. DCe is more common than DcE and DCE is extremely rare. Only put C and E together on the same chromosome if no other combinations are possible.

Most Common Rh Genotypes. The following genotypes are listed as the most common (R^1r) among caucasians and while (R^or) is the most common among blacks. R^z and r^y are so rare they are not included in the following table.

Antigens Present		Genotype		Incidence (%)	
		DCE	Weiner Haplotypes	Whites	Blacks
1	D, C, c, e	DCe/ce	R1r	31.1	8.8
		DCe/Dce	R1Ro	3.4	15
		Dce/Ce	Ror	0.2	1.8
2	D, C, e	DCe/DCe	R1R1	17.6	2.9
		DCe/Ce	R1r′	1.7	0.7

3	Ce	ce/ce	Rr	15	7
4	DCcEe	DCe/DcE	R1R2	11.8	3.7
		DCe/cE	R1r"	0.8	<0.1
		DcE/Ce	R2r'	0.6	0.4
5	DcEe	DcE/ce	R2r	10.4	5.7
		DcE/Dce	R2Ro	1.1	9.7
6	Dce	Dce/ce	Ror	3.0	22.9
		Dce/Dce	RoRo	0.2	19.4
7	DcE	DcE/DcE	R2R2	2.0	1.3
		DcE/cE	R2r"	0.3	< 0.1

Incidence of the most common Rh genotypes

Applications of Rh genotyping

1. Paternity testing of the blood group antigens is based on a process of exclusion. Since the RHD and RHCE are closely linked and Ce, ce, cE are produced by a single gene, there are limited combinations that the father can provide.

2. It is helpful in HDN predictability by determining the father's Rh genotype. This helps predict likelihood of of the foetus being Rh positive and by extension the risk for HDFN due to Rh incompatibility between mother and baby particularly when the mother has a high titre of immune anti-D (>15iu). The Rh genotype of the father will indicate whether the baby has a O%, 50%, or 100% chance of being D positive.

3. If the father is also D negative (ce/ce), the baby will be D negative as well and there is a 0% probability of the baby suffering from Rh_o HDFN.

4. If the father's Rh genotype appears to be either, R^1r, R^2r or R^or, the baby has a 50% probability of being D positive and suffering from Rh_o HDFN.

On the other hand if a father's Rh genotype appears to be any of the following, R^1R^1, R^2R^2, R^1R^2, R^oR^o, R^1R^o, or R^2R^o, the baby has a 100% probably of getting a D gene from his father and therefore being D positive and suffering from Rh_o.

Rhesus D Haemolytic Disease of the Foetus and Newborn (HDFN). The hemolytic condition occurs when there is an Rh incompatibility between the the mother and the foetus. The disorder in the fetus due to Rh D incompatibility is known as erythroblastosis fetalis. Hemolytic (blood lysis or destruction) or breaking down of red blood cells. Erythroblastosis refers to the release of immature red blood cells into the peripheral blood to compensate for HDFN assocaited anaemia. Foetalis refers to the foetus. When the condition is caused by the Rh D antigen-antibody incompatibility; it is called Rh D Hemolytic disease of the newborn (often called Rhesus disease). The sensitization to Rh D antigens usually result from feto-maternal transfusion during pregnancy or during delivery and often lead to the production of maternal immue (IgG) anti-D antibodies which have a low molecular weight and thus can pass through the placenta barrier. The first baby is usually unaffcted. This is of particular importance to D negative females at or below childbearing age, because any subsequent pregnancy may be affected by Rhesus D hemolytic disease of the newborn if subsequent babies are D positive. The sensitization is preventable in by injections of prophylactic IgG anti-D antibodies (Rho(D) Immune Globulin) given following any potentially sensitizing events during pregnancy and within 72 hours after delivery of a Rh positive baby.

Symptoms and signs in the fetus

1. Hepatosplenomegaly (enlarged of liver and spleen).
2. Anaemia that results in newborn's pallor.
3. Jaundice or yellow discoloration of the newborn's skin, sclera or mucous membrane. This may be evident right after birth or after 24–48 hours after birth. This is caused by hyperbilirubinaemia (one of the end products of red blood cell destruction).
4. Enlargement of the newborn's liver and spleen.
5. The newborn may have severe oedema of the entire body.
6. Dyspnea or difficulty breathing.
7. Anaemia may be severe enough to warrant a top up transfusion
8. Hyperbilirubinaemia may be severe enough to warrant an exchange blood transfusion to prevent kinecterus (an encephalopathy associated with degeneration and yellow pigmentation of basal ganglia and other nerve cells in the spinal cord and brain, caused by the severe unconjugated bilirubinemia occurring in newborn infants with HDFN).

D Variants

Weak D (D^u). D^u or weak D is a weakly expressed D antigen that can only be demonstrated after incubation at 37°C followed with antiglobulin testing (Coombs technique). Weak D often occur as a result of the presence of few D antigen sites per red cells compared to normal D positive individuals. Most monoclonal anti-D reagents give a normal strength reaction with weak D compared to polyclonal anti-D reagent. When there is discrepant results with 2 different anti-D typing reagents, it is safer to treat such patient as Rh-negative and give them Rh-negative red cell until the Rh Sstatus is confirmed by the referene laboratory. If confirmed as a weak D, the person should be treated as Rh positive whether as a donor or receipient. Individuals who are weak D are not capable of producing anti-D if transfused with Rh-positvie red cells. An Rh control must always be run along with the weak D test. Always consult the product insert to determine if Rh control needs to be run when performing the immediate spin D testing.

Immediate spin		**37°C Anti D**		**Anti-Human Globulin Test (AHG)**		**Rh Group**
Anti-D	Rh control	Anti-D	Rh control	Anti-D	Rh control	
4+	0					Positive
0	0	0	0	4+	0	Weak
0	0	0	0	0	0	Negative
0	0	0	0	4+	4+	Indeterminate. Result not interpretable. Repeat

Table: Results obtained when performing the D testing

Testing for Weak D. It is recommended that all donor blood that originally fails to react with anti-D at immediate spin must be tested for weak D. Units that test positive for weak D should be labeled D positive and should be transfused only to D positive individuals. When performing testing on prenatal and postnatal mothers, D-negative blood at immediate spin should be tested for weak D as well to determine if they are eligible for prophylactic D immune globulin. Why do weak D's exist. There are three explanations for weak D's.

1. Quantitative Weak D. There are individuals that quantitatively produce fewer D antigen sites. This is more common in Blacks and is often seen with the Dce haplotype. On rare occasions among Whites an unusual DCe or DcE may also produce a quantitatively decrease weak D.

2. Position effect Weak D. In this case the D is weakened by the position of a C on the opposite haplotype which is called the trans position. The two Rh genotype combinations where this type of weak D is seen are: Dce/Ce and DcE/Ce. Today this type of weak D would type as a regular D due to the use of IAT cards.

3. Partial D antigen (Mosaic D). It has been found that some D-positive individuals make an alloanti-D that reacts with other D positive cells but not their own. Many of these will demonstrate a weak D type of reaction. In this type of weak D, the individuals lack some of the components of

the D antigen and therefore are able to make allantibodies to those specific components if they are transfused with D positive blood containing the specific components that they lack.

D Variants. Some individuals have a variant D protein as a result of changes in their inherited D gene. These changes are often as a result of a change in the amino acid sequence of the D carrier molecule. This changes results in variable reaction with the anti-D reagent. Based on reactictivity these variant are categorised into ; II, IIIb,IIIc, Iva, IVb, Va, Vb, VI and VII. Other additional minor variations continue to be described. Anti-D reagents used for typing must be capable of detecting these variants D antigens except category VI and above. Individuals in category VI and above have the least amount of D antigen and capable of producing immune anti-D if transfused with red cells containing the portion of the D antigen which they lack. These individuals should be treated as Rh negative and transfused only with Rh D negative red cells.

Other Rh System Variants

Anti- C^{w}. Originally thought to be produced by an allele of C and c genes. C^{w} is a relatively low frequency antigen found in approximately 2% of Whites and 1% of Blacks. It is not an allele of C and c. Its allele is MAR, which is found in 99.9% of the population. C^{W} positive red cells are often C+. However the antigen associated with C^{W} is weaker than normal C. Anti- C^{W} is not an uncommon antibody often thought to be naturally occurring may be clinically significant in causing a mild type HDFN.

V and VS. V and VS are low frequency alleles found in 1% or less of caucasians but are more common in Blacks. V is found in 30% of the Blacks and VS in 32%.

G and anti-G. G is present when D or C present due to the presence of the amino acid serine at the 103 position of the Rh polypeptide. Anti-G will recongnizes the the serine amino acid at position 103 and react with both D+ and C+ cells. Red cells that are weak C and D also react weakly with anti-G. Anti –G has been separated by adsorption-elution techniques from sera containing anti-C+D. Cases have been described of Rh negative (rr) patients who have produced anti-C+D when her partner was D+ AND C- (cDE or cDe) or D- or C= (Cde or CdE) or when they have been delivered of C+ and D- babies (Cde/cde). Those antibodies have actually been found to be either anti-G or Anti-C+G. G antigen is highly immunogenic particularly in Rh negative (cde/cde) individuals.

Rh deletions and suppressions. A number of variants resulting from deletions or suppressions involving various part of the Rh complex have been described. Examples include; (-D-/-D-, Rh_{null}, cD-/cD- and C^{W}D-). In some of these cases some or all of the Rh antigens are missing on the red cell membrane. The –D- phenotype is heterozygous is occurs either as a result of the deletion or suppression of the CE gene. The red cell of –D- phenotype expresses both D and G antigens. These red cells express more D antigens than normal D+ individuals and are readily immunized by common Rh phenotype red cells via pregnancy and or transfusion to produce anti-Hr_0 or anti-RH17. These antibodies are clinically significant, capable of reacting with all Rh positive excluding Rh deletion and Rh_{null} and are capable of causing HDFN. Patient with these antibodies must only receve red cells that are –D- or Rh_{null}

Rh deficiency syndrome (Rhnull phenotype). Rh_{null} has no Rh antigens on their red cells but these individual can transmit normal Rh antigens to their offspring. In the most common type the core Rh polypeptide is missing. A less common type has the regulator gene that turns off the expression of Rh. There have been at least 43 individuals in 14 families that are Rh_{null}. In these individuals the red blood cell membrane is abnormal has a shortened red cell survival and some of these have been identified when it was observed that they had hemolytic anemia and abnormal red cell morphology (Rh_{null} disease). If these individuals develop an Rh antibody following a transfusion or pregnancy, it is considered a anti-total Rh antibody. The amorphic type of Rh_{null} is caused by the absence of silent alleles at the Rh locus (---/---). The parents and children with amorphic Rh_{null} are heterozygous for the silent gene. Pregnancy and transfusion can stimulate Rh_{null} people to produce an antibody (anti-Rh29) or anti-total Rh which reacts with (Rh29 antigen which is a high frequency antigen present in all red cells except Rh_{null}) all red cell phenotypes except $Rh_{null.}$

Rh antibodies. The Rh genome is made up of a mosaic of D, C, E, d, c, e alleles. You can produce antibodies to any one of D, C, E, c and e (anti-D is usually the most clinically significant and common also known as Rh disease). Rh antibodies are produced through exposure to and of these mosaic antigens during previous blood transfusion or pregnancy. It is important to determine a baby father's Rh group and genotype. If positive for the antigen for which mother has developed antibodies; the child runs the risk of being positive for the antigen and being affected by HDFN. If he doesn't have the antigen, the baby won't have it and won't be affected by HDFN. Testing dad is often the first and important step. If baby is positive for the offending antigen, it may be important to closely monitor mother's antibody titers for the mother to be under the care of an obstetrician. Rising titres is a way of assessing the likely severity of disease. Antibody- D titres of 4-15 iu are often associated with moderate HDN risk. However titres of > 15 iu are often associated with hish risk of HDN. It may be important in cases where the father is positive for the offending antigen to determine the feotal genotype at 16 weeks gestation. If baby is positive for the offending antigen and titre continues to rise, it may be important to access for that suggest hydrophic changes and foetal anaemia by carrying out amniocentesis and analysing the amniotic fluid for product of haemoglobin brakedown. Severely affected babies may need intrauterine blood transfusion and may need to be delivered earlier. Rh immunoglobulin prevents Rh sensitization to "D" the major Rh protein, but may not prevent sensitization to the other Rh antigens antigen (C, E, c and e). Characteristics of Rh antibodies include:

1. They are generally IgG although some particularly anti-C may have an IgM component.

2. React optimally at 37°C

3. They are generally immune although some so called naturally occurring anti-E, C^W and anti-c have been described.

4. They are enhanced by enzyme treatment and react optimally by anti-human globulin (AHG) technique.

5. They are clinically significant antibodies and are often incriminated in HDFN and transfusion reactions.

6. They do not activate complement but can destroy incompatible red cells invivo. Rh antibody coated red cells are detected by macrophages and removed from circulation by the spleen.

7. Some Rh antibodies occur as antibody mixtures (anti C+D, anti-c+E, anti-D+K, anti D+Fy^a).

Anti-D. Produced when Rh negative patients are transfused with Rh positive red cell in emergency as a result of lack of Rh negative red cells or by D negative mothers exposed to Rh positive foetal red cells during pregnancy or delivery. Anti D show dosage effect and may occur with other antibody specificity such as anti-D+ Fya or anti-D+ K. Is a clinically significant antibody and can cause transfusion reaction and HDFN.

Anti-c. Usually produced by R1R1 (CDe/CDe) and other phenotypes such as R^1r' (CDe/Cde) and r' r' (Cde/Cde). Occur either singly or in combination with E (anti-c+E). Is the most clinically significant antibody after anti-D and can cause transfusion reaction and HDFN. Anti-c titers of > 7.5 iu are associated with moderate and high risk HDFN.

Anti-C. It is a rare antidoby and commonly produced in combination with anti-D by (cde/cde pregnant women). It can also be produced in combination with anti-e by R_2R_2 (cDE/ cDE) individuals. It is usually a combination of IgG and IgM antibodies. Anti-C seldom causes HDFN and when it does, the disease is usally mild.

Anti-E. Anti-E is a more common antibody compared to anti-C. Immune antibody but may sometimes be so called naturally occurring. Some reacts only in enzyme technique. Commonly produced in R_1R_1 individuals exposed to R_2R_2 or R_2r red cells and exist mostly in componation with anti-c. Individuals positive for anti-E are obviously e/e genetically. Reacts variable in LISS-IAT in sensitive IAT and enzyme technique. Seldon causes HDFN and when it does the disease is usually mild.

Anti -e. Anti-e is a rare antibody and the antigen that stimulates its production is a weak immunogen. Antibody reacts optimally in enzyme techniques. Seldon causes HDFN and when it does the disease is usually mild. Your red blood cells must be little e negative or you wouldn't be able to make anti-e antibodies. Patients with anti-e may have been exposed to e antigens in a prior pregnancy or during a blood transfusion. Itis important to determine if baby's father is e positive. If positive, it is likely he may have passed that characteristic to your baby. If he doesn't have the e antigen, the baby won't have it and won't be affected at all by the e antibodies. Testing dad is often the first and important step. If baby may have e antigen, it may be important to closely monitor mother's antibody titers.

No	Forward grouping with ABO antisera			Red cell reaction with Anti Rh (D) antisera		Reagent control	Back Group with standard cells				ABO and Rh (D) Group
	Anti A	Anti B	Anti A,B	D (1)	D(2)		A_1	A_2	B	O	
1	4	0	4	0	0	0	0	0	4	0	A Negative
2	0	4	4	4	4	0	4	4	0	0	B Positive
3	4	4	4	4	4	0	0	0	0	0	AB Positive
4	4	0	4	4	4	0	0	0	4	0	A Positive
5	0	4	4	0	0	0	4	4	0	0	B Negative
6	4	4	4	0	0	0	0	0	0	0	AB Negative
7	4	4	4	4	4	0	0	0	4	0	? Acquired B
8	0	4	4	4	4	0	0	0	4	0	? Acquired B
9	4 mf	0	4 mf	4	4	0	0	0	4	0	Indeterminate (? A_1+A_2).
10	4	4	4	4	4	4	0	0	4	4	Indeterminate. ? positive DAT

ABO and Rh (D) Grouping result
Key: 4 = Positive, 0 = Negative and MF= Mixed field reaction

Rh grouping and Phenotyping. An individual may or may not have the *"Rhesus factor"* on the surface of their red blood cells. This term strictly refers only to the most immunogenic D antigen of the Rh blood group system. Rh grouping is performed by reacting the red cells of an individual with 2 potent and highly specific monoclonal anti-Rh D reagents. The status is usually indicated by *Rh positive* (Rh+) to indicate the presence or *Rh negative* (Rh-) to indicate the absence of the D antigen. Rh phenotyping is performed by reacting the red cell sample against 2 specific anti- Rh reagents (anti-D, C, E, c and e). The detected Rh antigen combination determine the Rh phenotype of the individual. It is impossiblle to determine the genotype of an individual from the phenotype result. The phenotype cannot indicate if the red cell is homozygous (DD) or heterozygous (Dd) since there is no d gene antigenic product.

Reaction with antisera					Antigen present/Rh phenotype
Anti-C	Anti-D	Anti-E	Anti-c	Anti-e	
4	4	0	4	4	CcDe
0	4	4	4	4	CDEe
4	4	0	0	4	CDe
0	4	4	4	0	Cde
0	0	0	4	4	Cde

Rh Phenotyping Result
Key: 4 = Positive and 0 = Negative

Applications of Rhesus D grouping result

1. All new blood donors and transfusion receipient should be tested routinely for their Rh (D) group using two examples of monoclonal anti D reagent obtained from same or different clones. Donors and transfusion receipient's red cells (particularly those that have Rh-alloantibodies) may be further tested to identify their Rh phenotypes to allow for selection of appriopriate red cells antigen for patients with alloantibodies to ensure that thet receive red cells negative for the alloantibody they have developed. It is very important that the reagent used for grouping are controlled by reacting them against known D + and D – samples.

2. Patients found negative should be transfused with Rh D negative red cells only while those found positive should be transfused with Rh D positive red cells. Certain D negative males and women who have no child bearing potential may be transfused in certain situation with Rh D positive red cells (when stock level are low, in emergency situation such as massive haemorrhages and liver transplant when a large volume of red cells are required and the blood bank is unable to meet the Rh D negative red cell requirements). All effort must be made to ensure that Transfusion-dependent patients receive preferable bloods that are Rh and Kell compatible with the receipient to prevent them fro developing antibodies to these antigens. Rh antibodies are capable of causing severe transfusion reactions and HDFN. The aim of Rh (D) grouping and phenotyping of donors and reciepients includes; To prevent the stimulation

of anti-D antibbodies as a result of transfusion by ensuring that D negative individuals are transfused with D negative red cells and to detect the presence of Rh alloantibodies in the recipients's plasma and to ensure that such patient receive red antigen negative and crossmatch compatible red cell transfusion.

False Positives. When following through to AGT for weak D a positive reaction is observed in the Rh control. This is commonly seen in patients/donors whose DAT are strongly positive. These red cells are coated with antibody (not necessarily Rh antibody) in vivo. Albumin is potentiating medium that enables reagent Anti-D to overcome the zeta potential allowing cells coated with IgG Anti-D to get close enough together to agglutinate. Cells coated in vivo with any IgG antibody will also agglutinate in the presence of albumin. These false positives are corrected by using form of Anti-D that does not require albumin. False positive can also be caused by rouleaux formation, which will look like agglutination macroscopically. Rouleaux would be identified microscopically due to the "coin-stacking" appearance of the red cells. This false positive reaction can be obviated by washing cells 3 to 4 times in saline and then retesting. There are two types of alternative types of anti-D:

1. Monoclonal (IgM) anti-D which is capable of agglutinating D positive cells without the presence of albumin at room temperature. A number of facilities normally use this type of anti-D and therefore do not routinely use Rh control.

2. Use of chemically modified anti-D reagents (modified with albumin) to break the disulfide bonds closest to the hinge region so antibody can reach cells that are farther apart.

False Negatives. False negatives are not readily identifiable, but can occur in the following circumstances. Antigen and antibody reaction occur in optimum proportion. The most common cause of a false negative reaction is the use of too heavy a cell suspension. In such cases there are to too many cells for the amount of antibody in the antisera. They may also rarely be caused by extremely strong positive DAT. In this case a patient's D antigen sites are coated in vivo and there are no sites left for commercial anti-D to attach to. This can be corrected by heating cells gently to elute off antibody off the red cell surface without damaging cells and then re-testing.

24. Lewis Blood Group System

The Lewis antigen system first discovered in 1946 (ISBT 007) is a human blood group system based upon genes expressed on chromosome 19 q13.3, (FUT2) and 19p13.3 (FUT3). Both genes have fucosyltransferase activity. Two main types of Lewis antigens exist (Lewis a and Lewis b). Lewis red cell antigens which are not produced by the erythrocyte itself. Instead, they are a component of exocrine epithelial secretions (glycolipid plasma secretion), and are subsequently adsorbed onto the surface of the erythrocyte. Absorption can only take place if the Se (secreter) gene is also present in the individual. It is often possible to have any combination of Lewis a, Lewis b, both or neither antigens. The most common are Lewis a negative and Lewis b positive Le (a-b+). Having both antigens present on red cells Le (a+b+) is extremely rare and is thought to be caused by a weak expression of the secretor gene. Unlike ABO blood group antigen, the Lewis antigens are not present at birth. They develop during the first 15 months of life. Lewis antibody seems to be naturally occurring IGM antibodies and react optimally in saline normally up to 20°C. It may also react at 37°C by AHG technique. They do not cause HDFN and are rarely implicated to cause transfusion reactions. They may activate complement and cause haemolysis of test red cells. Patients with Lewis alloantibody do not require antigen negative red cell transfusion. The link between the Lewis blood group and secretion of the ABO blood group antigens was possibly the first example of multiple effects of a human gene. The presence of fucosyltransferase converts the Lewis a antigen to Lewis b. This is the same fucosyltransferase which can convert membrane bound A, B or H antigens into soluble A, B and H, allowing the person to secrete them into body fluids. Therefore, people with Lewis a antigens will not secrete the A, B or H antigens (and are called ABH non-secretors), and the presence of the Lewis b antigen is only found in people who are ABH secretors. Lewis negative (Le a-, Le b-) can be either secretors or non-secretors. People who are heterozygous are either Le(a+b+) or Le(a-b-). The latter is more common. Le(a-b-) individuals are capable of producing anti Lea +Leb. Due to the fact that these antigen are adsorbed onto red cells from the plasma, it is posible for the Lewis antigen of an individual to be weak or even temorary disappear. It is also possible for a person Lewis phenotype to change from Le(a-b+) to Le(a-b-) particularly during pregnancy or in patients on steroid treatment.

Basic chemical structural relationship between H and Lewis blood group antigens

Precursor Substance (PS): Glycoprotein + Gal +GlcNAc +Gal

H Substance: Glycoprotein + Gal +GlcNAc +Gal----Fuc

Le^a Substance: Glycoprotein + Gal +GlcNAc-----Fuc +Gal

Le^b Substance: Glycoprotein + Gal +GlcNAc-----Fuc +Gal---Fuc

Key

GalNAc:N-acetyl-D-galactosamine

GlcNAc: N-acetyl-D-glucosamine

Fuc: L- Fucose

Gal:G-galactose

Distinct characteristics of antigens of the Lewis Blood Group System

1. Manufactured by the tissues
2. Lewis antigens are secreted into body fluids
3. Absorbed onto red cells from the plasma

Lewis Antigens

The development of the Lewis antigens is controlled by two alleles of the Lewis blood group system; Le is dominant and results in the presence of Lewis Antigen and the recessive le (absence of Lewis gene) is recessive and therefore 2 le/le needs to be inherited.

Genotypes. Both Le/Le and Le/le result Lewis positive antigen. Lewis antigen exists as either Lewis a (Le^a) or Lewis b (Le^b).

Lewis negative results from le/le.

Formation of Lewis Antigens

What Lewis antigens are formed depends on interaction between Lewis (Le/le), Secretor (Se) and H genes in the tissues to produce Lewis antigens in the secretions. Lewis antigens have a similar structure to ABO antigens. They are formed at terminal sugars of Type I precursor substance made by tissue cell in plasma. If person has the Lewis gene, it adds fucose to second sugar from the end = Lea. If a person is also a secretor, H gene adds fucose to terminal sugar of precursor substance = Leb antigen. If person NOT a secretor, no H added to precursor substance made by tissue cell, so it remains as Lea.

Not part of red cell membrane but are synthesized by tissue cells, carried by plasma, adsorb onto red cell surface. Not present on newborn red cells and it can disappear during pregnancy and in patients on steroid therapy.

Characteristics of Lewis antibodies (Anti-Le^a and Le^b)

Lewis Antibodies can either be Anti-Le^a or Anti-Le^b. Almost always produced by Lewis a negative; Lewis b negative people. Naturally occurring but not regularly occurring (unexpected antibodies). Frequently seen in pregnancy (due to loss of Lewis antigen during pregnancy). IgM, therefore usually not clinically significant. Does not cross placenta. Reacts optimally at room temperature, but some may react at 37°C. If anti-Lea present at 37°C, may cause hemolytic transfusion reaction. Anti-Leb is usually clinically insignificant. There is variation in the trequency of Lewis antigen in black and white population with Le (b+) more common in whites than blacks and Le (a+) more common in blacks than whites.

Lewis group antigen	Frequency in population (%)	
	Whites	Blacks
Le(a+b-)	22	23
Le(a-b+)	72	55
Le(a-b-)	6	22

Variation of Lewis antigen in various population groups

Red cell reaction		Phenotype	Genotype
Anti -Le^a	Anti-Le^b		
4	0	Le(a+b-)	H Le sese
0	4	Le(a-b+)	H Le Se
0	0	Le(a-b-)	H lele

Reaction of Lewis antibodies

Features	Anti-Lea	Anti-Leb
Immune/Naturally occurring	Naturally occurring in Le(a-b-) individuals	Naturally occurring in Le(a-b-) individuals but rarely in Le(a+b-)
Immunoglobulin class	IgM	IgM
Complement binding capacity	Bind complement and cause the haemolysis of Le(a+) red cells	Some examples bind complement
Haemolytic transfusion reaction	May cause HTR	Do not cause HTR
Ability to cause HDFN	Does not cause HDFN	Donot cause HDFN
Agglutination pattern	Show stingy agglutination reaction	Show stingy agglutination reaction
Detection method	Readily detected in enzyme technique, usually a cold agglutinin and may react at 37°C	Readily detected in enzyme technique, usually a cold agglutinin and may react at 37°C

Differences between Anti-Le^a and Le^b antibodies

Secretor Status

1. Secretor status controlled by Secretor (Se) gene
2. Secretor = Se/Se or Se/se (80%)
3. Non-secretor = se/se (20%)
4. Secretors have soluble A, B and H antigens in body fluids (plasma, tears and saliva)
5. Can test saliva for presence of ABH antigens

Practical application of saliva testing

1. Determine ABO type in patients with ABO discrepancies
2. Determine ABO type in patients massively transfused with another blood type

3. Can also use Lewis types to determine secretor status:
4. Lewis a positive, Lewis b negative = non-secretor
5. Lewis a negative, Lewis b positive = secretor
6. Lewis a negative, Lewis b negative = can't tell secretor status from Lewis types
7. Can only use this method if patient has not been heavily transfused recently

Testing for Secretor Status. Secretor status investigation is based on the principle of agglutination inhibition. The procedure include;

1. Patient's saliva boiled and cleared.
2. Cooled saliva mixed with reagent anti-A, anti-B and anti-H.
3. If soluble A, B, or H antigens present in saliva, these will react with antibodies in reagent antiserum, and neutralize it, so no antibody available to agglutinate test cells.
4. If no soluble A, B or H antigens in saliva, antibodies in reagent antiserum will not be neutralized, and will be free to react with test cells.

Group A Secretor. Have A antigens in saliva. Addition of reagent anti-A: antibodies tied up by soluble A antigens. Addition of known A cells results in no agglutination (no free A antibody to cause agglutination). No agglutination indicates = Positive test for secretor status

Group A Non-Secretor. No ABO antigens in saliva. Addition of reagent Anti-A leaves free antibody in serum. Addition of known A cells causes agglutination. Agglutination reaction indicates a negative reaction for secretor status

25. MNS blood group system

The genes that control the expression of antigens of the MNS system is located on chromosome 4. The antigens M and N are co-dominant alleles that are closely linked to the S and s antigens, which are also co-dominant. These antigens are inherited by a complex pattern similar to the Rh system.

The Ms and Ns linkage is more common than the MS and NS linkages. M+ and N+ RBCs are common (75% of population) and M+N+ cells are the most common genotype (50% of population). These antigens were an early discovery and are some of the oldest blood antigens known after the ABO system.

They were first described by Karl Landsteiner and Philip Levine in 1927. Anti-M and anti-N antibodies are usually IgM and are rarely associated with transfusion reactions. Anti-N is sometimes seen in dialysis patients due to cross-reactions with the residual formaldehyde from sterilizing the dialysis equipment. This is usually irrelevant for transfusion since this variant of the antibody does not react at body temperature. The S antigen is relatively common (55% of the population) and the s antigen is very common (89% of the population). Anti-S and anti-s can cause hemolytic transfusion reactions and HDFN. The U antigen is a high incidence antigen, occurring in more than 99.9% of the population. The U was originally referred to as "Universal", though this is not the case. U negative RBCs can be found in people of African descent. This mutation in red cell surface structure also makes the RBCs S- and s-. Anti-U has been associated with both hemolytic transfusion reactions and hemolytic disease of the newborn. The other 41 identified antigens in the MNS group are low incidence.

They include the He (0.8% of the population) or high incidence, such as EN^a (>99.9% of the population). All the antigens of the MNS blood group system are fairly frequent in the population with the following overall frequencies:

- M = 78%
- N = 72%
- S = 55%
- s = 89%
- U = Greater than 99%

U antigen is a high incident antigen NOT seen in individuals who lack both S and s antigens. Individuals who lack this antigen (<1%) have a high likelihood of forming anti-U as well as anti-S and anti-s.

Biochemistry of the MNS antigens. The M and N antigens are glycoproteins containing sialic acid that cross the cell membrane. Carboxyl terminus extends into the red cells interior, a hydrophobic segment as part cell membrane and an amino terminal segment on the external environment of the red cell. The external components of the antigens are destroyed by the enzymes like fiacin, typsin and papain. The antigens of the MNSU blood group system are well developed in newborns. Therefore a mother who is negative for one of these antigens could be stimulated to make antibodies that may cause HDN. The antibody would have to be an IgG immunoglobulin that reacts at 37°C).

MNS System Antibodies. Anti-M is frequently seen as a saline agglutinin if testing is done at room temperature. It is predominantly IgM and can be naturally occurring. It will show dosage and therefore M homozygous cells will react with antibody more strongly than heterozygous cells. Therefore the predominant form of the antibody is not clinically significant. There are instances where some or the entire antibody is IgG in nature. If you have an anti-M that strongly at 37°C and/or AHG, it should be considered to be potentially clinically significant. Mild to severe cases of hemolytic disease of the new born have been reported. Since the M antigen can be removed by enzyme, the reactivity of anti-M can be destroyed by enzyme.

Phenotype	Frequency (%)	
	Whites	Blacks
M+N-	28	26
M+N+	50	44
M-N+	22	30
S+s-U+	11	3
S+s+U+	44	28
S-s+U+	45	69
S-s-U-	0	Less than 1

Ethnic distribution of antigens of the MNS blood group system

When performing a crossmatch on a recipient's specimen that contains anti-M, a pre-warmed crossmatch should be preformed. Anti-N is very rare and has similar reactivity as anti-M. Most often seen in kidney dialysis patients as cross-reacting antibody to formaldehyde. Formaldehyde is used to sterilize Dialysis equipment. Anti-S anti-s and anti-U usually form following red cell immunization due to transfusions and pregnancies.

They are usually IgG and react best after 37°C with AGT (Coombs) technique. All are capable of causing haemolytic transfusion reactions (HTR) (delayed) and Hemolytic Disease of the Newborn (HDN). S is usually destroyed by enzyme but s is variable and U is not destroyed by enzyme treatment. Anti-U is rare but should be considered if a previously transfused or pregnant Black patient has an antibody to a high-incident antigen

Characteristics	Anti-M	Anti-M
Immune/naturally occurring	Naturally occurring	Naturally occurring
Immunoglobulin class	IgM and IgG	IgM and IgG
Frequency of detection	Fairly common	Rare
Detection	Cold agglutinin but may react in IAT at 37°C. Not detectable with enzymes. Rxn enhanced at Ph <6.5	Cold agglutinin but may react in IAT at 37°C. Not detectable with enzymes
Ability to bind complement	Unlikely to bind complement	Unlikely to bind complement
Haemolytic transfusion reaction (HTR)	May cause HTR at 37°C	May cause HTR at 37°C
Haemolytic disease of foetus and newborn	May cause HDFN	May cause HDFN

Diferences between anti-M and N Properties of the MNS blood group system

Characteristics	Anti-S	Anti-s
Immune/naturally occurring	Immune	Immune
Immunoglobulin class	IgG and IgM	IgG and IgM
Frequency of detection	Rare	Rare
Detection	May act as a cold agglutinin. React optimally in IAT at 37°C. Show variable reaction with enzymes	React optimally in IAT at 37°C. Show variable reaction with enzymes
Ability to bind complement	May bind complement	May bind complement
Haemolytic transfusion reaction (HTR)	May cause HTR	May cause HTR
Haemolytic disease of foetus and newborn	May cause mild to severe HDFN	May cause mild to severe HDFN

Diferences between anti-M and N Properties of the MNS blood group system

26. Kell blood group system

The Kell blood group system was first discovered in the serum of a number of mothers; Mrs Kallacher in 1945 (K1), and Mrs Cellano(K2) who were believed to have babies with hemolytic disease of the newborn. One of the reactions was not due to Anti-D. "The non-Rh antigen involved in this case was that subsequently known as Kell. Thus at the very outset the test had detected a previously unknown blood group system which has since proved to be of some clinical importance. The K_0 phenotype was first described in 1957 and the McLeod phenotype was found in Hugh McLeod, a Harvard dental student, in 1961. The Kell antigen system (Kell-Cellano system) is a group of antigens on the human red blood cell surface which are important determinants of blood type and are targets for autoimmune or alloimmune diseases which destroy red blood cells. Kell can be noted as K, k, or Kp.

The Kell antigens are peptides found within the kell protein, a 93 kilodalton transmembrane zinc-dependent endopeptidase which is responsible for cleaving endothelin-3. The KEL gene encodes a type II transmembrane glycoprotein that is the highly polymorphic Kell blood group antigen. The Kell glycoprotein links via a single disulfide bond to the XK membrane protein that carries the Kx antigen. There are several alleles of the gene which creates Kell protein. Two such alleles, K_1 (Kell) and K_2 (Cellano), are the most common. The kell protein is tightly bound to a second protein, XK, by a disulfide bond. Absence of the XK protein leads to marked reduction of the Kell antigens on the red blood cell surface. Absence of the Kell protein (K_0), however, does not affect the XK protein. Kell antigens are important in transfusion medicine, autoimmune and hemolytic disease of the newborn (anti-Kell). Individuals lacking a specific Kell antigen may develop antibodies against Kell antigens when transfused with blood containing that antigen. Subsequent blood transfusions may be marked by destruction of the new cells by these antibodies (haemolysis). People without

Kell antigens (K_0), must be transfused with blood from donors who are also K_0 to prevent transfusion-related hemolysis of Kell positive red cells. Autoimmune hemolytic anemia (AIHA) occurs when the body produces an antibody against a blood group antigen on its own red blood cells. The antibodies lead to destruction of the red blood cells with resulting anemia. Similarly, a pregnant woman may develop antibodies against fetal red blood cells, resulting in destruction, anemia, and hydrops fetalis in a process known as HDN.

Both AIHA and HDFN may be severe when caused by anti-Kell antibodies, as they are the most immunogenic antigens after thoseof the ABO and Rhesus blood group systems. McLeod phenotype (or McLeod syndrome) is an X-linked anomaly of the Kell blood group system in which Kell antigens are poorly detected by laboratory tests. The McLeod gene encodes the XK protein, a protein with structural characteristics of a membrane transport protein but an unknown function. The XK appears to be required for proper synthesis or presentation of the Kell antigens on the red blood ell surface. There are three pairs of alleles within the Kell system. Each pair has a high frequency and low frequency gene that is co-dominated if present.

The three pairs are;

1. K (Kell), or K1, and k (Cellano), K2
2. Kp^a (K3) and Kp^b (K4)(Penney)
3. Js^a (K6)and Js^b (K7)(Sutter)

K, Kp^a and Js^a are low frequency antigens and k, Kp^b and Js^b are high frequency antigens. There is a Kell phenotype, K null (K_o or K5), is very rare and K, k, Kp^a, Kp^b, Js^a, Js^b antigens are not expressed. The Kell Systems antigens are found in only small amounts on the red cell carried on a single protein. K has approximately 3500 sites and k has between 2000-5000. The function of this protein is unknown.

Phenotype	**Phenotype Frequency %**	
	Whites	**Blacks**
K+k-	0.2	Rare
K+k+	8.8	2
K-k+	91	98
Kp(a+b-)	Rare	0
Kp(a+b+)	2.3	Rare
Kp(a-b+)	97.7	100
Js(a+b-)	0.0	1
Js(a+b+)	Rare	19
Js(a-b+)	100.0	80
Ko [K-,k-,Kp(a-b-),Js(a-b-)]	Extremely rare	

Variation in the distribution of Kell phenotypes in different population groups

Kell System Antibodies. Anti-Kell is the most clinically significant antibody within this system. The Kell antigen is considered the next most antigenic after the D antigen of the Rh system. Individuals lacking the K antigen can make anti-Kell after only two exposures to Kell-positive blood. Because over 90% of the population are Kell negative it is not difficult to find donor blood that is compatible with the recipient. Antibodies to other antigens in Kell system are very rare.

Antibody Characteristics of the antibodies to the Kell System

1. IgG
2. Cause HDN and HTR (delayed)
3. React best in Coombs after 37°C incubation. Enzyme has no effect
4. Does not show dosage (homozygous KK and heterozygous Kk cells react with the same strength)

Antibody	Reactivity				Bind comple-ment	Haemo-lysis	HTR	HDN
	< RT*	37	AHG	Enzymes				
K	Some	Some	Most	No	Some	No	Yes	Mild-Severe
K	Few	Few	Most	No	(Some)	No	Yes	Mild
Kpa	Some	Some	Most	No	(Some)	No	Yes	Mild
Kpb	Few	Few	Most	No	(Some)	No	Yes	Mild
Jsa	Few	Few	Most	No	(Some)	No	Yes	Moderate
Jsb	(No)	(No)	Most	No	(Some)	No	Yes	Moderate

Properties of antibodies of the Kell blood group system
HT = Room Temperature
HTR = Haemolytic Transfusion Reaction
HDFN = Hemolytic Disease of the Foetus and Newborn

27. Duffy Blood Group System

The Duffy antigen is located on the surface of red blood cells and is named after the patient in which it was discovered. The protein encoded by this gene is a glycosylated membrane protein and a non-specific receptor for several chemokines. The protein is also the receptor for the human malarial parasites Plasmodium vivax and Plasmodium knowlesi. Polymorphisms in this gene are the basis of the Duffy blood group system. It was noted in the 1920s that black Africans had some intrinsic resistance to infection with malaria but the basis for this remained unknown. The Duffy antigen gene was the fourth gene associated with the resistance after the genes responsible for sickle cell anaemia, thalassemia and glucose-6-phosphate dehydrogenase. In 1950 the Duffy antigen was discovered in a multiply transfused hemophiliac whose serum contained the first example of anti-Fya antibody. In 1951 the antibody to a second antigen, Fyb, was discovered in serum. Using these two antibodies three common phenotypes were defined: Fy(a+b+), Fy(a+b-), and Fy (a-b+). Several other types were later discovered bringing the current total up to six: Fya, Fyb, Fy3, Fy4, Fy5 and Fy6. Only Fya, Fyb and Fy3 are considered clinically important. Reactions to Fy5 have also rarely been reported. The Duffy antigen /chemokine receptor gene (gp-Fy; CD234) is located on the long arm of chromosome 1 (1.q22-1.q23) and was cloned in 1993. The gene was first localised to chromosome 1 in 1968 and was the first blood system antigen to be localised. It is a single copy gene spanning over 1500 bases and is in two exons. It encodes a 336 amino acid acidic glycoprotein.

The gene carries the antigenic determinants of the Duffy blood group system which consist of four codominant alleles—FY*A and FY*B—coding for the Fya and Fyb antigens respectively, FY*X and FY*Fy, five phenotypes (Fy-a, Fy-b, Fy-o, Fy-x and Fy-y) and five antigens. Fyx is a form of Fyb where the Fyb gene is poorly expressed. Fya and Fyb differ by in a single amino acid at position 42: glycine in Fya and aspartic acid in Fyb (G in Fya and A in Fyb at position 125). A second mutation causing a Duffy negative phenotype is known: the responsible mutation is G -> A at position 298. The genetic basis for the Fy(a-b-) phenotype is a point mutation in the erythroid specific promoter (a T -> C mutation at position -33 in the GATA box). This mutation occurs in the Fyb allelle and has been designated Fyb^{Es} (erythroid silent). Two isotypes have been identified. The Fy-x allelle is characterized by a weak anti-Fyb reaction and appears to be the result of two separate transitions: Cytosine265Threonine (Arginine-89Cysteine) and Guanine298Adenosine (Alanine100Threonine). Another rare genotype is the Fyb^{Wk}. Most Duffy negative blacks carry a silent Fy-b allele with a single T to C substitution at nucleotide -46, impairing the promoter activity in erythroid cells by disrupting a binding site for the GATA1 erythroid transcription factor. The gene is still transcribed in non erythroid cells in the presence of this mutation. The Duffy negative phenotype occurs at low frequency among whites (3.5%) and is due to a third mutation that results in an unstable protein (Arg89Cys: C -> T at position 265). Differences in the racial distribution of the Duffy antigens were discovered in 1954, when it was found that the overwhelming majority of blacks had the erythrocyte phenotype Fy(a-b-): 68% in African Americans and 88-100% in African blacks (including more than 90% of West African blacks). This phenotype is exceedingly rare in whites. Because the Duffy antigenis uncommon in those of Black African descent, the presence of this antigen has been used to detect genetic admixture. Overall the frequencies of Fya and Fyb antigens in Caucasians are 66% and 83% respectively, in Asians 99% and 18.5% respectively and in blacks 10% and 23% respectively. The frequency of Fy3 is 100% Caucasians, 99.9% Asians and 32% Blacks. Phenotype fequencies are: Fy(a+b+): 49% Caucasians, 1% Blacks, 9% Chinese Fy(a-b+): 34% Caucasians, 22% Blacks, <1% Chinese Fy(a+b-): 17% Caucasians, 9% Blacks, 91% Chinese. A Duffy negative blood recipient may have a transfusion reaction if the donor is Duffy positive. Since most Duffy-negative people are of African descent, blood donations from people of black African origin are important to transfusion banks. The Duffy antigens Fya and Fyb are a pair of co-dominant alleles found on chromosome 1. The phenotypes Fy (a-b+), Fy (a+b+), Fy(a-b+) are very common among the US white population. Fy (a-b-) is very rare in the white population but makes up 68% of the black population of the United States. Biochemically the Duffy antigens are glycoproteins that have an external loop. This external loop can be destroyed by enzymes such as ficin, papain, and trypsin. The Fya and Fyb antigens are receptors for the malarial parasite, *Plasmodium vivax.* Therefore individuals that are phenotypically Fy(a-b-) have a resistance to malaria. This particular phenotype is found up to 100% of Western Africa and of course 68% of the American Blacks.

Phenotype	Phenotype Frequency %	
	Whites	Blacks
Fy(a+b-)	17	9
Fy(a+b+)	49	1
Fy(a-b+)	34	22
Fy(a-b-)	Very rare	68

Phenotype and frequency of the Duffy blood group system

Properties of Duffy System Antibodies

1. Duffy antibodies frequently seen in multiply-transfused Blacks.
2. Anti-Fy^a much more common than anti-Fy^b and is more likely to cause HTR and HDN.
3. They are of the IgG immunoglobulin class
4. Anti-Fy^a can cause HDN and HTR (delayed) and anti-Fy^b is milder and no HDN cases have been reported but could possibly be a cause.
5. React best in Coombs after 37°C incubation
6. Reactions destroyed by enzyme of the red cells

Antibody	Reactivity				Bind Complement	Hemolysis	HTR	HDN
	< RT	37	AHG	Enzymes				
Fya	Rare	Rare	Most	Destroy	Some	No	Yes	Mild- Severe
Fyb	Rare	Rare	Most	Destroy	Some	No	Yes	(Yes)

Properties of antibodies of the Duffy blood group system
RT = Room Temperature
HTR = Hemolytic Transfusion Reaction
HDFN = HAemolytic Disease of the Foetus and Newborn

28. Kidd Blood Group System

The Kidd antigen system (also known as **Jk antigen**) is present on the membranes of red blood cells and the kidney and helps determine a person's blood type. The Jk antigen is found on a protein responsible for urea transport in the red blood cells and the kidney. The gene encoding this protein is found on chromosome 18. Two common Jk alleles are Jk(a) and Jk(b). Jk (a) was discovered by Allen et al in the year 1951. Whereas Jk (b) was discovered by Plant et al in 1953. Individuals who lack the Jk antigen (Jk null) are unable to maximally concentrate their urine. The Jk antigen is important in transfusion medicine. People with two Jk(a) antigens, for instance, may form antibodies against donated blood containing two Jk(b) antigens (and thus no Jk(a) antigens). This can lead to hemolytic anemia, in which the body destroys the transfused blood, leading to low red blood cell counts. Another disease associated with the Jk antigen is hemolytic disease of the newborn (HDN), in which a pregnant woman's body creates antibodies against the blood of her fetus, leading to destruction of the fetal blood cells. HDN associated with Jk antibodies is typically mild, though fatal cases have been reported. Jk^a and Jk^b antigens are inherited on chromosome 18 where urea transport mechanisms are located. Cells that are Jk(a-b-) are less likely to to lyse in the presence of high concentration of urea. These antigens are inherited by the co-dominant alleles Jk^a and Jk^b that are high frequency antigens. The Kidd antigens are thought to be grouped very close together in clusters on the red cell membrane. Due to the close proximity of the antigens when the antibodies are attached complement can be activated. The activation of complement can cause intravascular transfusion reactions. Approximate frequencies among the white US population are the following; Jka = 75%, Jk^b = 75% and approximately 50% of the white population is Jk^a and Jk^b positive. The more specific frequencies are listed in the table below for both whites and blacks.

Phenotype	Phenotype Frequency %	
	Whites	Blacks
Jk(a+b-)	28	57
Jk(a+b+)	49	34
Jk(a-b+)	23	9
Jk(a-b-)	Extremely rare	

Phenotype and frequency of the Kidd Blood Group System

Kidd System Antibodies

Both anti-JK^a and anti-Jk^b are hard to detect and identify since they are very weak and are detected primarily at the antiglobulin phase of testing. These antibodies are usually low titer as well as being weak reactions. The antibodies disappear rapidly from circulation and also in stored serum since their recognition is enhanced if complement is present. These antibodies will often show dosage. Enzyme can enhance the reaction as well as PEG enhancement solution. Characteristics of anti-Jk^a and anti-Jk^b are as follows; They are of the immunoglobulin class IgG. React best after 37°C with Coombs technique. Can cause HDFN. Can cause Hemolytic Transfusion reactions that are acute intravascular reactions, or they may be delayed transfusion reactions that show up after the patient's immune system is re-exposed and the memory cells quickly produce antibodies to the antigens. While most of the antibodies discussed in newsletter are more likely to cause extravascular hemolytic transfusion reactions, the Kidd antibodies can activate complement and therefore cause intravascular hemolytic transfusion reactions.

Anti-body	Reactivity				Bind Complement	Hemolysis	HTR	HDFN
	< RT	37	AHG	Enzymes				
Jka	Few	Few	Most	Enhance	All	Some	Yes	Mild
Jkb	Few	Few	Most	Enhance	All	Some	Yes	Mild

Characteristics of the Kidd Blood Group antibody
RT = Room Temperature
HTR = Hemolytic Transfusion Reaction
HDFN = HAemolytic Disease of the Foetus and Newborn

29. Bg Antibodies

The Bg antibodies were first described by Bennett and Goodspeed. They are not considered clinically significant, but may mask clinically significant antibodies. They are antibodies to white cell antigen remnants on red cells. Anti-Bg^a reacts with Human Leukocyte Antigen (HLA)-B7. Anti-Bg^b reacts with Human Leukocyte Antigen (HLA)-B17. Anti-Bg^c reacts with Human Leukocyte Antigen (HLA)-A28. Reactions relating to these antibodies are weak, react possibly at room temperature or more commonly in the antiglobulin (Coombs) phase. They react with only a few cells in a cell panel.

They do not cause hemolytic disease of the newborn or hemolytic transfusion reactions. They are seen frequently seen in multiply transfused patients or in multiparous women (multiple pregnancies).

HTLA Antibodies (High Titer Low Avidity antibodies)

High Titer Low Avidity antibodies are not clinically significant, but serological reactions make them look like they are High Titer if the antibodies are titered. The titers are usually at least 1:64 and often will be over 1:1000. Reactions are very weak and will break apart very readily due to the weak attraction between the antigens and antibodies (low avidity). These antibodies basically have a high titer but a very weak reaction. Some institutions actually score the strength of the antigen reaction in points which will allow them to differentiate some of the differences seen in various reactions.

Score = strength of reaction given points or score ; 4+ (12 points), 3+(10 points), 2+ (8 points), 1+(5 points) and negative (0 points). Specific serologic characteristics of the HTLA antibodies are; IgG, react best in Coombs after 37°C incubation, react with most cells (antibodies to high-frequency antigens), not clinically significant since they are not known to cause hemolytic disease of the newborn or haemolytic transfusion reactions. Since they are antibodies to high-frequency antigens they may mask clinically significant antibodies that are also in the serum.

30. I Blood Group Systems

I Blood Group System. The I antigen is found on almost all adults and is part of the precursor component of the oligosaccharide that forms the A, B, and H antigens. There are two types of oligosaccharides: type 1 and type 2. These chains that are part of the ABH antigens form the I antigen found in infants. All cord bloods form i antigen from straight-line sugar chains on precursor substance of the A, B, and H antigens. As indicated: in most children i is converted to I by the age of 2 years.

Anti-I, Anti-IH, and Anti-i Antibodies. Anti-I antibodies are the most common antibodies found if antibody screenings are done at immediate spin, room temperature. Their are IgM immunoglobulins and therefore are saline agglutinins with their optimal temperature at 4°C. Since they are IgM they also do not cross the placenta. Anti-I is naturally occurring often due to a Mycoplasma pneumoniae infection or some lymphomas and leukemias. These antibodies are usually not clinically significant Anti-I reacts with all adult cells (including patient's own, all reagent cells, all donor cells). Anti-I does not react with cord cells. Auto-anti-I is a common cold agglutinin.

High titers of auto-anti-I can interfere with serological testing:

In ABO typing, the forward grouping may have patient cells coated with IgM autoantibody, so all cells agglutinate. When this happens all results are positive and the group looks like AB+. On the reverse grouping anti-I in serum reacts with all adult cells, so A1 and B cells always agglutinate. All results are positive and the group looks like an O.

Anti-A	Anti-B	Anti-A,B	A1 cells	B cells	Cells + anti-D	Cells + Rh Cont	Interpretation
4+	4+	4+	4+	4+	4+	4+	Unknown ABO Group

Method to resolve these Problems

1. Correct forward typing by washing cells in warm saline and re-testing.
2. Correct reverse by warming the serum before testing, or adsorbing the cold autoantibody out of the serum.

3. Crossmatch results will indicate that all donors are incompatible. This anomaly can be correct by:
4. Warming the donor cells and patient's serum before crossmatching,
5. Omitting potentiators like LISS
6. Using monospecific anti-IgG. Anti-IH antibodies directed against both I antigens and H antigens.
7. Therefore they react most strongly with group O adult cells, least with cord cells or A1 cells.

Antibody	Adult A Cells	Adult O Cells	Cord A Cells	Cord O Cells
Anti-I	2+	2+	0	0
Anti-IH	2+	4+	0	2+
Anti-H	0	2+	0	2+
Anti-i	0	0	2+	2+

Table : Comparison of Anti-I, Anti-IH, and Anti-H Reactions

Anti-IH is seen most often in A1 adults and is not clinically significant but may cause problems with the ABO grouping and crossmatch results just as anti-I does. Follow the same steps for resolving the problem as indicated for anti-I.

Disease predisposition

Anti-I and anti-IH are only clinically significant when they cause Cold Hemagglutinin Disease (CHD). In this disease a strong autoanti-I is present. The blood in patient toes, fingertips, ear-lobes is cooler than than 37°C and the antibody coats cooled cells, binds complement, and causes hemolysis. This disease is treated by keeping the patient's extremities warm so the blood is not allowed to cool. High-titer anti-I also commonly associated with Mycoplasma. Pneumoniae infections. Treatment would be giving the patient appropriate antibiotics. Anti-i, which is fairly uncommon and transient, is associated with infectious mononucleosis.

31. P Blood Group System

Antigens of the P system include; Pk, P and P1. Basic structure is the precursor substance, but is called globoside (P) or paragloboside (p) in the P system. P antigens are poorly developed at birth and therefore do not usually cause Hemolytic Disease of the newborn. They are present in variable amounts on different red cells and seem to diminish in storage. Like ABO and Ii antigens; they are composed of sugar chains. Like A and B antigens, they are present on tissue cells as well as red cells. Similar antigens found in nature (bird droppings, pigeon eggs, hydatid cyst fluid) and these substances can be used to neutralize anti-P in a patient's serum. These similar antigen solutions can be useful when the antibody is interfering with ABO and crossmatch testing. The Pk antigen occurs when the Pk antigen does not convert to P. 80% of people with P antigen are P1 phenotype (have P and P1 antigens) and 20% of people with P antigen are P2 (P antigen only - no P1). The P2 phenotype merely signifies absence of P1 antigen in people with P antigen (globoside). Individuals who are Pk consistantly have an alloanti-P that is an IgM antibody. The absence of the P antigen is very rare and is designated as p.

P- antibodies

Alloanti-P1 is the most common of the antibodies in the P system. This antibody is commonly seen in P2 people. Alloanti-P1's characteristics includes; IgM class and therefore is saline reactive, enhanced by cold incubation, may bind complement. Not clinically significant naturally occurring but not regularly occurring. It is formed with no known red blood cell stimulus - either pregnancy or transfusion. If individuals are P1 negative, they do not automatically have anti-P1 i, but it is fairly common. Antigen-antibody reactions in P system enhanced by adding albumin to system, or by treating red cells with enzymes. Auto anti-P is an IgG antibody seen in P1 or P2 persons and causes clinically significant Paroxysmal Cold Hemoglobinuria (PCH). The Donath-Landsteiner Test helps diagnose PCH. It is designed to detect biphasic anti-P. A biphasic antibody reacts with the antigen on the red blood cell at colder temperature, binding complement. When antigen-antibody-complement complex warms up, the red blood cells are hemolyzed. Donath-Lansteiner test is performed by incubating patient's serum with his own cells first at 4°C, then at 37°C, and then looking for hemolysis. A positive Donath-Landsteiner = no hemolysis at 4°C, no hemolysis at 37°C, hemolysis only in the tube that was incubated at both temperatures. A negative Donath-Landsteiner = Negative at both temperatures or hemolysis at 4°C as well as 37°C

Donath-Landsteiner Test

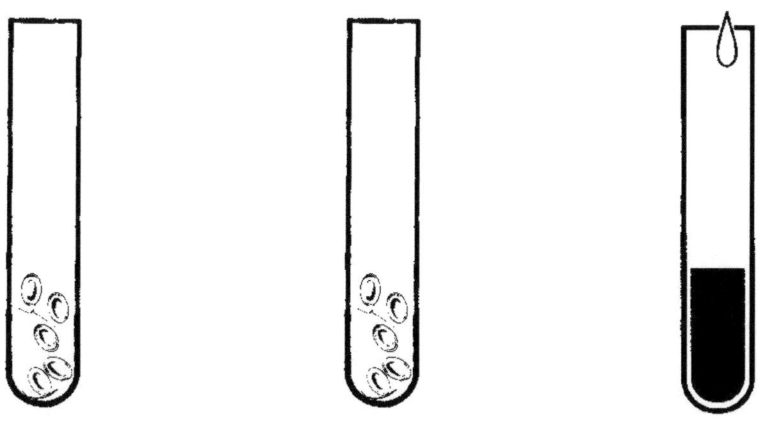

4°C incubation: No hemolysis = Negative	37°C incubation: No hemolysis = Negative	4°C + 37°C incubation: hemolysis: = POSITIVE

32. Lutheran Blood Group System

Lutheran antigen system is a human blood group system based upon genes on chromosome 19. This system is a single locus system, with antigens Lua and Lub. The Lu (b) negative phenotype is very rare. Antibodies to Lutheran antigens are IgG. The genes of the Lutheran group are linked to the genes responsible for the secretion of ABH substances. Lutheran blood group system, classification of human blood based on the presence of substances called Lutheran antigens on the surfaces of red blood cells. There are 19 known Lutheran antigens, all of which arise from variations in a gene called BCAM (basal cell adhesion molecule). The system is based on the expression of two codominant alleles, designated Lua and Lub. The antigens Aua and Aub, known as the Auberger antigens, were once thought to make up a separate blood group but were later shown to be Lutheran antigens arising from variations in the BCAM gene. The phenotypes Lu(a+b–) and Lu(a+b+) are found at various frequencies within populations. The Lu(a–b+) phenotype is the most common in all populations, whereas the Lu(a–b–) phenotype is extremely uncommon. Though present in the fetus, Lua is seldom the cause of erythroblastosis fetalis or of transfusion reactions. Lutheran antigens are weakly expressed on cord red cells. They are destroyed by enzyme treatment (papain and trypsin). They are thought to play a role in red cell adhesion. The Luthran null phenotype Lu(a-b-) which occur from either recessive or dorminant genetic background. The incidence of The Luthran null (Lunull) phenotype is rare (0.02% in the UK). Lutheran antibody Anti-Lua and Anti-Lub are rarely found in serum. They are often found in the serum of patients who have developed other alloantibodies. Anti-Lua is not a clinically significant antibody. It is an IgM antibody and react optimally in saline at 4-20°C and seldom react at warm temperature of 37°C. Anti-Lub is an IgG antibody and reacts optimally at a warm temperature of 37°C and show variable clinical significance.

33. Minor Blood Group systems

There are other minor less clinically significant but important blood group system. Their frequency varies from one ethnic group to the other. Their occurrence is low in certain population and is virtually restricted to specific ethnic groups. Information on patient ethnic group often plays a role in identification. These minor antigens are often not Included in antibody screening and identification panels. Samples in which antibody to these system is suspected should be referred to the reference laboratory. Antibodies to these systems are often seen in patients that have developed other clinically significant antibodies.

Blood Group System	Antibodies
Diego	Anti-Dia/Anti-Dib/Anti-Wra/Anti-Wrb
Cartwright	Anti-Yta/Anti-Ytb
Dombrock	Anti-Doa/Anti-Dob
Colton	Anti-Coa/Anti-Cob
Indian	Anti-Ina/Anti-Inb

Examples of Minor Blood Group Systems

System	Antibody	Origin	Ig class	Medium of reactivity			
				Sal 200C	Sal 370C	AHG 370C	Enz 370C
ABO	Anti-A	NO/I	IgM	Y	Y	Y	Y
	Anti-B	NO/I	IgM	Y	Y	Y	Y
	Anti-A,B	NO/I	IgM(G)	Y	Y	Y	Y
	Anti-A1	NI/I	IgM(G)	Y	R	R	R
Rh	Anti-D	I	IgG/M	Rare	Some	Y	Y
	Anti-C	I	IgG/M	Rare	Some	Y	Y
	Anti-c	I	IgG	Rare	Rare	Y	Y
	Anti-E	NO/I	IgG/M	Some	Some	Y	Y
	Anti-e	I	IgG	Rare	Rare	Y	Y
MNS	Anti-M	NO/I	IgM	Y	Rare	Some	N
	Anti-N	NO/I	IgM	Y	Rare	Rare	N
	Anti-S	I	IgG	Rare	Rare	Y	N
	Anti –s	I	IgG	Rare	Rare	Y	N
P	Anti-P1	NO/I	IgM	Y	Rare	Rare	Some
Kell	Anti-K	I	IgG	Rare	Some	Y	Some
	Anti-k	I	IgG	Rare	Rare	Y	Some
Duffy	Anti-Fya	I	IgG	Rare	Rare	Y	N
	Anti-Fyb	I	IgG	Rare	Rare	Y	N
Kidd	Anti-Jka	I	IgG	Rare	Rare	Y	Some
	Anti-Jkb	I	IgG	Rare	Rare	Y	Some
Lewis	Anti-Lea	NO/I	IgM/G	Y	Y	Y	Y
	Anti-Leb	NO/I	IgM/G	Y	Y	Y	Y
Lutheran	Anti-Lua	NO/I	IgM/G	Y	Rare	Some	Some
	Anti-Lub	NO/I	IgM/G	Rare	Rare	Y	Some

Antibody reaction pattern of the clinically significant blood group systems.

Private antigens. Some individuals produce antibodies to a low incidence (1% of population and not part of an established blood group system) antigen (private antigens). These antigens are not clinically significant, rare, not included in antibody screening cells as well as antigen panels for antibody identification. They are often detected by chance during a crossmatch and in HDFN investigation and are often referred to the reference laboratory for identification. Examples of private antigens includes; Swa, Wu and Pta.

Public antigen. Private antigens are antigens that are found which are present in red cells of a vast majority of the population (>99%) and do not form part of any blood group system. Individuals with antibodies to these antigens are likely to react with all red cells included in antibody detection and identification panels. DAT and auto control in these individuals are often negative-an indication that the reaction is caused by an alloantibody rather than an autoantibody. Some antibodies to high frequency antigens are clinically significant and can cause HDFN and HTR. Examples of public antigens are; Vel, Lan, Jra, Oka. It is often difficult to get antigen negative red cells for these individuals. Some countries may hold blood of these rare phenotype in their frozen bank. Anti-Fy3, anti-U and anti-Jsb are common in Africans due to a large number of Africans having the rare Fy(a-b-), U and Js (a+b-) phenotypes while the anti-Jra and anti-Inb are frequent among Asian population due to Asian people having the rare Jr(a-) and In(a+b-) phenotype.

High titre low affinity antibodies (HTLA). High titre low affinity antibodies although not clinically significant and cause no red cell destruction, their identification can be quiet challenging. Examples are Kna (Knops). Antibodies to high frequency antigens (Chido/Rodgers) are directed to complement protein C4 which is commonly seen in varying amount on some red cells. These antibodies reacts with some red cells and not at all with others.

34. Complement

Complement helps fight off bacterial and viral infections, eliminates protein complexes, and helps in the immune response complex. The three major roles of complement are; promoting acute inflammation process that allow white cells and macrophages to migrate to the source of the problem, altering the cell surfaces to encourage phagocytosis (opsonization) and modifying the cell surface that will eventually lead to cell lysis. Complement is a series of proteins found in fresh, normal serum. It is in the beta region on protein electrophoresis and is categorized as a beta globulin. The complement component that is found in the highest concentration is C3. Terminology commonly used for the various complement components:

1. Complement components are identified by C and their number: C1, C2, C3 etc

2. Complement products resulting from the splitting of these proteins during the activation process are followed by a lower case letter: C3a, C3b, C1q

Characteristics of Complement: Complement cause cell destruction through lysis, can cause cell destruction through opsonization (enhanced phagocytosis) especially with C3b as well as chemotaxis via certain split products acting as chemical signals to the phagocytic cells. Anaphylaxis can also occur through the split products (C5a and C3a), which promote inflammation. C5a and C3a can bind with mast cells and basophils leading to the release of histamine. This is turn results in; increases vascular permeability, smooth muscle contraction to preserve blood for vital organs and increases cellular membrane adhersion. Complement is normally inactive in serum or if activated the activation pathways are inhibited by control mechanisms of other complement proteins. It becomes activated by; antigen-antibody reactions - most often IgM (classical pathway) and bacterial polysaccharides, virus particles, enzymes, endotoxins (alternate and lectin pathway).

Complement Cascade - (Classical Pathway). The complement cascade is made up of 9 protein molecules (C1-C9). These proteins act sequentially. Each protein once activated is able to activate others. The classic complement cascade is activated once one IgM (IgM molecule since it has 5 immunoglobulin subunits) or 2 IgG (certain IgG molecues are capable of binding with complement includes; IgG 1, 2, or 3) molecule attaches to the red cell membrane. Complement needs 2 IgG molecules bound to antigen sites that are within 30-40 nm of each other. The sequence of reaction is (C1- C4- C2- C3- C5- C6- C7- C8- C9). If the complement activation proceeds to completion, channels are formed through the red cell membrane at the site of the complement activation resulting in the flow of fluid (water) into the red cells and results in lysis (rupture) of the red cells.

The steps of the classical pathway

1. Antigen-Antibody reaction occurs
2. Complement senses adjacent Fc receptors
3. Complement is activated and forms C1qrs complex
4. C1qrs activates C4
5. Activated C4 breaks down to C4a and C4b
6. C4b activates C2 to form C4b2a complex
7. C4b2a complex is also known as C3 convertase
8. In presence of Ca+, C4b2a activates C3
9. Activated C3 breaks down to C3a and C3b
10. C3b attaches to RBC membrane and is sensed by Reticulo Endothelial (RE) system and removed from circulation.
11. Activated C3a activates many C5 molecules that lead to the development of the Membrane Attack Complex.

12. Each activated C5 activates many more C6 and C7 molecules
13. C6 and C7 conversion proceed rapidly to C8 and C9 activation
14. Activated C8 activates many more C9 molecules
15. Activated C9 attacks red cell membrane, boring holes in it.
16. Contents of red cell leak out into plasma leading to intravascular hemolysis. As the complement cascade results in biologic side-effects such as chemotaxis, opsonization, and anaphylaxis.

Phases of the classical complement pathway

Activation phase: This phase involves the activity of complement component C1 following the formation of an antigen-antibody complex and the subsequent activation of component C2 and C4. Complement component C1 is made up of 3 subunits (C1q, C1r and C1s). C1 is activated following an antigen-antibody reaction in the presence of free calcium ions. The use of EDTA and citrated plasma disrupt the activity of C1 and inhibit complement activation. The C1q portion of the C1 molecule is made up of 6 immunoglobulin-binding sites. This facilitate the interaction between the C1 molecule and the CH2 domain of the Fc portion of the IgG (1 ansd 3) as well as the IgM-antigen bound immunoglobulin. Binding of two Fc portion of the IgG (within <40nm of each other) or a single IgM molecule (have 5 Fc binding sites) to the red cell membrane activates C1q. The binding of C1q with the Fc portion of two IgG or one IgM bound to the red cell membrane activated C1. Acticvated C1 acts on C4 and C2 molecules. This results in the cleavage of C4 into two component (C4a and C4b). While the C4a is release into the fluid phase, the C4b covalently bind to the Fc region of the red cell bound immunoglobulin. The activation of C1 also result in the cleavage of C2 molecule into C2a and C2b. While C2a is released into the fluid state, the C2b in the presence of calcium ions bind to C4b to form the C4b2b complex (C3 convertase). The activity of C4 and C2 can be inhibited by either the C1 inhibitor (C1 INH) or by the short half life of C2b molecule.

Amplification phase: The amplication phase involves the activation of C3 by the C1 activated C4B2b complex (convertase). This results in the cleavage of C3 into C3a and C3b. The C3a is released into the fluid state acting as anaphylatoxin and causes increased vascular permeability. The C3b binds unto the C4b2b to form C4b2b3b complex. The binding of C3b on the red cell membrane facilitates immune adherence and promotes the binding of such C3b bound red cells to C3b receptor site of macrophages. This results in the sequesteration of such C3b bound red cells by macrophages in the spleen or liver. A positive reaction with and C3d AHG reagent in a positive DAT test is a sign that complement activation has taken place in the patient circulation. The amplification phase of complement activation can be inactivated bythe activity of C3b and / or C4b inactivator proteins (C3Bina AND C4bINA). The complement cascade frequently stops at the C3B stage.

Membrane attack phase: This involves the activation of C5 by C4b2b3b complex and subsequent activation of C6, C7, C8 and C9. This activation results in the cleavage of C5 into C5a and C5b. The C5a is released into the fluid state where it acts as an analphylatoxin and increases red cell permeability. The C5b binds to C6 and C7 to form a tri-molecular complex which is firmly inserted into the red cell membrane. C8 and C9 are the bound to the C5b67 complex in a circular fashion and produces a membrane lesion or hole of about 10nm diameter. This facilitates the flow of ions and water across the red cell membrane resulting in the loss of the osmotic gradient and red cell lysis

Facors affecting the clinical significance of an antibody. Not all red cell alloantibodies are capable of activating complements and causing red cell destruction invivo. The red cell destruction potential of an antibody depends on a number of factors:

Nature of antibody coating the cell. IgM antibodies are the best because they have more antigen-binding sites. They can achieve binding of two adjacent antigens by single IgM molecule. Only certain IgG subclasses are capable of activating complement: IgG subclasses 1, 2, and 3 of these IgG subsets, IgG 3 are the best. IgG subclass 4 does not activate complement.

Number of antigen sites on red cell. The more antigen sites found on the red blood cell, the more likely two adjacent ones are bound by antibody. The A and B antigens are in very high concentration on the red blood cells. The natural-occurring, expected antibodies (anti-A, anti-B, and anti-A, B) are IgM. ABO incompatibilities are the most likely to result in intravascular transfusion reactions from the activation of the classical pathway. Other factors include; ability of the antibody to activate complement, the blood group specificity and the temperature of optimum reactivity of the antibody. Generally antibodies that react optimally at 37°C are mostly clinically significant. They are capable of causing haemolytic transfusion reaction (resulting from incompatible red cell transfusion) and or HDFN.

Possible Outcomes of Complement Activation in Blood Banking. The signs and symptoms of complement activated –related invivo red cells destruction similar to that seen in haemolytic transfusion reaction include; intravascular hemolysis (complement cascade goes to completion) and the cells are lysed, extravascular hemolysis where the complement cascade stops at C3b step. Cells coated with C3b are removed from circulation via macrophages and neutrophils, "Damaged cells" (spherocytes and stroma fragments) lead to decreased cell survival and possible activation of Hageman factor that in turn leads to coagulation activation, unexplained Disseminated Intravascular Coagulation (DIC)-related bleeding may also occur due to small clumps of agglutinated cells in the blood stream, fibrinogen consumption, activation of fibrinogen system and fibrin destruction, when leukocytes are exposed to various antigen-antibody complexes they will also respond by secreting various cytokines that will lead to: fever, a drop in blood pressure and additional release of white blood cells from the bone marrow as well as a number of other activities; renal failure (anuria and renal damage) is the most common complication of an untreated hemolytic transfusion reaction, hypotension, contraction of the blood vessels in the kidney since it is one of the smooth muscles that respond in anaphylaxis, intravascular clots, fever (>10c rise in temperature), toxic effects of free haemoglobin, flushing of the face, chest and lumbar pain, nausea and haemoglobinuria.

Non-Immune Hemolysis. Physical factors that can cause haemolysis include; temperature extremes (outside body), hypotonic solutions (IV solutions), mechanical (pumps, intravascular clots) and chemical- toxins. Causes of immune-mediated cell destruction (Hemolysis) include; antibodies that bind complements, antibodies that do not bind complement and Complement activation only.

Types of Immune-Mediated Hemolysis

Intravascular Hemolysis. Antigen–antibody reaction often results in complement actication. When such activation proceeds to completion, the red cell membrane are damaged and lyses within the circulation. Intravascular hemolysis is complement mediated since the hemolysis is due to activation of the complement pathway by the classical pathway. Intravascular indicates the cell destruction takes place within the blood vessels. This type of hemolysis can be life-threatening due to both the possibility of anaphylaxis and renal failure. The lyses of the red cells releases haemoglobin into the circulation resulting in haemoglobinaemia and haemoglobinuria. Examples of antibodies that can cause haemolysis invivo includes anti-A, anti-B and most particularly anti A,B. These antibodies are often incriminated in haemolytic transfusion reactions resulting from the transfusion of ABO incompatible red cells (Acells to a group B patient, Bcell to a group A patient or A or B cells to a blood group O individual).

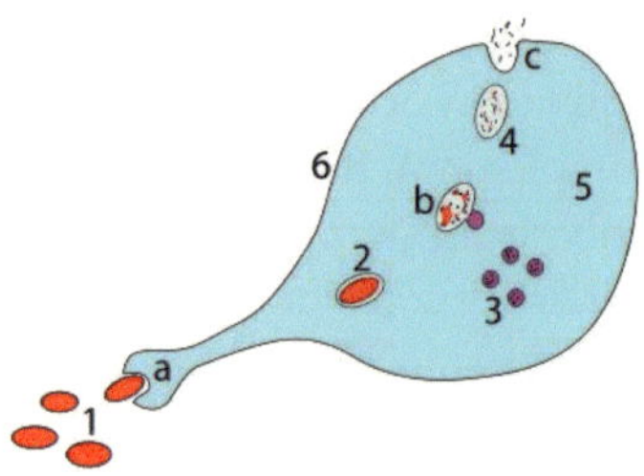

Figure: Steps of a macrophage ingesting an antibody coated red cells
a. Ingestion of the antibody caoted red cells through phagocytosis (a phagosome is formed)
b. The fusion of lysosomes with the phagosome creates a phagolysosome. The antibody caoted red cell is broken down by enzymes.
c. Waste material is expelled

Extravascular Hemolysis. Anti- A, anti- B, anti-AB and most other antibodies can cause the destruction of red cells by macrophages outside the circulation. Not all IgG and IgM antibodies activates complement. Rhesus antibodies for example does not activate complement. The binding of such antibody to red cells can however be recongnised by macrophage IgG receptors. This binding often occurs in the spleen. The IgG coated red cells are not fit for circulation and are thus either engulfed or digested by the macrophage. This results in the digestion of the red cell membrane resulting in fluid loss leading to formation of a spherocyte. These sherocytes loses that permeability and are trapped as they go through the microcirculation of the spleen. Extravascular hemolysis may be antibody mediated or complement mediated. The cell destruction takes place within RE system (sinusoidal lining cells of the spleen) and is generally not life-threatening. The survival rate of the transfused cells will be decreased. Red cells coated with C3b are recongnized and selectively removed by macrophages in the liver (kupffer cell). Red cells coated with IgG and C3b aere removed in either the spleen and /or the liver. The rate of extravascular haemolysis however depends on the number of antibody bound red cells present as well as the volume of incompatible red cell transfused. The haemolysis may sometimes be rapid enough to result in haemoglobinuria. A condition in which the oxygen transport protein haemoglobin is found in abnormally high concentrations in the urine. The condition is often associated with haemolytic anaemia, in which red blood cells are destroyed, thereby increasing levels of free plasma haemoglobin. The excess hemoglobin is filtered by the kidneys, which release it into the urine, giving urine a red color. Management of haemolytic transfusion reaction include; maintaining a good fluid balance by infusing saline to support the kidney fuction and replacing coagulation factors and platelet in cases of DIC-related consumption coagulopathy by transfusing fresh frozen plasma (FFP), cryoprecipitate and platelet concentrate.

Immune Response Following a Blood Transfusion Leading to Alloimmunization. Donor red cells carrying foreign antigens die normally and are phagocytized by RE system. Foreign antigens are processed and stimulate immune response. IgM antibody produced after several weeks, probably produce no cell destruction. Gradual decline of red cells results in continuous re-exposure of the antigen to the immune system. Primary and secondary responses can overlap each other. IgG antibodies can be produced while IgM antibody productions is going on, from the same blood transfusion (same "stimulating event"). Low-titer IgM antibodies may not cause cell destruction, but higher-titer IgG antibodies will eventually lead to extravascular hemolysis.

Intravascular Hemolysis (complement mediated)

Mechanism of intravascular hemolysis. Complement is activated when two adjacent antigen sites are bound by antibody. The activated complement rapidly proceeds through several chemical changes to membrane attack complex. The membrane attack complex bores a hole through red cell membrane, causing hemolysis. The rate of complement activation and amount of complement activated determines whether complement cascade goes to completion.

Signs of intravascular hemolysis. Sudden drop in blood pressure due to the anaphylactoxins: C5a and C3a. Hemoglobinuria due to the lysis of of the red blood cells. If more hemoglobulin is released that can be carried by albumin. Hemoglobinemia (plasma hemoglobulin levels) occurs again due to the lysis of red blood cells in the blood vessels. Decreased haptoglobin since haptoglobin can also carry hemoglobin. There are limited amounts of haptoglobulin produced so once it is used, it will be removed by the liver and the haptoglobulin levels decreased. No rise in hematocrit following blood transfusion since the donor blood is destroyed. Anaphylactic shock, death may result if large amounts of complement activated. Antibodies that bind complement (classical pathway) includes IgM antibodies (anti-A, anti-B, anti-I, anti-Lewisa) as well as IgG antibodies (anti-A, B, auto anti-P, anti-D, anti-Kidd, anti-Kell and others).

Mechanism of antibody-mediated hemolysis. Antibodies attach to antigens on red cell membrane and are sensed by phagocytes in RE system. The the antibody-coated red cells are ingested by the phagocytic cells and destroyed at a rate faster than normal cell destruction. RE system plucks antibody off cells, leaving damaged membrane. Cell becomes a spherocyte with shorter lifespan. Antibodies that do not bind complement but promote extravascular cell destruction. Extravascular hemolysis processes are caused by IgG antibodies:

1. Rh antibodies (anti-D, anti-C, anti-c, anti-E, and anti-e)
2. Anti-Kell (anti-K, anti-k, anti-Kpa, anti-Jsa etc.)
3. Anti-Kidd (anit-Jka and anti-Jkb)
4. Anti-Duffy (anit-Fya and anti-Fyb)
5. Anti-S

Signs of extravascular hemolysis include;

1. A falling hematocrit
2. Increased bilirubin (unconjugated)
3. Increased LD
4. Abnormal peripheral smear (polychromasia, spherocytes and fragments).

Extravascular Hemolysis - Complement Mediated. In extravascular hemolysis that is complement mediated the breakdown products of activated complement attach to red cell membrane (primarily C4b and C3b and C3d). Presence of C3b coated cells are sensed by phagocytes in RE system. Complement-coated cells are ingested and destroyed at a rate faster than normal cell destruction.

Causes of Complement-Mediated Extravascular Hemolysis. Any of the IgM or IgG antibodies that are capable of activating complement can cause this type of hemolysis. Besides the classical pathway the alternate pathway of complement activation can also occur due to the presence of various components like cell walls of bacteria and yeast, dialysis membranes, dextran, and some tumor cells. Certain drugs can also activate complement and can lead to a complement-mediated extravascular hemolysis.

Complement reaction invitro. Sometimes a serum sample used in an antigen-antibody reaction in the transfusion laboratory may activate complement and result in the binding of C3 onto the red cells. The anti-human globulin test will often detect such binding. In such cases the C3 coated red cell may be lysed if the complement activation goes to completion. In such cases lysis is often noted as a positive reaction. Complements can be inactivated in the following ways; heating the plasma at 56°C for 30 minutes (complement components C1 and C2 are heat labile) and use of calcium binding anticoagulants (EDTA and citrate). The activity of complement component C1 is dependent on the presence of free calcium ions. Antibodies present in EDTA and citrate plasma unlike serum will not produce the binding of C3 onto red cell neither will they cause lysis of red cells. Broad spectrum AHG reagent contains anti-C3 and anti-IgG and can detect the presence of C3 and IgG coating on red cells.

35. The antiglobulin test

The antiglobulin test, which is also referred to as the anti-human globulin test (AHG) or the Coombs test, is the cornerstone of detecting clinically significant unexpected antibodies that have coated cells either in vivo or in vitro. Red cells coated with complement or IgG antibodies do not agglutinate directly when centrifuged. These cells are said to be sensitized with IgG or complement. Antiglobulin test is one of the most important serological tests done in a routine blood transfusion laboratory. It utilizes the anti-human globulin (AHG) reagent to bring about agglutination of red cells coated with immunoglobulin or complement component, which do not show any agglutination in saline. Red cells which are coated with incomplete (IgG) antibodies show agglutination on addition of anti-human globulin (AHG or Coombs reagent). The coating can occur either in vivo or in vitro following incubation with serum containing the antibody. The majority of incomplete antibodies are IgG which attach to the red cell membrane by the Fab portion. The two arm of IgG molecule are unable to bridge the gap between red cells which are separated from each other because of the negative charge on their surface. While this results in sensitization of the cells, agglutination is not seen as the RBCs do not form lattice. Addition of AHG reagent results in the Fab portion of the AHG molecule combining with the Fc portion of two adjacent IgG molecules, thereby bridging the gap between the red cells and causing agglutination.

Types of Antiglobulin Tests

There are two types of antiglobulin tests:

- Direct Antiglobulin Test (DAT). Detects antibodies or complement coating patient's cells in vivo.
- Indirect Antiglobulin Test (IAT). Uses a 37oC incubation step so antibodies in serum can react with antigens on cells in vitro after washing the cells antiglobulin reagent is used to detect antibody coating of cells.

Anti-Human Globulin (AHG) Reagent.

Anti-human globulin reagent is produced by immunizing rabbits, goats or sheep with human serum or purified add type antigen. Animals are bled after a specified period and the reagent is purified by absorbing unwanted antibodies. Anti-human globulin reagent can be polyspecific and monospecific. Polyspecific antiglobulin reagent contains antibodies to human IgG, C3 and C4 components of the complement. Monospecific antiglobulin reagent may be against any one of the human IgM, IgG, and IgA or complement component C3 or C4. Monoclonal AHG is now available against IgG or complement components. Monoclonal technology may be used to make monoclonal antiglobulin reagent. Specificity types include; polyspecific An-

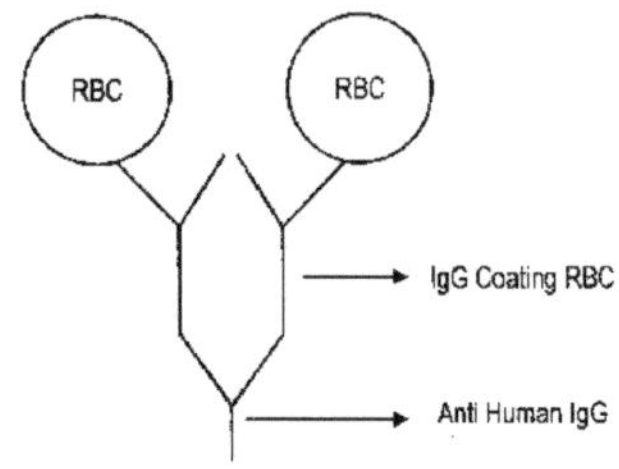

ti-human Globulin: blend of Anti-IgG & Anti-C3b, -C3d and monospecific reagents: Anti-IgG alone or Anti-C3b,-C3d alone.

Direct antiglobulin test (DAT/DCT)

Direct antiglobulin test is used to detect in-vivo sensitization (coating) of red cells with immune antibody (IgG) or the complement component (C3d or C3c). It is a useful test in the diagnosis of haemolytic disease of the newborn (HDFN), diagnosis of autoimmune haemolytic anemia (AIHA), investigation of haemolytic transfusion reaction and in the investigation of drug induced red cell sensitization. If antigen-antibody reaction has taken place in vivo, cells becomes coated with IgG antibody and/or complement. If the cells are washed 3-4 times to remove unbound or free antibody or complement, the only antibody or complement left attached to red cells will be those thar are bound to the red cells. Addition of AHG (Coombs serum) causes the anti- human globulin in Coombs serum reacts with anti human globulin (antibodies or complement) coating on red cells resulting in agglutination. If no visible agglutination occurs, the test is negative. Coombs Control Check Cells must be added to all negative samples to ensure that the reagent is performing optimally. The Direct Antiglobulin Test uses a polyspecific reagent (anti-IgG or anti C3) and detects in vivo coating of patient cells by either IgG antibodies, complement, or both. Within the patient's blood stream antibodies attach to their specific antigens on the red blood cells. This happens in Hemolytic Disease of the Foeus and Newborn (HDFN), in transfusion reactions, and in autoimmune hemolytic anemia. Certain drugs are also known to activate complement and it can also coat the cells in vivo. DAT is one of the investigations carried out to effectively diagnose immune red cells and sometimes platelet destruction. To confirm a suspected autoimmune haemolytic anaemia in which the DAT is positive with a polyspecific reagents, it may be necessary to use monospecific reagents (anti-IgG, anti-C3b, anti-IgM and anti-IgA) to identify the class of antibody responsible. Evidence of red cell destruction includes; falling haemoglobin without any other cause, haemolytic anaemia –associated reticulocytosis, reduced haptoglobins, elevated serum bilirubin (unconjugated), excess urinary urobilinogen, raised serum lactic dehydrogenase (LDH), haemosiderinuria, methemalbuminemia, polychromasia, erythroid hyperplasia of the bone marrow and positive DAT.

Sample collection

Blood sample for DAT should be collected in EDTA (Na2 or K2) to prevent in-vitro uptake of complement.

Reagents

Anti-human globulin reagent (AHG)

Positive Control: Sensitized 0 Rh (D) positive cells

Negative Control: Unsensitized 0 Rh (D) positive cells

Preparation of 0 Rh (D) positive sensitized red cells

1. Take 0.5 ml of 5-6 times washed and packed 0 Rh (D) +ve red cells in a test tube.
2. Add 2-3 drops of IgG anti-D (select a dilution (titre 1:4) of anti-D which coats the red cells but does not agglutinate them at 37°C).
3. Mix and incubate at 37°C for 30 minutes. If there is agglutination, repeat the procedure using more diluted anti-D.
4. Wash 3-4 times and make 5% suspension in saline for use.
5. Perform a Direct antiglobulin test which should give a 2+ reaction. If no agglutination occurs, repeat the test by using less diluted anti-D serum.
6. 0 Rh (D) negative sensitized red cells are also prepared by treating 0 Rh (D) negative cells in the same manner. The preparation should give a negative direct antiglobulin test (DAT).

Procedure (DAT)

1. Place 1 drop of 2-5% suspension of red cells in a clean labeled test tube.
2. Wash the red cells 3-4 times with saline and decant the final wash completely.
3. Add 1-2 drops of Al-IG reagent.
4. Mix and centrifuge at 1000 rpm for 1 minute.
5. Shake the tube gently to dislodge the cell button and read the results using a concave mirror.
6. If result is negative, incubate the test for further 5 minutes at room temperature, centrifuge and look for agglutination and record the results.
7. Add 1 drop of 5% IgG-sensitized red cells to the negative test. Look for agglutination, if a negative result is obtained the test result is invalid and the test should be repeated.
8. Appropriate controls are run with the test.

Interpretation: Agglutination of red cells indicates a positive result. DAT Controls tubes should be read before final interpretation. A positive reaction after immediate spin indicates presence of IgG coating antibodies. Reactions due to IgG become weaker after incubation. A positive reaction after 5 minute incubation indicates coating by complement component.

Indirect antiglobulin test (IAT/ICT)

This test is used to detect the presence of incomplete antibodies and complement-binding antibodies in the serum after coating on to the red cell in-vitro in. It is useful in the screening and identification of unexpected (irregular) antibodies in serum, compatibility testing and detection of red cell antigens using specific antibodies reacting only in antiglobulin test (K, Fya, Fyb, Jkb, e.t.c.) and in the investigation of haemolytic disease of the newborn. Add equal volume of serum to 3-5% red cell suspension. If no antigen-antibody reaction occurred, no attachment of antibody or complement to red cells occurs. Cells washed three to four times. This causes all plasma or serum antibodies not attached to the red cells are washed away. Anti-human globulin (Coombs serum) is added, which would react with antibody-coated cells if present to give agglutination. No agglutination will occur if no antibodies or complement has been attached to the red cells for the anti-human globulin (Coombs serum) to react with. To confirm a negative reaction, Coombs Control Check Cells must be added. Coombs Control Check Cells will react with antibodies in Coombs serum still "floating around" in the tube to give a positive reaction. Agglutination following addition of CCC verifies negative result. Blood sample for IAT should be collected in plain labeled test tube (serum). EDTA anticoagulated plasma sample can also be used.

Reagents. Anti-human globulin reagent. In order for agglutination to occur an additional antibody, which reacts with the Fc portion of the IgG antibody, or with the C3b or C3d component of complement, must be added to the system. This will form a "bridge" between the antibodies or complement coating the red cells, causing agglutination. The light-colored antibody molecule represents the anti-globulin reagent that binds with the Fc portion of the IgG antibody attached to the red blood cells. The light-colored antibody molecule represents the anti-globulin reagent that binds with the complement attached to the red blood cells. Traditionally rabbits were immunized with human gamma globulin to make this antibody to IgG or C3d.

Preparation of reagent 0 cells. Obtain pooled 0 Rh (D) positive cells (reagent O cells) in 2 test tubes X and Y. Each tube should contain at least 2 donor's samples. Reagent cells should preferably be homozygous (double dose) for antigens and must contain the main clinically significant antigens (Rh, Kell, Kidd, Duffy, MNS and Lewis). Wash 3 times with normal saline. Prepare a 5% suspension for use. Reagent 0 cells, commercially available or prepared in the laboratory.

Controls

- Positive Control: Sensitized 0 Rh (D) positive cells.
- Negative Control: Unsensitized 0 Rh (D) positive cells

Procedure (IAT)

1. Centrifuge the tubes at 3000 rpm for 5 minutes to separate the serum.
2. Add 2 drops of serum in each of the tubes labeled C and D (sample should be fresh for detecting complement - binding antibodies).
3. Add 1 drop of 5% suspension of X cells to tube labeled 1 and I drop of Y cells to tube labeled 2.
4. Mix and incubate both tubes at 37°C for 30-60 minutes.
5. Spin at 1000 rpm for 1 minute and examine for agglutination. Record the results. Agglutination will not occur if incomplete antibodies are present.
6. Wash the cells in each of the tube 3-4 times with warm saline. Decant the saline completely after the last wash over a filter paper.
7. Add 1-2 drops of AHG reagent to each tube. Centrifuge immediately and look for centrifugation.
8. If negative, incubate at room temperature (22°-24°C) for further 5 minutes.
9. Re-centrifuge and look for agglutination.
10. Confirm negative test by adding a drop of IgG sensitized 0 Rh (D) positive cells. Agglutination should be seen. Autocontrol must be kept with IAT.

Interpretation. Agglutination in one or both the tubes indicates presence of unexpected antibody in the test serum. If no agglutination occurs, use enhancing techniques. Results of control tubes should be considered before final interpretation.

Factors Affecting the Sensitivity of IAT

Temperature. The optimal temperature of reactivity of IgG antibodies is 37°C. Incubation at higher or lower temperature may give false results.

Serum: red cell ratio. Increasing the ratio of serum to cells increases the antibody coating. Commonly used ratio for for IAT 2:1 but for cells suspended in LISS use equal volume of serum and 2% cell suspension.

Incubation time. Optimum incubation time for saline, albumin or enzyme technique is 30-60 minutes. For red cells suspended in saline incubation time is routinely 15 minutes while in emergency cases the incubation time is about 5 minutes

Suspension medium. The sensitivity of IAT can be increased with addition of 22% bovine albumin, enzyme or by using red cells suspended in LISS.

Reasons for false negative results include:

1. Inadequate washing of the cells in the Coombs phase. Residual serum neutralizes AHG.
2. A small fibrin clot has formed in the tube, neutralizing AHG. Be sure sample has thoroughly clotted.
3. Coombs reagent was omitted or is inactive.
4. Weak or questionable reactions may be enhanced by:
5. Increasing the amount of serum used to 3-4 drops. PEG must be omitted, and the incubation time extended to 30 minutes.
6. Omitting PEG and adding albumin to the test mixture. Extend the incubation time to at least 20 minutes.
7. Using enzyme treated cells. See manufacturer's directions.
8. Repeat testing using PEG to the test mixture. See manufacturer's directions.
9. Occasionally you may get a moderately strong reaction at room temperature that persists weakly in Coombs. This may not be clinically significant if it is due to complement binding at room temperature from a cold-reactive antibody. To determine if the reaction is due to complement binding, do a pre-warmed screen

Examples of alloimmune hemolysis

1. Hemolytic disease of the foetus and newborn (HDFN or erythroblastosis fetalis).
2. Rh D haemolytic disease of the newborn (Rh disease).
3. ABO hemolytic disease of the newborn (may only be weakly positive)
4. Anti-Kell hemolytic disease of the newborn
5. Rh c hemolytic disease of the newborn
6. Rh E hemolytic disease of the newborn
7. Other blood group incompatibility (RhC, Rhe, Kidd, Duffy, MN, P and others)
8. Alloimmune hemolytic transfusion reactions

Examples of autoimmune hemolysis

1. Warm antibody autoimmune hemolytic anemia
2. Idiopathic
3. Systemic lupus erythematosus

4. Evans' syndrome (antiplatelet antibodies and hemolytic antibodies)
5. Cold antibody autoimmune hemolytic anemia
6. Idiopathic cold hemagglutinin syndrome
7. Infectious mononucleosis
8. Paroxysmal cold hemoglobinuria

Drug-induced immune-mediated hemolysis

1. Methyldopa (IgG mediated type II hypersensitivity)
2. Penicillin (high dose)
3. Quinidine

Forward (Cell group)				Back (Serum group)	
Anti-A	Anti-B	Anti-A+B	Auto control	A1 cell	B cell
2+	2+	2+	2+	4+	4+

Polyagglutinable effect of positive DAT on RBC typing

Forward (Cell group)			Back (Serum group)	
Anti-A	Anti-B	Anti-A+B	A1 cell	B cell
0	0	0	4+	4+

Effect of positive DAT obviated by washing of red cells prior to testing

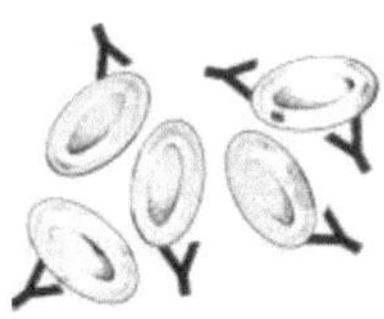

IgG-coated red blood cells

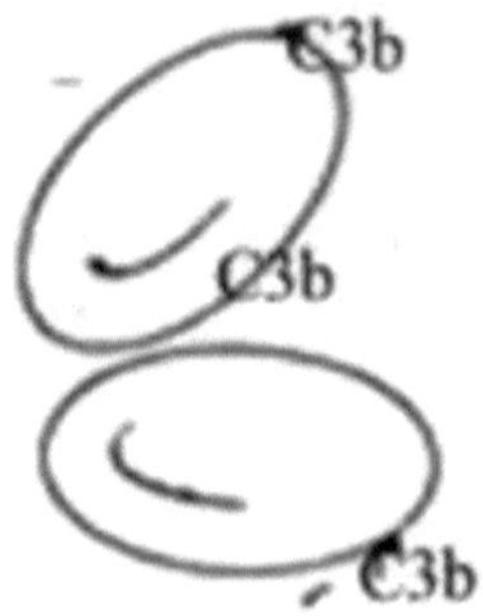

Complement-coated red blood cells

False-Negative Reactions. False-negative reactions can occur when antigen-antibody reactions have occurred but washing is inadequate and free antibody remains when the anti-human globulin is added. Anti-human globulin (Coombs) antibody prefers to react first with free antibody and then with antibody-coated cells. If the free antibody has already reacted with the anti-human globulin, no free Coombs serum to react with Coombs Control Check Cells (CCC). False negatives that are detected by negative Coombs control cells include; inadequate cell washing will lead to unbound antibody remaining in the red cell suspension that are available to neutralize the AHG (Coombs serum) so it will not react with red cells bound with antibody, delay in adding Coombs serum after washing step will lead to antibody eluting off, detaching from the cells while cells are sitting in saline. Now free antibody present in the saline neutralizes the Coombs, serum so it will not be able to react with the cells bound with antibody, small fibrin clot among the cells that were not washed away will have immunoglobulins and complement present. The antibodies and complement in the fibrin clot neutralizes AHG, Coombs, serum leading to a negative test, inactive AHG (Coombs serum) or the failure to add AHG (Coombs serum) will also be detected by a negative reaction when adding Coombs Control Check Cells. There are also false negatives NOT detected by negative Coombs Control Cells that include; too heavy cell suspension, delay during cell washing procedure, which can lead to antibody eluting off cells while they are sitting in saline and then the antibody is washed away during the remaining washes, improper centrifugation can either lead to lost of cells during the washing or the need to shake too hard during resuspension.

False positives. False positive reactions can also occur when performing this test. These would not be detected by the use of Coombs Control Check Cells. Reasons for a false positive reaction could be the following; using improper sample (clotted cells instead of EDTA for Direct Antiglobulin Test, DAT), spontaneous agglutination (cells heavily coated with IgM), non-specific agglutination (sticky cells). All of these reactions would be the result of cells appearing to agglutinate, or actually agglutinating. Using a clotted tube for the DAT may allow complement to become activated in the test tube since calcium ions are free to be part of the complement cascade.

Causes of positive DAT

Autoimmune Haemolytic Anaemia (AIHA). Autoimmune hemolytic anemia (AIHA) refers to a collection of disorders characterized by the presence of autoantibodies that bind to the patient's own erythrocytes, leading to premature red cell destruction. Specific characteristics of the autoantibodies, especially the type of antibody; its optimal binding temperature; and whether it binds complement can play a role in its diagnosis. In all cases of AIHA, however, the autoantibody leads to a shortened red blood cell survival (haemolysis) and when the rate of haemolysis exceeds the ability of the bone marrow to replace the destroyed red cells anaemia with its attendant signs and symptoms reuslts. AIHA affect an estimated annual incidence of 1 in 80,000 persons in the general population. Positive DAT has been reported (IgG and /or C3) have been reported in patient with Plasmodium falciparum malaria. AIHA can be subdivided into

1. Warm AIHA
2. Cold AIHA
3. Cold Paroxysmal Cold Haemoglobinuria (PNH)
4. Drug associated AIHA

Warm Type Autoimmune Haemolytic Anaemia (WAIHA). Warm AIHA is the most common of the autoimmune hemolytic diseases. About half of the cases are idiopathic the second half are attributable to other predisposing factors such as medications. The most common antibody involved in warm antibody AIHA is IgG. Sometimes the C3 component of complement and IgA is also incriminated. Diagnosis is often by the use of monospecfic anti-IgG reagents. These IgG antibodies attach to a red blood cell, leaving their FC portion exposed. The FC region is recognized and grabbed onto by FC receptors found on monocytes and macrophages in the spleen. These cells will bite off portions of the red cell membrane. The loss of membrane causes the red blood cells to become spherocytes. Spherocytes are not as flexible in micro circulation as normal biconcave RBCs, and will be singled-out for destruction by the reticuloendothelial system including the spleen. The red blood cells trapped in the spleen cause the spleen to enlarge (splenomegaly). Two models have been postulated to explain this immune-related red cell destruction: the hapten model and the autoantibody model.

1. The hapten model proposes that certain drugs (penicillin, cephalosporins, tetracyclines, antihistamines, sulphonamides, ibuproten, levodopa and methyldopa) bind to certain proteins on the red cell membrane and act as haptens. A hapten (in this case the drug) is a small molecule that can elicit an immune response leading to the production of an antibody only when attached to a large carrier such as a protein (red cell membrane protein). Antibodies are created against the protein-drug complex, leading to haemolysis of the patient's RBCS.

2. The autoantibody model proposes that, through a mechanism not yet understood including certain drugs can cause antibodies to be made against red blood cells and leads to red cell destruction. It is possible for it to occur in an immunocompromised patient

WAIHA may be idiopathic (without any known cause), secondary to another disease such as systemic lupus erythematosus or rheumatoid arthritis or a haematological malignancy such as chronic lymphocytic leukemia (CLL) and Myelo Dysplastic Syndrome (MDS). It may also be associated with receiving a drug. Laboratory findings in WAIHA include

1. Severe anemia

2. Increased mean corpuscular volume (MCV) due to the presence of a large number of young erythrocytes

3. Hyperbilirubinemia (from increased red cell destruction) conjugated or unconjugated type.

4. Diagnosis is made by a positive direct Coombs test

5. Clinical examination and history.

Treatment. Commonly used treatments for warm antibody AIHA includes; initial medical treatment consists of prednisone, corticosteroids, immunoglobulins, splenectomy should be considered if other treatments are ineffective. If refractory to both these therapies other options include rituximab, danazol, cyclosphosphamide, azathioprine and cyclosporine. High dose intravenous immune globulin may be effective in controlling hemolysis but the benefit is short lived (1–4 weeks).

Cold Type Autoimmune Haemolytic Anaemia. Cold AIHA or cold agglutinin disease, caused by IgM antibodies most active at <30oC, is a hemolytic anemia characterized by RBC agglutination and hemolysis in acral cold exposed areas of the body. An IgM complement fixing antibody binds to RBCs at 28-31oC. In cold type AIHA, IgM antibodies which react optimally at low temperatures below that of the core temperature of the body. They are therefore called "cold agglutinins. Usually C3 is often present. At lower body temperature these cold antibodies bind to red cells and initiate the complement cascade. As RBCs are warmed in the central organs the bound IgM is lost leaving only bound C3. The complement cascade already triggered can go to completion with resultant intravascular haemolysis and associate haemoglobinuria. Cold agglutinin disease is associated with; lymphoma (antibodies against anti-i), mycoplasma pneumonia (antibodies against anti-I), rarely infectious mononucleosis (antibodies against anti-i), people with cold agglutinin disease have a chronic hemolytic anemia with periods of jaundice, and hemoglobinuria. Cold agglutinin disease with RBC agglutination may be associated with Raynaud's phenomenon.

Paroxysmal cold haemoglobinuria. Paroxysmal cold hemoglobinuria (PCH) (Donath-Landsteiner syndrome) is a cold type AIHA characterized by the sudden presence of hemoglobin in the urine (hemoglobinuria) typically after exposure to cold temperatures. In people with PCH, a polyclonal IgG usually with anti-P autoantibody binds to red blood cell surface antigens in the cold. This can occur in a susceptible individual as blood passes through cold extremities in cold weather. When the blood returns to the warmer central circulation, the red blood cells are lysed with complement causing intravascular hemolysis. PNH is often associated with hemoglobinuria and anemia. The anaemia may be mild or severe. PCH is a rare autoimmune haemolytic anaemia that can occur following an infection, when a microorganism triggers the formation of antibodies that cross-react with the P antigen on the red blood cell membrane. Treatment with prednisone may be used in individuals with PCH and severe anemia. Viral infections that can cause PCH include:measles, mumps, influenza, adenovirus, chickenpox, cytomegalovirus, and Epstein-Barr virus. Bacterial infections that can cause PCH include syphilis, Haemophilus influenzae and Mycoplasma pneumoniae. Chronic PCH associated with syphilis resolves after the syphilis is treated with appropriate antibiotics. PCH can also be a side effect of some vaccinations. People with PCH are advised to avoid exposure to cold temperatures. If anemia is severe, blood transfusion may be needed. Careful compatibility testing by the blood bank is necessary because autoantibodies may interfere with blood typing. P positive red cells is normally tolerated by a number of patient and in other it may be necessary to transfuse rare P negative if P positive red cell transfusion results in haemolysis and non-increment of the patient haemoglobin after transfusion of P positive red cells. The Donath-Landsteiner test is used to confirm PCH. In the test you incubate group O cells with serum at 00C and the 37°C. The contrl is incubated only at 37°C. In a positive test haemolysis is observed in the tube incubated at 00C and then 37°C but not in the tube incubated at 37°C alone.

Drugs that can cause a positive DAT test. A number of drugs are capable of binding to red cells and initiating an immune response leading to the stimulation of antibodies to the drug. These antibodies can react with the drug or the drugs, the drug and red cell membrane component or the red cell membrane component. The DAT in most cases are positive with IgG and sometimes with C3. The antibodies can either be; drug –dependent antibodies which react with the drug coated red cells and may cause haemolysis of the drug coated red cells. Drug –related immune complexes that attach to surface of RBCS causing haemolysis, haemoglobinuria and renal failure. Re-adminstration of the culprit drug can cause severe haemolysis, positive C3-related DAT. Drug can independently stimulate an antibody that reacts with the red cell membrane without the drug. Drugs such as methyldopa causes this type of DAT positive. Eluates react with the RBCS without the drug. Some drugs (cephalosporins) can alter the red cell membrane and cause a non-immunological uptake of IgG or IgM proteins. Autoimmune and drug associated immune destruction is not confined to red cells alone. Destruction of platelet can also occur and result in auto immune thrombocytopenia. Drugs commonly incriminated in drug-related positive DAT include; penicillin, cephalosporins, tetracyclines, antihistamines, sulphonamides, ibuproten, levodopa and methyldopa. When the blood is drawn the antibodies and/or complement have already attached to the red cells. Those red cells from the EDTA tube will be washed 3 or more times and a 3% cell suspension is made. A drop of cell suspension and the anti-human globulin are mixed in a tube and then centrifuged. If agglutination occurs, it indicates the patient has a positive Direct Antiglobulin

Test due to antibody coating the cells in vivo. If IgM antibodies involved, DAT will be identified by complement binding since the polyspecific antisera has both anti-IgG and anti-C3.

Technique for DAT Test

1. Add 1 drop of patient cells from EDTA tube to tube
2. Wash these drops of blood 3-4 times to remove plasma antibodies (human globulin) and make a 3% cell suspension.
3. Add a drop of 3% cell suspension to a clean, labeled tube.
4. Add drop of Polyspecific AHG (Coombs serum) to the tube.
5. If test is positive with polyspecific reagent, set up again using monospecific reagents to see if it is antibody or complement or both coating the cells.
6. We want to make the test as sensitive as possible, so allow all negatives to incubate 5 minutes to enhance complement coating.
7. Read all negatives microscopically to detect weak coating.
8. False positives may occur if sample is collected in EDTA tube.
9. In-vitro complement coating frequently happens when sample clots or cools down due to weak cold-acting auto-antibodies like anti-I
10. Complement coating is prevented by using a lavender.
11. Whenever positive DAT is obtained, obtain the following information on the patient:
12. Diagnostic in cases of autoimmune hemolytic anemia, hemolytic disease of the foetus and newborn and transfusion reactions.
13. Medications
14. Recent transfusion history of both red cell and plasma components
15. Other lab values that may indicate red cell destruction (hematocrit, bilirubin, LDH)

Clinical challenges of a positive DAT

1. Normal patient with unexplainable reasons for a positive DAT

2. Transfusion reaction work-ups require that a DAT be performed on the post-transfusion specimen since the patient's antibodies and/or complement may coat the transfused donor cells. These reactions are usually weak positive or mixed field agglutination since you are testing a mixed population of patient and donor cells.

3. Warm-acting autoimmune disease can lead to patient antibodies coating their own cells. This results in a strong positive result. A cold-acting autoimmune haemolytic anemia would be due to IgM antibodies that in turn activate complement. The complement-coated cells would then be detected by the antiglobulin reagent.

4. Haemolytic disease of the foetus and newborn is due to the mother's IgG antibodies crossing the placenta and coating the antigens on the fetal red blood cells. Cord blood collected at the time of birth would be tested, but may need to follow up by a heel stick of EDTA blood. The reaction is usually a strong positive.

5. Complement on the red cells may be the result of antigen-antibody reactions which may involve the lysis of red cells. Complement can also be activated if immune complexes are present in the plasma and the activated complement attaches to the red cells. Complement can also become activated by the C3 by-pass mechanism and the lectin activation process.

6. Passive transfer of antibody from donor units of plasma or platelets may attach to the patient's red cells since recipients are given ABO compatible blood but other unexpected red cell antibodies may not have been detected. These antibodies in donor plasma can coat antigens on patient cells when group AB, A, or B receive group O plasma products (platelets)

7. ABO mismatched transplants of particularly bone marrow can occur if a universal "O" donor bone marrow is given to an A, B, or AB recipient. Passenger lymphocytes from group O donor organ make antibody to group AB, A, or B recipient cells and these in turn can activate complement. It is also more common for "O" individuals to make an IgG anti-A,B, which would also contribute to a positive DAT.

8. Sensitization of red cells due to medications like penicillin and cephalosporins that usually involves non-specific coating of red cells. Other drugs like tetracyclines, antihistamines and sulphonamides cause the development of immune complexes that are capable of activating complement. Some drugs, like ibuproten, levodopa and methyldopa, are also known to cause autoimmunity. If a patient has a positive DAT, drug-induced problems should be considered.

Indirect Antiglobulin Testing

The indirect antiglobulin test is one of the most important and commonly used techniques in immunohematology. It is used commonly for the detection of; weak D's in donor bloods and pregnant females of individuals who type D (-) at room temperature when doing ABO and Rh typing, the presence or absence of antigens on a person cells from particularly the Kell, Kidd, and Duffy Blood Group systems and the presence of unexpected, clinically significant antibodies in the patient's serum during the antibody screening procedure and the antibody identification procedure. The purpose of the indirect antiglobulin test is to detect In vitro sensitization of red cells. This is done when sensitization does not lead to direct agglutination. This occurs when there are too few antigens on the red cell, too few antibodies in the serum and those antibodies are in the IgG class. In summary, we incubate cells containing most clinically significant antigens with test serum at 37oC for 15 to 30 minutes. After incubation wash the cells three to four times in saline. Add AHG (Coombs reagent), centrifuge and read for agglutination. If the test is negative, add Coombs Control Check Cells to check for false negatives.

Uses. Screening serum for unexpected antibodies usually Involves patient serum plus reagent red cells (screening cells) I and II or I, II and III depending on manufacturer. The patient's serum potentially has unknown antibodies. Screening cells contain known and common clinically significant antigens. If there is agglutination after Coombs step with the screening cells, it means that the patient has an unexpected antibody. If antibody screen positive, the serum is further reacted against a panel of cells containing known antigens (IAT and Enzyme panel) to allow for the antibody to be specifically identified.

The importance of antibody screen. Testing donor plasma to make sure no unexpected antibodies will be transfused to the recipient. Testing recipient serum before transfusion to make sure patient has no unexpected antibodies to react with donor cells and to enable those with alloantibody to receive antigen negative red cell transfusion. Testing maternal serum to make sure pregnant mother has no antibodies to react with fetal cells causing hemolytic disease of the foetus and newborn.

Red Cell Antigen Typing. Red cell antigen typing involves patient cells plus reagent antiserum. The patient's cells are the unknown antigen and the reagent antiserum is the known antibody. The antiglobulin technique is used for antigen typing for a weak D and a number of other clinically significant antibodies like the Kell, Kidd, and Duffy antibodies. If there is agglutination after the addition of anti-human globulin, or Coombs step, patient cells had that corresponding group specific antigen. The specific procedure varies depending on what antigen is being tested for, and what brand of antiserum is being used. Remember you must always read and follow manufacturer's standard operating procedure in the product insert carefully.

Uses for red cell antigen typing. Typing donors for antigen if patient has antibody. You would want units that are negative for that antigen. Verifying that patient is negative for an antigen. For example the husband of a pregnant woman with a clinically significant alloantibody (anti- D and K) will need to have his red cells typed to determine the likelihood of the developing foetus being positive for the antigen for which the mum has the corresponding group specific antibody. Typing patient to see what antigens he/she lacks can help predict what antibodies he/she is capable of producing if they seem to be particularly likely to make additional antibodies. An individual as a rule only make antibody when exposed to red cell antigen which they lack.

Controls. When performing red cell antigen testing always run known positive and negative controls. This will verify that antiserum is acting properly and helps you interpret your test results. The positive control should be heterozygous for the antigen to ensure antiserum is capable of detecting weaker antigens. *For example, when performing antigen typing for K, you would want a cell that is K+ and k+.*

PositiveControl	Negative Control	Patient Control	Patient Test
Heterozygous cells	Cells with no antigen	Patient Cells	Patient cells
4	0	0	4, 0 or MF
Reagent Antiserum	Reagent Antiserum	Rh control	Antiserum.

Key
Positive = 4, Negative = 0 and MF = Mixed Field Reaction

36. Good Manufacturing Practice (GMP)

What is GMP. Good Manufacturing Practice (GMP) is that part of the quality system that ensures that blood products are consistently produced and controlled to the quality standards appriopriate to their intended use. It is used to describe a group of practical activities and controls put in place to facilitate the production of blood products that meet the required specification and is fit and safe for use. GMP covers all aspect of manufacturing;collection, transportation processing, storage, quality control and delivery of the finished product. The basic principle of GMP is that the responsibility for quality control should be held by an independent person from the people who are responsible for the production of the product.

Quality. Quality is defined as the totality of the features and characteristics of a product or service which shows that it meet the stated or required specification. Quality Programs includes; quality control, quality assurance and quality improvement. For Blood Banking Quality Programs are essential requirements of agencies such as the Food and Drug Administration (US), MHRA (UK), CPA (UK) and MLSCN (Nigeria). These agencies has the following responsibilities: Responsibilities of the blood product requirements (anticoagulants and preservatives, shelf life of blood products and clinical indication for use). Specific requirements related to independent quality control and quality assurance for overall quality of blood products and the processes related to storage, testing and transport of blood products.

Quality Assurance. The sum total of organised arrangement put in place by an organisation to ensure that medicinal products meet the quality required for their intended use. Quality control is a process of measuring actual quality performance and comparing it with a standard and taking action whenever there is a deviation from the standard. This comparism must take place during the production stages and before the product is released for use to ensure that the specification required is met.

Why GMP. GMP is important because it ensures that a quality system is built into an organisation and the processes involved in the manufacturing of blood and blood products. The control of quality begins even before the blood product is collected (designing of laboratory, equipment specification and defining of procedures). The principle of GMP recommends that there are clear written specification for the product, the packaging of the products, testing and processing, handling and storage, receipt and despatch, suitable premises, equipment and trained workforce. Every blood transfusion laboratory is required by law and on the bais of the principle of Good Laboratory Practice (GLP) and Good Manufacturing Practice (GMP) to actively support the quality systems in place for the following procedures.

1. Standard Operating Procedures (SOP's)
2. Training plans, competencies and development of procedures
3. Approval of lot release of reagents, quality control of reagents and maintenance of equipment.
4. Review and approval of practices relating to personnel, equipment, selection of suppliers, process control, final inspection and handling of non-conforming components, methods in place for handling incidents, errors, and accidents.

GMP requirements. The principle of GMP requires that the following factors that play a role in ensuring that the quality of a product are consistently met and that the product meet the quality required for it's intended use.

1. Quality management
2. Personnel
3. Premises and equipment
4. Documentation
5. Production
6. Quality control
7. Contract manufacture and analysis
8. Complaints and product recall
9. Self inspection

Quality Management. Manufacturer must ensure that product is fit for intended use and will not put the recipient of blood product at risk. Ensure that senior management staff of the organization takes responsiblility for ensuring product quality and safety as well commitment of staff responsible for production and supply of product. A blood transfusion organisation must have in place and implement an effective and comprehensive Quality Assurance system based on the principles of good manufacturing and good laboratory practices as well as quality control. The quality assurance system must be supported by adequate material endowment (premises, equipment and facilities) as well as supported by adequate staffing by trained and competent personnel.

Personnel Requirements. Any successful quality assurance system will depend on personnel. Robust method must be in place for hiring of qualified personnel. Job descriptions and responsibilities for all positions need to exist and be available. Every staff must engage in Continuing Professional Development (CPD) activities and must have a Personal Development Plan (PDP) that is reviewed annually. Training program and full documentation of that training for new and continuous employees. Whenever a new procedure or instrument is implemented a training program needs to be in place. Regular competency evaluations including direct observation and documentation of such must occur as well as appraisal should be carried out at least anually. All staff must be aware and work on the principles of GMP. Ensure that all staffs exposed to infective agents (viral infective agents such as HBV) are up-to-date with their vaccination.

Premises and Equipment- related requirements. Premises and equipment must be built and proactively maintained to suit the task being carried out. The premises must be adequate, health and safety considerations must be made. Layout and design must be optimum to minimize errors and facillitae maintenance and effective cleaning and disinfection. Work must be done accurately and precisely, keeping the work area clean and uncluttered. Validation of new equipment must be carried out before its certification for use. Calibration and preventative maintenance must be carried out on all equipment including standard equipment like refrigerators, complex equipment and computer systems. Continual monitoring of blood bank refrigerators extremely important in both blood centers and transfusion services. Equipment must be kept cleaned and proactively maintained, should have an equipment operating procedure (EOP) for every equipment, maintenance log and evidence of quality control report run daily on equipment. There should be no entry for unauthorized persons. Production and storage areas must not be used as right of way. Defective equipment should be removed or appriopriate labelled as defective with a do not use sign. Although both transfusion services and blood centers are primarily concerned with safe transfusions and related issues, there also needs to have processes in place related to employee safety. The following needs should be met; Compliance with (control of substances hazardous to health) COSHH requirements: chemical and biologic, disaster preparedness, adequate space and ventilation, adequate sanitation and water systems as well as evaluations of limitations of physical structure prior to implementation of new equipment or processes.

Documentation and document control requirements. Clearly written documentation prevents errors from spoken communication. Therefore the following must be standard operating procedures for carrying out test. These documents should be written in ink, be unambiguous and must have a clear and concise content, title and purpose and must be reviewed regularly. Each document must have a unique identifier. Every laboratory organization must have a document control policy defining how documents (SOPs, forms, worksheet and others) in use in the laboratory must be uniquely identified (including document number and version), written, validated, approved and issued for use, reviewed and what should instigate a document change or review. Documents used in the transfusion laboratory fall into 5 levels/categories; policies (relates to "What to do" in response to various situations), processes (relates to "how it happens"), procedures (relates to "How to do it"), forms/records, supporting documents that need to be completed when you are performing the procedures and following the processes and policies and documentation of incidents, errors, near misses and accidents. In order to build a continually improving system, methods need to be in place to detect incidents, errors, near misses and accidents. Therefore the following should be in place; A process to capture incidents and errors. If incident occurs, the severity of the incident must be determined by the facility. If it is a one-time incident or multiple similar incidents. There should be a system in place to carry out a root cause analysis (What might be the root cause?) to determine the likelihood is that it will re-occur again and determine what process (corrective action) is be put in place to ensure that it does not happen again. Develop processes for continuous improvement to help eliminate both one-time incidents and multiple similar incidents. Audit the process from time to time. Develop a robust process to get things right first time and all the time avoid defects and repeats. Documentation requirements vary from hospital to hospital but there is requisite information that must be documented by the transfusion laboratory and on the patient's medical record. This is important in order to allow for tracability of transfusion of blood components should an adverse event occur in future, or a new threat to the blood supply is identified or becomes required for litigation purposes. Documentation must include information on component type (RBC, pooled platelet, FFP or cryoprecipitate). Other information required include;

1. Donation (unit) number, including centre code.

2. ABO/Rh of the component, if applicable;

3. Time transfusion of each unit was started and completed including a note of any adverse events observed.

4. Signatures of the individuals (requester, nursing staff that did the bed side check and set up the transfusion).

5. Time the transfusion was started, discontinued, and completed.

6. Volume of blood product administered and whether a reaction to the transfusion occurred.

7. Clear and accurate records of daily temperature monitoring of blood bank and reagent fridges, proficiency testing of staff, equipment main-

tenance, validation, reagent records, quality control checks, crossmatch documentation must be stored for a set period of time (30 years in the UK). These records must show what was done and by whom.

8. Clear and accurate record keeping provides a complete audit trail which facillitates the investigations of complaints, defects, problems and incidents and help the laboratory take necessary corrective and preventive action.

9. As a rule the compatibility label must remain on blood component until the transfusion is discontinued.

Production. Production activities must follow clearly defined standard procedures and must only be performed by designated, qualified, trained and competent staff. All materials used for the production process must be stored optimally and in an expiry date order to allow for materials closest to expiry to be use first in preference with longer expiration date. Effort must be made to prevent microbial contamination of the product. Production process must strictly follow the standard operating procedures. Changes can be made to the document but this must be approved by a competent person in charge of quality. All equipment used for the production process must be validated, regularly maintained to ensure that activity produces expected results. Process control include;development of SOP, control of changes in policies, processes or procedures, acceptance testing to new/revised software involved in blood bank procedures, validation of new policies, processes or procedures, monitoring and control of production processes, participation in proficiency testing appropriate for each testing system in place, established QC procedures for supplies and equipment, supplier qualifications and product specification need to be in place and control processes for non-conforming blood and blood components and products.

Quality control requirements. Quality control is associated with independent sampling and testing to ensure that a process meets the stated specification. A Quality control program includes both internal quality control (IQC) and External Qaulity Assessment (EQA). Internal assessment includes daily QC checks of reagents used in the laboratory and must be managed by the department quality team. IQC is a measure of precision. External Quality Assessments includes inspections, surveys, and proficiency surveys performed by Quality Assessment agencies like the MLSCN, CPA, MHRA, NEQAS and AABB. EQA ensures that diagnostic laboratory results are accurate reliable and comparable. The principles of quality control requires that: All reagents in use in the transfusion laboratory are adequately controlled (IQC) before use. Internal QC testing is a measure of precision. It is a quality control requirement that every transfusion laboratory registers and partakes in external quality assurance (EQA) scheme (NEQAS and WEQAS in the UK). Participation in EQA facilitates optimal patient care ensuring that the results of investigations are reliable and comparable wherever they are produced. Enrolment in an EQA scheme can help the laboratory to; improve their process and increase profitability, improve customer satisfaction, comply with current legislation (MLSCN, CPA, MHRA) and improve the laboratory's credibility with potential customers. When a new shipment of reagents is received, the product insert needs to be reviewed and any changes in the standard operating procedure needs to incorporated into the laboratory procedure before the reagents are used by the laboratory. Total compliance with the manufacturer's directions must be followed. Blood bank reagents must never be used after the expiration date. Daily quality control testing needs to be done for ABO, Rh, and Antibody Screening. Typing antisera for other red cell antigens will be tested when performing the antigen testing on the patient and donors since this test is not done each day. Prior to use of incoming supplies they need to be tested. Each manufacturer is required to provide a product insert for each reagent. The product inserts needs to include the following; reagent's description, proper use procedures, what to expect in regards to performance and limitations of reagents. Determination needs to be made relating to whether they are satisfactory for intended use. Documentation of package, storage and transportation. Documentation of testing that needs to done by facility before being put into use.

Contract, Manufacture and analysis. Contract manufacture and analysis must be correctly defined, agreed and controlled in order to avoid misunderstandings which could result in a product or work of unsatisfactory quality. There must be a written contract between the Contract Giver and the Contract Acceptor which clearly establishes the duties of each party. The Contract Giver (transfusion laboratory) is responsible for assessing the competence of the Contract Acceptor (contractor) to carry out successfully the work required and for ensuring by means of the contract that the principles and guidelines of GMP as interpreted in this Guide are followed. The Contract Giver should provide the Contract Acceptor with all the information necessary to carry out the contracted operations correctly in accordance with the marketing authorisation and any other legal requirements. The Contract Giver should ensure that the Contract Acceptor is fully aware of any problems associated with the product or the work which might pose a hazard to his premises, equipment, personnel, other materials or other products. The contract giver should ensure that all processed products and materials delivered to him by the Contract Acceptor comply with their specifications or that the products have been released by a qualified person. The contract acceptor must have adequate premises and equipment, knowledge and experience and competent personnel to carry out satisfactorily the work ordered by the contract giver. The contract acceptor should ensure that all products or materials delivered to him are suitable for their intended purpose. The contract acceptor should not pass to a third party any of the work entrusted to him under the contract without the contract giver's prior evaluation and approval of the arrangements. Arrangements made between the contract acceptor and any third party should ensure that the manufacturing and analytical information is made available in the same way as between the original contract giver and contract acceptor.

The Contract. A contract should be drawn up between the Contract Giver and the Contract Acceptor which specifies their respective responsibilities relating to the manufacture and control of the product. Technical aspects of the contract should be drawn up by competent persons suitably knowledgeable in transfusion technology, analysis and Good Manufacturing Practice. The contract should describe clearly who is responsible for purchasing materials, testing and releasing materials, undertaking production and quality controls, including in-process controls, and who has responsibility for sampling and analysis. Any records relevant to assessing the quality of a product in the event of complaints or a suspected defect must be accessible and specified in the defect/recall procedures of the Contract Giver.

Complaints and product recall. GMP principle stipulates that all complaints and other information concerning adverse events and potentially defective product must be investigated. There should a procedure in place for recall of defective blood and blood products. Recall process should be free from any ambiguity and could be initiated promptly by all qualified staff and should be regularly reviewed. A process should be in place to carry out a root cause analysis in cases of complaints and any adverse events to enable a corrective and preventive action to be taken to prevent a re-occurrence of the root cause. The quality control officer should be involved in all cases of complaints, defects and near –misses.

Self inspection (Internal Audits). An audit is defined as a systematic, independent & documented process for obtaining evidence and evaluating objectively the extent to which audit (GMP principles) criteria are fulfilled. Audits can either be horizontal, vertical or examination. Horizontal audit involves the assessment of one element of the quality system. Examination audit involves a process whereby the assessor watches a test being performed, to ascertain if SOP is being followed. It is a method used to confirm competence of the staff and level of training. Vertical audit: involves a process whereby a sample is tracked from sample receipt to the issue of result. Regular audits are essential to sustain or improve a quality system. Non -compliance notes raised against identified short falls are being addressed and will be reviewed in subsequent audits. All identified non-compliances must be resolved. Root cause analysis must be carried out and all appropriate corrective actions must be implemented. Internal audits vertical and horizontal as well as examination audits should be conducted regularly to monitor the implementation and compliance with GMP principles. All internal audits must be carried out by an independent and designated persons. It must be as objective as possible

37. Principle of Good Laboratory Practice (GLP) and its application in transfusion

Good Laboratory Practice (GLP) embodies a set of principles that provides a framework within which studies are planned, performed, monitored, recorded, reported and archived. Laboratory testing carried out by Biomedical Scientist are generally recognized as affecting decisions literally concerned with life and death issues. There is therefore the need to adopt sound laboratory practices directed at assuring the quality of service delivered. The primary product of a transfusion laboratory is laboratory results of analysis carried out on a blood specimen. Quality assurance (QA) of such a laboratory must include all of the activities associated with ensuring that biologic testing is done properly, interpreted correctly, reported with appropriate estimates of error and confidence levels and communicated effectively and timely to the requesting clinician to facilitate the offering of best possible care to customers. QA activities also include those maintaining appropriate records of sample origins and history (sample-tracking), as well as procedures, raw data, and results associated with each sample. The various elements of good laboratory practice includes; use of standard operating procedures (SOP's), statistical procedures for data evaluation, availability and use of personal protective equipment, availability and use of infection control equipment, effective management of waste including sharps, availability of post exposure prophylaxis, provision protective vaccination, instrumentation validation, reagent/materials certification, analyst certification, laboratory facilities certification, specimen/sample tracking and availability of audit process and investigation of incidents.

Standard Operating Procedures (SOP's)

SOPs are a written document or instruction detailing all steps and activities of a process or procedure. ISO 9001 principles essentially require the documentation of all procedures used in any manufacturing process that could affect the quality of the product. Standard Operating Procedure (SOP) is a set of written instructions that document how a routine or repetitive activity should be a laboratory. The development and use of SOPs are an integral part of a successful quality system as it provides individuals with the information to perform a job properly, and facilitates consistency in the quality and integrity of a product or end-result.

SOP Preparation. Those SOPs should be written by individuals knowledgeable with the activity and the organization's internal structure. These individuals are essentially subject-matter experts who actually perform the work or use the process. A team approach can be followed, especially for multi-tasked processes where the experiences of a number of individuals are critical. Characteristic of a good SOP includes; should be written with sufficient detail so that someone with limited experience with or knowledge of the procedure, but with a basic understanding, can successfully reproduce the procedure when unsupervised, should be reviewed (validated) by one or more individuals with appropriate training and experience with the process. It is especially helpful if draft SOPs are actually tested by individuals other than the original writer before the SOPs are finalized. The finalized SOPs should be approved as described in the organization's Quality Management Plan. Signature approval indicates that an SOP has been both reviewed and approved by management, need to remain current to be useful. Therefore, whenever procedures are changed, SOPs should be updated and re-approved. If desired, modify only the pertinent section of an SOP and indicate the change date/revision number for that section in the Table of Contents and the document control notation and SOPs should also be systematically reviewed on a periodic basis (every 1-2 years) to ensure that the policies and procedures remain current and appropriate, or to determine whether the SOPs are even needed. The review date should be added to each SOP that has been reviewed. If an SOP describes a process that is no longer needed, it should be withdrawn from the current file and archived.

General format for standard operating procedures (SOP)

Title Page and table of content. The first page or cover page of each SOP should contain the following information: a title that clearly identifies the activity or procedure, an SOP identification (ID) number, date of issue and/or revision, the name of the laboratory to which this SOP applies, and the signatures and signature dates of those individuals who prepared and approved the SOP as well as signature of those who have read, been trained and are committed to following the SOP in carrying out the process/task. Electronic signatures are acceptable for SOPs maintained on a computerized database. A Table of Contents may be needed for quick reference, especially if the SOP is long, for locating information and to denote changes or revisions made only to certain sections of an SOP.

Text. Well-written SOPs should first briefly describe the following; the purpose of the work or process and the scope to indicate what is covered, denote what sequential procedures should be followed, divided into significant sections; possible interferences, equipment needed responsible person, personnel qualifications, limitation, calculations, reporting, manual handling issues, risk assessment and health and safety considerations and describe all appropriate QA and quality control (QC) activities for that procedure, and list any cited or significant references.

Statistical procedures. Data generated by a laboratory will need to be evaluated for the purpose of; showing a trend in workload, justification for employment of more staff, justification of need for a higher throughput equipment procurement, scientific research, quality and process improvement, maintenance of optimum stocking of reagents, consumables and blood products. Laboratories may adopt certain standards which are deemed acceptable within that field (for example using 95% or 99% confidence levels for particular tests) or they may adopt specific statistical analysis procedures for defining detection limits, confidence intervals, analyte measurement units.

Availability and use of personal protective equipment. GLP principle stipulates that laboratory staff wear appriopriate personal protective equipment (PPE) when working with biological agents and all potentially infectious materials. Personal protective equipment (PPE) is specialized clothing or equipment worn by a worker for protection against a hazard. The hazard in a health care setting is exposure to blood, saliva, or other bodily fluids or aerosols that may carry infectious materials such as Hepatitis C, HIV, or other blood borne or bodily fluid pathogen. PPE prevents contact with a potentially infectious material by creating a physical barrier between the potential infectious material and the healthcare worker. Personal protective equipments includes:

Laboratory coats. Anyone working in a containment laboratory should wear a laboratory coat. The lab coat must be fastened at one side, to the neck with close fitting cuffs. Coats should be flame retardant and sufficiently impermeable to protect clothing underneath. Laboratory coats must be removed before leaving the laboratory and hung on appropriate hooks. Contaminated laboratory coats should be autoclaved before being sent for washing. Personal clothing must not be hung on the same hooks used for hanging lab coats.

Gloves. Gloves should be worn if indicated in the risk assessment for the task being performed. Gloves should be worn for all work with biological agents or potentially infectious material (cell cultures, HIV, HBV, HCV, and TB). Gloves must be worn when working in a category 3 laboratory. A range of sizes and materials (latex and nitrite) should be available for users to use. Latex gloves must not be used unless justified in a written risk assessment. Gloves should be removed before leaving the laboratory, and before using items that may be used by others not wearing gloves such as telephones and computers. Heat resistant gloves must be worn when using the autoclave or handling a hot material.

Eye goggles. If the risk assessment indicates that splashes of blood or body fluids are likely, and work is not carried out in a microbiological safety cabinet, then suitable eye and/or face protection (goggles) or a visor should be worn to protect mucous membranes. Eye protection may also be required for work with chemicals that can harm the eyes.

Respiratory protective equipment (RPE). Suitable RPE, that has been fit-tested, must be worn when working with airborne hazardous substances. Exposures to airborne hazardous substances can be reduced by either: substituting with less toxic material, enclosing the process and ventilating the laboratory where the task takes place to ensure an acceptable concentration. Important point to note with use of RPE equipment include;must be used if other means of controlling substances hazardous to health are inadequate, should be used in addition to using other means of control. RPE equipment is only effective if used and maintained properly. The following must be in place; training should be given to all persons performing task on its use and maintenance, the type of protection used should have an appropriate protection factor in relation to the anticipated concentration of hazardous substance(s), the PPE should be comfortable for users to wear and a good seal to the face and all RPE equipments (except single use disposable types) should be tested regularly and must be in optimum stock levels at all times.

Disposable aprons. Aprons must be worn over laboratory coats when carrying out a task that is associated with risk of spillages.

Availability and use of infection control equipment. Infection control addresses factors related to the spread of infections within the health-care setting (whether patient-to-patient, from patients to staff and from staff to patients, or among-staff) including prevention (via good hand hygiene/ hand washing, cleaning/disinfection/sterilization, vaccination, surveillance), monitoring/investigation of demonstrated or suspected spread of infection within a particular health-care setting (surveillance and outbreak investigation) and management. It is well documented that the most important measure for preventing the spread of pathogens is effective handwashing. Hand washing is mandatory in most health care settings. Employers must provide readily accessible hand washing facilities, and must ensure that employees wash hands and any other skin with soap and water or flush mucous membranes with water as soon as feasible after contact with blood or other potentially infectious materials (OPIM). Drying of hand is also an essential part of the hand hygiene process. Warm air hand dryers and modern jet-air hand dryers are required.

There is effective management of waste including sharps. Infectious waste (Clinical waste) and is mainly produced by hospitals, health clinics, doctors' surgeries and veterinary practices, but can come from residential homes, nursing homes and collection of blood for transfusion, which may cause infection to any person coming into contact with it. Laboratory or clinical waste is made up completely or partly of, human or animal tissue, blood or other bodily fluids, excretions, drugs or other pharmaceutical products, swabs or dressings, syringes, needles or other sharp instruments and also includes drugs or other pharmaceutical products. All sharps must be appriopriately disposed into sharps bin. Sharps bins should not be overfilled must have information on source, the signatute of staff that put the sharps bin together and the staff that closed it for final incineration and must be kept in a safe place, disposal should be through a registered waste carrier. Sharps are items that can cause cuts or puncture injuries and include; needles, syringes, lancets, scalpels, stitch cutters, razor blades, glass ampoules and sharp instruments. All producers of waste, their employees and service carriers, have a duty of care to ensure all waste is being disposed of legally. A duty of care is imposed on all those who produce, carry, keep, treat and dispose of controlled waste or have control of such waste.

Post exposure prophylaxis. Post-exposure prophylaxis (PEP) is any prophylactic treatment started immediately after exposure to a pathogen (such as a disease-causing virus) in order to prevent infection by the pathogen and the development of disease. In some cases where vaccines do not exist, Post Exposure prophylaxis is another method of protecting the health care worker exposed to a life threatening infectious disease. In case of exposure to blood and body fluid of an HIV –infected patient through needle stick injury, HIV infection can be prevented by giving the exposed heathcare worker post-exposure prophylaxis made up of a course of antiretroviral drugs. This reduces the risk of seroconversion after events with high risk of exposure to HIV. The antiretroviral regimen used in PEP is the same as the standard highly active antiretroviral therapy used to treat AIDS. It requires close compliance and can have unpleasant side effects including malaise, fatigue, diarrhea, headache, nausea and vomiting. Human Normal Immunoglobulin (HNIG) or hepatitis A vaccine may be used as PEP for staff exposed to blood and body fluid of an hepatitis A positive source patient depending on the clinical situation. If a health care worker who is not previously vaccinated or a non-responder is exposed to an HBsAg positive source patient blood or body fluid, HBV vaccine and hepatitis B imune globulin (HBIG) can be administered. But for those already vacinated and are responders, a booster dose should be given. Persons exposed to Hepatitis C should get monthly PCR test. If seroconversion occurs, then interferon +/- ribavirin must be started.

Staff must up-to-date for the protective vaccination. Health care workers may be exposed to certain infections in the course of their work. Vaccines are available to provide some protection to workers in a healthcare setting. Depending on regulation, recommendation, the specific work function, or personal preference, healthcare workers may receive vaccinations for hepatitis B; Influenza, Measles, Mumps, Rubella, Tetanus, Diphtheria, Tetanus, Pertussis, Nieseria meningitidis and varicella. In general, vaccines do not guarantee complete protection from disease, and there is potential for adverse effects from receiving the vaccine. Staff must be up-to-date for their protective vaccination.

Instrumentation validation. Instrument validation is a process that is very important for any analytical laboratory. Instrument validation ensures that an instrument is fit for its intended use (fit for purpose). Data produced by faulty instruments may give the appearance of valid data. These events are particularly difficult to detect with modern computer-controlled systems which remove the analyst from the data collection and instrument control functions. Important points on instrument validation includes:

1. It is essential that some objective procedures are implemented for continuously assessing the validity of laboratory instrument and the data they provide.
2. These procedures must be executed on a regular basis to establish the continuing acceptable operation of laboratory instruments within manufacturers prescribed specifications.
3. Time-related graphical records of the results of these instrument validation procedures (control charts) must be documented either electronically or as a soft copy.

Reagent/materials certification. GLP guidelines emphasize that all reagents intended for use in the analysis of patient sample must be tested and quality controlled and certified fit for it intended use. Certification must follow accepted procedures, and must be adequately documented. Each container of laboratory reagent must be labeled with information related to its certification value, date, and expiration time. Time expired reagents must never be used for diagnostic purposes on patients samples. Reagents must by quality controlled daily before use. Equipment must be quality controlled with reagents after every major maintenance work is done on it. Reagents including temperature dependent reagents must be appriopriately stored. Most temperature dependent reagents are stored optimally between 2-8°C. Evidence of temperature monitoring of fridges used for storage of reagents must be kept to show remedial action to be taken when temperature is not maintained within the optimum temperature range.

Certification of analysts. Certification of analyst is a required part of QA. Some acceptable proof of satisfactory training and/or competence with specific laboratory procedures must be established for each analyst. Because the American Chemical Society does not currently have a policy regarding "certification" of chemists or analysts, the requirements for "certification" vary, and are usually prescribed by the laboratory in question. These standards would have to be accepted by any agency or client obtaining results from that laboratory. For our biomedical scientist in the laboratory, the requirement is the completion of a degree course in Biomedical Science, certification by the Health Professions Council (UK), the Medical Laboratory Science Council of Nigeria (MLSCN) and other related regulatory authorities as well as training and competency on the task being performed.

Certification of laboratory facilities. Laboratory certification is normally done by some external agency. For example, an analytical laboratory might be audited by representatives of a federal agency with which they have a contract. An independent laboratory might file documentation with a responsible state or federal agency. The evaluation is concerned with such issues as space (amount, quality and relevance), ventilation, equipment, storage, hygiene, etc. Student chemistry laboratories are generally evaluated by the American Chemical Society, as part of the process of granting approval for the overall chemistry program presented by the college or university.

This latter approval process is not as detailed regarding analytical facilities as the certification processes pursued by agencies concerned specifically with quality assurance.

Specimen/sample-tracking. Specimen tracking is an aspect of quality assurance which has received a great deal of attention particularly with the advent of computer-based Laboratory Information Management Systems (LIMS). GLP principle stipulates that; procedures should be in place for assuring adequate specimen/sample-tracking may vary among laboratories; the procedures must however maintain the unmistakable connection between a set of analytical results and the specimen from which they were obtained. In addition, the original source of the specimen must be recorded and likewise unmistakably connected with the set of analytical data. Finally, in many cases there must be information or an audit trail of a sample (to include when sample was receive, booked on the LIMS, when sample was loaded on analyzer, when results was technically validated on the analyzer, when result was clinically validated and available to the requesting clinician. At every stage of this trails all responsible laboratory staff must make comments on what was done and why.

Documentation and Maintenance of Records. A central feature of GLP guidelines is the maintenance of records in a clear, accurate and auditable form. Documentation is important for several reasons:

1. Specimen origins, chain-of-custody, raw analytical data, processed analytical data, SOP's, instrument validation results, reagent certification results, analyst certification documents and other relevant records must be available and kept safe for a specified period of time.
2. Maintenance of instrument and reagent certification records provides for post-evaluation of results, even after the passage of several years.
3. Maintenance of all records specified provide documentation which may be required in the event of legal challenges due to repercussions of decisions based on the original analytical results.
4. Many vendors are now providing many of these capabilities as part of computer packages for operating modern instruments. For example most modern computer-based instruments will provide for the indefinite storage of raw analytical data for specific samples in a protected (tamper-proof) environment as well as maintenance of historical records of control chart data establishing the operational quality of instruments during any period during which analytical data have been acquired by that instrument.
5. The length of time over which laboratory records should be maintained will vary with the situation. The general guidelines followed in regulated laboratories are to maintain records for at least five years. In some countries these records are being maintained much longer. The development of higher density storage devices for digitized data is making this kind of record-keeping possible.

Accountability. GLP procedures inherently establish accountability for laboratory results. A laboratory organization, the analysts and manufacturers of instruments and reagents are responsible to a larger extent for laboratory results generated by the laboratory. Responsibility for all aspects of the laboratory processes leading to technical results and conclusions must be clearly defined and documented. Laboratory organization have the responsibility to ensure that a robust process is in place to assure the quality of results emanating from the laboratory. This situation should place appropriate pressure on analysts to conduct studies with adequate care and concern, laboaratory organization to put a process in place to assure quality and instrument manaufacturers to ensure that their instruments and reagents are fit for purpose. Moreover justify that a process should be in place in the laboratory that ensures the possibility of identifying more quickly and succinctly the source(s) of error(s), identifying the root causes and taking corrective and preventive action to maintain acceptable quality of laboratory data.

Other GLP general rules

1. Develop SOP for all task, ensure that all staff performing the task are tranied to the SOP, sign to the SOP and infact are following the SOP strictly.

2. Ensure that correct equipment and reagents are being used. Outdated reagents, malfunctioning equipment and equipment that have not been adequately cleaned, calibrated, maintined and quality controlled must not be used for diagnosis on patient sample.

3. Put a robust method in place to avoid mix up of samples as well as labelling errors.

4. Report and root cause every mistakes, near misses, errors and bad practices and come up with corrective and preventive action to prevent such errors (Never cover up. Cover up is dangerous and can cause loss of lives).

5. Put in place a mechanism for implementing corrective and preventive action (re-training of staff with deficiencies, modification of process. Records must be clear, accurate and securely kept for several years depending on regulation. Records must identify person responsible, confirm what was done.

38. Quality Issues in Transfusion Medicine

Quality assurance is a vital topic in transfusion medicine. Quality management system (QMS) is the sum total of all the processes that allow for the effective control of the whole operation. It is not just an added-on to the process but it is a very vital part of the process control in the transfusion laboratory. It includes the use of a documented set of policies and procedures which define how you achieve a defined quality of product or service. In the laboratory, a quality product or service is a service that meets the customer requirements. It is providing the right result on the right specimen from the right patient that is cost effective (value for money), reliable, accurate, reproducible (best possible care), timely (improving health), effectively and appropriately communicated by a highly motivate laboratory professional (joy and pride at work) to the users of the service, enhances the quality of care offered to customer. To achieve our goal of making the availability of safe blood at all times without shortage, a uniform and updated national blood policy should be introduced all over Nigera. This will definitely give confidence in introducing good quality control, quality assurance and accreditation at all levels of transfusion practices. Standard Operating Procedures (SOP) are needed for the blood banks.

Quality management system

Quality management system (QMS) is the sum total of all the processes that allow for the effective control of the whole operation. It includes the use of a documented set of policies and procedures which define how you achieve a defined quality of product or service. In the lab, a quality product or service is a service that meets the customer requirements. It is providing the right result on the right specimen from the right patient that is cost effective (value for money), reliable, accurate, reproducible (best possible care), timely (improving health), effectively and appropriately communicated by a highly motivate laboratory professional (joy and pride at work) to the users of the service, enhances the quality of care offered customer. A simple definition of quality is 'fitness for a purpose'. In blood transfusion service, the primary goal of quality is 'transfusion of safe unit of blood.' The objective is to ensure availability of a sufficient supply of blood, blood components of high quality with maximum efficacy and minimum risk to both donors and patients. To achieve quality in a defined procedure, a laboratory may encounter constraints such as; organizational constraints in terms of staffing patterns, finances available, training of staff and technical constraints for example the ability of laboratory to perform a specific test.

Need for Quality

A failure in the quality of blood collected or screening of donated blood unit can be very serious and may result in fatal consequences. If appropriate quality systems are designed, implemented and monitored, the issue of an improperly tested unit can be avoided. Besides laboratory testing, a failure in the quality system can lead to numerous situations which may be potentially dangerous to the patient, i.e.

1. failure to identify the patient correctly
2. wrong sample labelling
3. mix-up of results amongst different patients
4. Failure to detect presence of an abnormality in the patient's sample.
5. issue of unscreened blood due to faulty laboratory procedures

Therefore, it is very important to recognise the need for quality and implementation of quality assurance scheme in all laboratory procedures. The difference between these two terms may be unclear to many people and the terms cannot be used interchangeably. Quality assurance deals with the maintenance of a system to ensure that the performance in a laboratory is of the required quality. In a blood transfusion centre, it means that a management system should exist to look into provision of a safe unit of blood and, if any errors are identified, these should be corrected. Quality control is the inspection system which involves specific actions performed to monitor the effectiveness of the system and checks that the mistakes have not occurred.

Indicators to monitor the quality of your laboratory's performance

1. Turnaround times.
2. Internal quality assessment.
3. External quality assessment.
4. It is not sufficient to sit back and assume that we are doing fine quality wise.
5. In fact, since no system is perfect, there is every tendency that we do make mistakes. If we do, then;
6. How many do we make and why? Are there trends.
7. How often do we exceed our turnaround times?
8. How often does our LIMS go down?
9. How often do we produce an incorrect result, or send the correct result but for the wrong patient?
10. We need to measure our performance.
11. Measuring our performance is the only was to monitor and measure improvements.

What constitutes quality from a customer's perspective?

1. Customer see the response time for lab test as critical to the quality of care.
2. Want to be informed about the turnaround times.
3. Expect that laboratory results are reliable.
4. Expect a simple and easy to follow instructions on sample collection and handling.
5. Require a prompt, customer focused and friendly phlebotomy service.

6. Want a continually improving service.
7. Require a cost effective quality service
8. Want a safety, environment and infection control conscious lab service.
9. Customers like a process oriented service with a feedback system.

What is quality assurance?. All arrangements in place to ensure that products and services meet the quality required. It includes; staff training, equipment maintenance, use of internal quality, enrolment in external quality programmes, use of STD operating procedures, objective performance of audits, submission to accreditation and carrying out user satisfaction survey.

Benefits of a quality system includes

1. Achieving accreditation.
2. Achieving better control of processes.
3. Drives improvement (documented quality system is mechanism for improvement).
4. Proof those adequate procedures are in place in the event of legal proceedings.
5. Improved service for the customer.
6. Increased efficiency through reduction of mistakes and waste.

Internal quality control and external quality assurance. Internal quality control (IQC) is the analysis of material of known content. Confirms that the procedures are performing within predetermined specifications. Day-to-day monitoring of reproducibility or precision but not accuracy. Detect errors in any one analytical run. Qualitative assays include internal controls to validate run. Use of QC run on analyzers requires control charts (or Shewhart plots) using Westgard rules. Control material for use in control charts must:

1. Behave like real samples
2. Be sufficient for a period of time.
3. Be stable over time period of use.
4. Be appropriately apportioned for convenient use.
5. Vary little in concentration between aliquots.

Internal Quality Assessment (IQA) and External Quality Assessment (EQA). Quality assurance in clinical laboratories is for the provision of precise and accurate analyses to support optimal healthcare. The importance and value of internal quality control and external quality assessment have gained a higher professional profile particularly with the introduction of the new Clinical Pathology Accreditation standards. Quality assurance improves test reliability through helping to minimise the variability arising from biological or analytical sources inherent in all qualitative and quantitative measurements. An important contribution to the reliability of laboratory results however lies in ensuring correct specimen collection, handling and identification. Although most modern analytical systems are apparently simple to use, the quality of results does not come automatically with the equipment. Appropriate quality assurance measures that include; analytical quality control measures (IQA and EQA) need to be taken, including of course staff motivation, training and assessment. Internal and external quality assessments are vital components of a quality system that offers valuable insights into the effectiveness of the quality system.

Internal quality assessment (IQA): Internal quality assessment assesses in real time whether the performance of an individual laboratory or testing site is sufficiently similar to their previous performance for results to be used. It controls reproducibility or precision and facilitates continuity of patient care overtime. Most IQA procedures employ analysis of a control material and compare the results with pre-determined limits of acceptability. Discrepancies in results are investigated, with major discrepancies requiring repeat testing, possibly with request for another specimen. Larger numbers of samples can be handled in IQA than in EQA schemes. There is also flexibility of sample types to be assessed. External quality assessment (EQA) by contrast looks at differences between sites testing the same analyte, so there can be continuity of testing over geography. This usually involves the analysis of identical specimens at many laboratories and the comparison of results with those of other sites. While IQA controls the precision of investigations, EQA should be providing an assessment of their accuracy since it lack bias with respect to other test sites. EQA is done periodically and retrospectively. EQA also provides assessment of the overall standard of performance, the relative performance of the analytical procedures (method principle, reagents and instruments) as well as the specimen distributed. EQA is likely to help stimulate needed quality improvement. EQA may also indicate analytical procedures showing excellent performance characteristics and which can be recommended and also identify unsatisfactory procedures which should be discouraged. Internal quality assurance is meant to allow laboratory scientist to check their performance by themselves and help them to monitor the reliability of their technique. In other words, it deals with the measures taken by a local laboratory to maintain laboratory standards. IQA includes procedures designed for continuous evaluation of the work of the laboratory concerned and it aims at achieving high level of safety and efficiency.

External quality assessment (EQA). This is the challenge of the efficacy of laboratory quality assurance procedures by specimens of known but undisclosed content. A central body periodically distributes EQA specimens to different testing sites, and compare individual laboratory results with that of other participating laboratories, and with the correct answer. It gives participants an insight into their routine performance so that they take appropriate corrective action where necessary. External quality assessment facilitates optimal patient care by providing a comprehensive external quality assessment service in laboratory medicine. Through education and the promotion of best services, it helps ensure that the results of investigations are reliable and comparable wherever they are produced. Assessment of IQA results can be more sensitive to local clinical and technical styles than it is possible with EQA schemes and scoring made more stringent than in EQA. External quality assurance involves a central reference laboratory which monitors the standards of local laboratories. EQA is a system whereby a set of reagents and techniques are assessed by an external source and the results of testing laboratory being compared with those of an approved reference laboratory. External quality assessment has the following merits:

1. Comparability: Participating laboratories are able to assess whether their results are comparable with those of other laboratories. This provides a means of detecting and checking whether such differences are affecting results of investigations of clinical specimens, hence patient care.

2. Educational stimulus: Participation in EQA can serve as an educational tool for laboratory staff, especially in the area of quality management.

3. Credibility: Participation in EQA scheme is a demonstration that the laboratory has a responsible attitude to quality issues.

4. Insight into National Performance levels: EQA results provide laboratory professionals, funding organisations, and health service administrators with an insight into national performance levels for informed decision making on the use of and support for laboratory services.

5. Improvement in national performance levels: Identification of problem areas enables laboratory professionals to take action to remedy deficiencies, which results in performance improvements over time.

6. External quality assessment schemes are standardised and has expert direction.

The EQA process is essentially retrospective and provides an assessment of performance rather than control for each test performed. Participating laboratories may give EQA samples special treatment to improve their chances of getting a high performance score. This practice does not give a fair reflection of the performance of the laboratory and may not give true insight into where there may be genuine problems in the process, therefore hinder improvements in the system. In contrast however, IQA results can be more sensitive to local clinical and technical styles than it is possible with EQA schemes and scoring made more stringent than in EQA. Internal quality assessment can be used to monitor the whole laboratory, from specimen registration to issue of reports. Performance standards can be derived from the process. Used together IQA and EQA provide a method of ensuring accuracy and consistency of results and are vital tools in the quality assurance of the clinical laboratory. IQA and EQA results should be reviewed at laboratory meetings and should be readily available information that could stimulate quality improvement in the laboratory.

Risk assessment. Think about all the steps involved from specimen collection to result availability to clinician. Think about all the critical control points. This is a form of risk assessment. At each step, there is a possibility that something could go wrong. Also at each step it is important to consider if specific conditions need to be met, e.g., incubation at 37°C. Identify the risks in all the steps and document what control measures in place in your lab to manage risks. Consider measures not being taken or inadequate in your own laboratory to manage a risk that you have identified. Risk analysis can play a role in continuous improvement.

Continuous quality improvement (CQI) in transfusion

Quality system can provide a mechanism for improvements by generating evidence based data to monitor quality improvements. By carrying out regular and objective audits and implementing corrective and preventive action. By building a culture of continual improvement. Only thing that adds value is transformation of raw material into something the customer wants. A continuous improvement process is an ongoing effort to improve products, services, or processes. These efforts can seek "incremental" improvement over time or "breakthrough" improvement all at once. Delivery (customer valued) processes are constantly evaluated and improved in the light of their efficiency, effectiveness and flexibility. Some successful implementations use the approach known as Kaizen (the translation of Kai (change) zen (good or improvement). This method became famous by the book of Masaaki Imai "Kaizen: The Key to Japan's Competitive Success."The core principle of CIP is the (self) reflection of processes. (Feedback). The purpose of continuous improving process (CIP) is the identification, reduction, and elimination of suboptimal processes (Efficiency). The emphasis of CIP is on incremental, continuous steps rather than giant leaps (Evolution). Key features of Kaizen include:

- Quality system can provide a mechanism for improvements by generating evidence based data to monitor quality improvements.
- By carrying out regular and objective audits and implementing corrective and preventive action.
- By building a culture of continual improvement.
- Only thing that adds value is transformation of raw material into something the customer wants.
- Improvements are based on many, small changes rather than the radical changes that might arise from research and development.
- As the ideas come from the workers themselves, they are less likely to be radically different, and therefore easier to implement.
- Small improvements are less likely to require major capital investment than major process changes.

- The ideas come from the talents of the existing workforce, as opposed to using R&D, consultants or equipment – any of which could be very expensive.
- All employees should continually be seeking ways to improve their own performance.
- It helps encourage workers to take ownership for their work, and can help reinforce team working, thereby improving worker motivation.

The elements above are the more tactical elements of CIP. The more strategic elements include deciding how to increase the value of the delivery process output to the customer (Effectiveness) and how much flexibility is valuable in the process to meet changing needs. The involvement of all workers require training, it is necessary to be able to distinguish between symptom and ailment so that efforts are spent solving the root causes of the problem.

Steps Involved In Using CQI. Quality is a cycle of continuous improvement. Proper CQI starts with planning and data collection. Statistical analysis on the wrong or incorrect data is not useful, the analysis must be appropriate for the data collected. Be sure to PLAN, and then constantly re-evaluate your situation to make sure the plan is correct. The key to any process improvement program is the PDSA cycle described by Walter Shewart.

Plan. Collect data and establish a baseline – what is the current process doing now? Identify the problem and the possible causes. The QC tools described in this manual can help organizations identify problems and possible causes, and to prioritize corrective actions.

Do. Make changes designed to correct or improve the situation. These changes often come form quality improvement suggestions made by staff or from feed back from service user's satisfaction surveys and findings from root cause analysis carried out following an incident or complaint from service users.

Study. Study the effect of these changes on the situation. Collect data on the new process and compare to the baseline. This is where control charts are used – they show the effects of changes on a process over time. Evaluate the results and then replicate the change or abandon it and try something different.

Act. If the result is successful, standardize the changes and then work on further improvements or the next prioritized problem. If the outcome is not yet successful, look for other ways to change the process or identify different causes for the problem. Control charting is one of a number of steps involved in CQI. The steps include discovery, analysis, prioritization, clarification, and then charting. Before using the Statit software, appropriate data must be collected for analysis. Then, you need to begin again and do it over and and over.

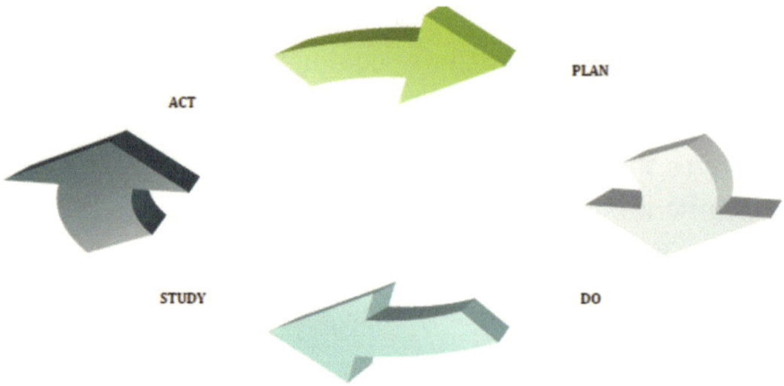

Figure: Plan, do, study and act (PDSA cycle)

Quality Audits in transfusion

A quality audit is a systematic, independent and documented process of evaluating selected elements of a quality system. Ensure that system being implemented is effective and is being complied with. There are 3 types of audits;

- Horizontal audit: Involves the assessment of one element of the quality system
- Examination audit: Involves a process whereby the assessor watches a test being performed, to ascertain if SOP is being followed. It is used to confirm competence of the staff and level of training.
- Vertical audit: Involves a process whereby a sample is tracked from sample receipt to the issue of result.

Quality audits re-emphasize the following:

1. The importance of proper record keeping and documentation.
2. The need to work to defined standards and procedures.
3. The importance for effective and appropriate storage and monitoring of temperature –dependent reagents.
4. The need for proactive maintenance of equipments.
5. The need to develop a culture of continuous improvement.

Examples of vertical and horizontal audits

Horizontal audits include an element of the quality process; equipment, staff training, document control, housekeeping, internal audit, evaluations. Important aspects to look at includes; associated records, SOPs, EOPs, visual appearance, suitability for use, staff interactions with the system & whether the system is achieving its intended result. Vertical audit cuts across the entire process from sample reception to result availability. It includes variables such as ; storage of reagents, health and safety issues, staff training, infection control, competences, equipment maintenance, internal and external quality assessments, premises, corrective actions, pre, examination and post examination.

Performing a quality audit

1. Preparation of a checklist.
2. The better the checklist is, the easier and more standardised audits become.
3. A checklist prepared for one audit may be updated and used for repeat audits of the same topic.
4. Organise a pre-audit meeting.
5. Consult relevant SOPs since you will need to ensure staff members are compliant to the SOP.
6. Draw up quality improvement notes arising from the audit to facilitate a continually improving process.
7. Organize a post audit meeting to discuss non-compliances & quality improvement issues arising.
8. Implement suggested change.

Example of an audit check list

Audit type/number and details (Verical audit/ AUD 100: General duties in transfusion)/Completed by/completion date: Dr Osaro/3/11/2011		
Number	**Audit question**	**Response**
1.	Identify test, processes, procedure being audited.	
2.	Are there SOP available for sample examination processes?	
3.	Have procedures been validated for use prior to introduction. List document examined	
4.	Are SOP current, signed and dated	
5.	Are SOP being followed by staff performing task	
6.	Is there evidence of document control in place. State last revision date	

7.	Are there COSHH (control of substances hazardous to health) risk and general assessment s available for all task.	
8.	Are there procedure in place for reporting and monitoring of accidents and incidents	
9.	Are staff responsible clearly identified and are there evidence of training and education.	
10.	Are there procedures for sample receipt, transport and booking in?	
11.	What is the specimen number of the sample being audited. Is there sufficient information to uniquely identify patient. Is there evidence of date and time of sample collection. Does request form contain required clinical information.	
12.	Is there process in place for handling urgent sample. Is there criteria for rejection of sample	
13.	Is there record available for each stage of the process such that there is complete audit trail of staff, equipment reagents and quality control procedures involved. List document examined?	
14.	Is there evidence that equipment used is routinely maintained, daily checks done and quality controlled. List equipment checked	
15.	Is the lab enrolled into and EQA. Are EQA report reviewed. indicate scheme	
16.	Does lab report contain time and date of report, results and reason if no examination done. Are there interpretive comments and are abnormal results highlighted	
17.	Does lab has turnaround time for test/process being audited. Is set turnaround time feasible and are target being met	

Examples of non-conformance notes

1. The internal quality control used for a test run was out of limits and there is no evidence that any action was taken.
2. Purpose is to convey findings in a clear and accurate manner to the auditee (what was wrong and what to do next)
3. Fridges used for storage of temperature dependent reagents have gone outside ambient temperature several times and there is no remedial action taken.
4. Incidents, near misses and complaint are not investigated
5. Staff satisfaction surveys are not being done
6. Staff performing task have not been trained or competency tested
7. There are no standard work for task being performed
8. The transfusion lab is not registered for any EQA scheme
9. Thre are no policy in place for infection control, manual handling and there are no personal protective equipment for staff
10. Staff occupational health-related vaccination is not up to date.
11. Someone is doing a routine test for which there is no SOP.
12. There is a bottle of clear liquid on the bench with no label on. A member of staff says it is only water.

Aim of non-conformance notes

1. To advise the next auditor what you have found so that they can follow it up.
2. To present a record that can be re-assessed at a later date during management review.
3. To enable auditee to determine root cause, determine remedial, corrective and prevention action to eliminate root causes.
4. Non-compliance notes (NCNs) are used to report any deficiencies found during an audit.

Dealing with non conformances

1. What remedial action (Quick fix) you would take.
2. Consider the further corrective action to eliminate root causes.
3. Implement corrective action.
4. Audit the process to ensure that root cause have been eliminated.

5. Continuously solving root problems drives organizational learning and improvement.

6. Sophisticated technique for solving problems is to: ask "why?" objectively five times.

Responding to audit findings – non-compliance

Audit criterion 1.

Guidelines require that patient records contain a record of the clinician's reason for prescribing each red cell transfusion.

Audit findings

A doctor's record of the reason for transfusing is found in only 20% of patients' files.

Root Causes

Failure in the oversight function by supervising clinical staff and consultants.

Corrective action

Obtain the agreement of clinical staff to achieve a target of 90% documentation of the reason to transfuse and to participate in education on the importance of clinical accountability for transfusion and to a repeat audit.

Audit Criterion 2

Guidelines require that all patients undergoing transfusion have observations of pulse, blood pressure, respiration and temperature recorded before and at specified time intervals during the transfusion.

Audit Findings

These routine observations are performed incompletely or not at all in a substantial proportion of transfusion episodes.

Root Causes

Failure in the supervisory function of clinical lead or consultants.

Corrective action

Obtain the agreement of clinical staff to achieve a target of 90% documentation of patient observations according to the guidelines and to a repeat audit. To overcome the problem that nursing staff believe that they do not have time to perform the task, consider action such as; review the priorities among nursing duties to make more nursing resource available and the clinical responsibility for the decision should be clearly defined, and the Hospital Transfusion Committee should decide if notification to other authority (ies) is required.

Audit Criterion 3

Directive requires that the final fate of all blood components issued for recipients is recorded by the hospital blood bank.

Audit finding

Hospital blood bank does not have data on the final fate of all components.

Root Causes

Failure in the oversight function by senior nursing managers.

Corrective action

Obtain the agreement of clinical staff to achieve an initial target of 98%. Inform staff that monthly reports will be provided to senior nursing managers, identifying the clinical areas not meeting the agreed target. These mangers will be required to identify how non-conformance will be addressed.

Quality Policy

Every transfusion laboratory must have a quality policy. The document should set out the laboratory stand on quality. A quality system provides service users the confidence that a laboratory has a system and procedure in place to allow for a continually improving quality service. It should include the following;

1. A statement on the type of quality service the lab intend to provide and over what hours of the day the service will be available
2. State the focal person or group responsible for quality issues in the lab.
3. The human and material resource required to run the quality service
4. Have a defined management structure
5. Should contain statement on quality elements; document control, compliant handling, incident handling, audits, staff training, health and safety.
6. Should include information on document control. Documents must be uniquely identified to include the number and version. It should be typed, validated, approved by authorized personnel, issued and reviewed regularly.

Example of a Quality policy

The laboratory management of the Nelson Laboratories shall establish a quality policy that includes the following:

1. The Blood transfusion Laboratory shall provide all the elements of routine blood transfusion service. This shall include shall provide blood transfusion services including; blood grouping, antenatal testing, compatibility testing, provision of routine antenatal anti-D prophylaxis, processing of blood components and plasma fractions for administration to patients and determination of Feto Maternal Haemorrhage and management. Blood transfusion services shall be provided on 24 hours a day by shift –working.

2. The transfusion laboratory is committed to providing the highest quality and timely diagnostic service. We shall strive to provide service that is continually improving and takes into consideration the needs and requirements of its users.

3. The laboratory shall operate a quality management system to integrate the organisation, procedures, processes and resources. Quality management shall be exercised using the lean principles in all her processes. It focuses on 4 elements of quality; no avoidable deaths, no defects, no waste and highest staff morale). We shall use continuous improvement and lean tools in delivering services that meets the needs of our patients and other service users.

4. The Department's management team shall provide a framework for setting quality objectives, ensuring that these objectives are reviewed regularly to ensure that quality policy commitment and customer requirements are being met.

5. Annual reviews of the quality management system by the laboratory management team will allow for a critical evaluation of current quality status to be compared with previous years. The responsibility for quality improvement shall reside with the department Board.

6. The department shall ensure that all personnel are familiar with the contents and work within the context of the quality manuals and all procedures relevant to their work. We shall ensure that our personnel are adequately trained, certified and maintain a Continuous Professional Development (CPD) profile.

7. The department shall ensure that all personnel uphold professional and ethical values and continues to show commitment to good professional practice and conduct.

8. The department is committed to the health, safety and welfare of its entire staff.

9. Visitors to the department will be treated with courtesy with due consideration given to their safety while on site.

10. Our personnel shall remain our greatest resource. The department is committed to supporting and appreciating our staff ensuring that staff morale is continually enhanced.

11. The department is committed to complying with all relevant environmental legislation. As required by environmental regulators, we shall implement the following best practices by training employees on proper procedures to reduce our facility's impact on the environment.

12. Employee training may include the following; spill response training for personnel who handle hazardous material and hazardous materials management.

13. We shall ensure that all staff has a legal obligation to take reasonable care of your own health and safety and that of others who may be affected by your acts or omissions.

14. All work will be carried out within current Health, Safety and environmental legislation. We will ensure that our employees understand the health, safety and environmental commitment of the department.

15. The department will comply with standards set by the Medical Laboratory Science Council and other regulatory authorities and is committed to the following;

16. Staff recruitment, training and development and retention of qualified staff at all levels to provide a full and effective service to our users.

17. Proper procurement and maintenance of equipments as are needed for the provision of the service.

18. The collection, transport and handling of all specimens in such a way as to ensure the correct performance of laboratory examinations.

19. The use of examination procedures that will ensure the highest achievable quality of all laboratory tests performed.

20. Reporting results of examinations in a ways that are accurate, timely, confidential and clinically useful.

21. The assessment of user satisfaction in addition to internal audits and external quality assessment, in order to produce continual quality improvement.

22. The quality policy shall be signed dated and issued by the Laboratory Medicine Department manager

23. The department is committed to ensuring that the quality policy is communicated in an understandable language and that it is readily available and being implemented throughout the laboratory.

24. The department is committed to ensuring that the quality objectives set for the department are reviewed regularly at annual laboratory depart-

ment management meetings to ensure that policy commitment and customer requirements are being meant.

25. The department is committed to ensuring that confidentiality shall be our watch word in the handling of patient personal information of patients held by the laboratory.
26. Document must be signed and dated by the Laboratory Medicine Department Manager

Quality System & Total Quality Management (TQM)

In a blood transfusion service, the quality system deals with all aspects to ensure that the product or the tested and 'safe unit of blood' is as safe as possible. Quality system must be applied to all laboratories, whether small or more advance. It should include the implementation, maintenance and monitoring of the quality assurance system. The introduction of a quality system in blood transfusion centre starts with:

- In-depth vision and knowledge of all the aspects of blood transfusion.
- Planning required for effective donor selection, donor screening, and laboratory work, issue of safe blood and transfusion of blood to the recipient.
- Formulating the mechanism for monitoring to ensure that quality is maintained.

Total quality management includes; Quality in procurement (donor, material, reagent), quality in preparation (efficient and effective blood component preparation), quality in design and development (improved techniques and procedures) and quality in supply (transportation and service). Laboratory quality assurance scheme include:

1. Proper identification of all samples.
2. Validation of the sensitivity, specificity and reproducibility of new batch of test kits and reagents.
3. Strict adherence to the recommended procedure.
4. Use of the appropriate test and internal controls.
5. Regular proficiency testing exercise.
6. Adherence to safety guidelines and safe disposal.

Quality Control of Equipments

Besides assessment of function immediately after installation and repair of equipment, day to day checks in routine use of equipment are necessary.

Equipment requirements:

1. All the equipment in blood transfusion laboratory should meet mandatory specifications.
2. A written record of periodic function checks and maintenance on each piece of equipment should be mandatory.
3. A preventive maintenance should be planned for trouble free operation.
4. Uninterrupted power supply should be maintained for all the equipment with efficient back-up system.
5. Annual maintenance contract with manufacturers and suppliers should be obtained.

Equipment	Maintenance Required
Refrigerator for storage of blood	Read recording temp chart frequent at least once a day (correct temp. range 2-6oC). Test alarm system weekly. Test accuracy of alarm cut-in temp., once in 4 months. Check counter temp inside the cabinet with precision thermometer periodically.
Deep Freeze	Similar to blood storage refrigerator. Check accurate temp by thermometer kept inside the cabinet, twice a day.
Bench centrifuge	Check accuracy of speed and time with precision rpm meter (incho meter & stop watch every three months. Check motor brushes at regular intervals
Refrigerated Centrifuge	Check accuracy of speed & time with tachometer and stop watch every three months. Check temp inside the centrifuge bowl by a temp. tester with the lid closed & head stationary. Check motor brushes every three months.

Water bath	Check temp 2-3 times a day. Check thermometer accuracy periodically. Change the water every week using only distilled water. Send the discarded water for culture to rule out any fungus/microbe contaminating the water bath. Use the stirrer for uniform maintenance of the temperature. If no stirrer is attached check temp. at diagonal end of bath periodically to ensure reasonable degree of uniformity.
Cell Washer	Check shortly before use. Check speed & time monthly. Check function 6 monthly. Check temp. monthly. Check volume dispensed by cell washer monthly
Incubator	Check the temp. 2-3 times in a day. Check accuracy of temp. periodically
pH meter	Two point calibration (check control solution pH 4-7 : 7-10) before each time of use. Full maintenance every six months
Weighing balance	Check the sensitivity of electronic balances using known weights once a week. Full maintenance every six months
ELISA reader	Check the reproducibility of results every 3 months Calibration graph six monthly. Full maintenance every six months. Check the filters for any fungal growth every 3 months. Keep the filters in the dessicator
Auto pipettes	Calibrate the pipettes regularly using mercury or water.
Whole blood collection equipment (Vacuum agitator, non-vacuum agitator, balance and scales for weight)	Check with known weights daily/day of use
Micro haematocrit	Check minimum packing time once every 3 month
Platelet incubator	Check temp and agitator. Check speed agitator daily
Thawing device	Check temp daily or day of use. Checks for cleanliness and replace water when contaminated

Table: Guidelines for quality control of equipment in blood transfusion service

39. Management Review Meetings in the transfusion laboratory

Management review meeting is an extremely important part of the success of a quality management system and it is an organization's most significant source for improvements. Management review can be used to tie together all the elements of an organization's program and bring cohesiveness to the quality management system. Management review meetings should ideally be focused on "trends, objective evidence, and data-based decisions," not on daily operations. The following topics should be included in the agenda of a typical management review meeting:

1. Follow-up actions: Discuss matters arising from previous management review meetings.
2. Update reports from managerial and supervisory personnel.
3. Quality Assurance Report: Discuss changes to the quality assurance standard, external quality assessment reports including non-conformance to standard procedures and regulatory issues.
4. Reports of assessment by outside regulatory authorities like the CPA and MHRA
5. Equipment/Maintenance: Discuss calibration information, repair & maintenance trending data, trend on equipment maintenance cost and equipment downtime as well as effect of equipment downtime on the laboratory set turnaround time.
6. Quality of Subcontractors: Subcontractor/suppliers performance, quality related subcontractor problems and actions, subcontractor trends.
7. Customer Complaints: Review results of audits, customer feedback service, summary of user satisfaction surveys, complaints for trending of feedback, issues and resulting actions.
8. Corrective and Preventive Actions: Status of previous preventive, corrective and improvement actions. Current type & source of corrective issues, areas most commonly having issues, trends of root causes, reoccurring problems and corrective improvement actions.
9. Internal Auditing of Quality management system: Discussion of internal audit results, audit schedule and non-conformances by units.
10. Quality Planning: Discussion on upcoming projects, status of ongoing projects, significant changes including staffing and staff morale boosting implementations.

11. Resources: Review major changes in organization, management, resource (staff, facility, and equipment) or process.

12. Improvement: Review of quality policy, quality objectives and overall quality system effectiveness and improvement of system and product.

13. Contribution to patient care: Discuss indicators that monitor the laboratory's contributions to patient care.

14. Date and Time of Next Meeting. The date and time for the next meeting should be fixed before the end of every management review meeting. The Quality Assurance Manager will produce documentation (including analyses, reviews, proposals, etc.) for circulation to participants before the next meeting. The content of the meetings will be formally documented and recorded by the Quality Assurance Manager. These records will be made available to External Assessors.

Other topics may be added as appropriate depending on the nature and scope of the laboratory. There may be some slight variations between laboratories (equipments or subcontracting used). Although there is no specific requirement for frequency of management review meetings, quarterly meetings are however most often recommended. This allows an organization to stay on top of upcoming issues and yet collect data between meetings that are meaningful. The disadvantage of annual meetings is that management may not be able to prevent issues or resolves issues in a timely manner. It is extremely important for management to try and keep good, detailed records of what was discussed, what conclusions were reached and what actions are needed. If meetings are set around an organization quality objectives, then for each topic at the meeting the following questions should be asked objectively:

1. What is our measurement?
2. What are our objectives?
3. How are we doing?
4. Are there any trends?
5. Is there any action needed? (e.g. people, process, materials, equipment)
6. Is there anything else we should consider?

These objective actions arrived at during management review meeting can help prompt laboratory management to ensure that actions are discharged within appropriate and agreed timescale. Management Review Meetings are designed to ensure that all quality -related functions are reviewed at the highest possible level so that all levels of management affecting quality are made aware of changes, updates revisions, verification activities and policies. Management review meetings allow for the coordination and Planning of changes in order to provide a continuously improving user requirement focused service and to maximize the productivity of persons involved in the planning, coordinating and implementation of "quality" changes.

40. Standard Operating Procedure

An SOP is a written document or instruction detailing all steps and activities of a process or procedure. ISO 9001 essentially requires the documentation of all procedures used in any manufacturing process that could affect the quality of the product. The aim is to ensure that a trained staff can perform task to achieve consistently the desire outcome. It should have a named author and must be validated by a second party, approved by the responsible manage and have information on date issued and statement that photocopied version is not controlled. It should be uniquely identified (document control number) and reviewed regularly. It is a useful tool in the training of new staff. All staff performing the task spelt in the SOP must sign the SOP as an attestation that they have read, have been trained on the SOP and are committed to work consistently following the SOP. The development and use of SOPs are an integral part of a successful quality system as it provides individuals with the information to perform a job properly, and facilitates consistency in the quality and integrity of a product or end-result. In addition, the best written SOPs will fail if they are not followed. Therefore, the use of SOPs needs to be reviewed and re-enforced by management, preferably the direct supervisor. Current copies of the SOPs also need to be readily accessible for reference in the work areas of those individuals actually performing the task, either in hard copy or electronic format, otherwise SOPs serve little purpose. The development and use of SOPs minimizes variation and promotes quality through consistent implementation of a process or procedure within the organization, even if there are temporary or permanent personnel changes. SOPs should be written in a concise, step-by-step, easy-to-read format. The information presented should be unambiguous and not overly complicated. SOPs need to remain current to be useful. Therefore, whenever procedures are changed, SOPs should be updated and re-approved. If desired, modify only the pertinent section of an SOP and indicate the change date/revision number for that section in the Table of Contents and the document control notation. SOPs should be also systematically reviewed on a periodic basis, e.g. every 1-2 years, to ensure that the policies and procedures remain current and appropriate, or to determine whether the SOPs are even needed. Each organization should develop a numbering system to systematically identify and label their SOPs, and the document control should be described in its Quality Management Plan. An SOP should include the following sections:

1. The first page or cover page of each SOP should contain the following information: a title that clearly identifies the activity or procedure, an SOP identification (ID) number, date of issue and/or revision, the name of the applicable agency, division, and/or branch to which this SOP applies, and the signatures and signature dates of those individuals who prepared and approved the SOP.

2. A table of Contents may be needed for quick reference, especially if the SOP is long, for locating information and to denote changes or revisions made only to certain sections of an SOP.

3. Well-written SOPs should first briefly describe the purpose of the process, including any regulatory information or standards that are appropriate to the SOP process, and the scope to indicate what is covered. Define any specialized or unusual terms.

4. Denote what sequential procedures should be followed, divided into significant sections; possible interferences, equipment needed as well as state cautions (indicating activities that could result in equipment damage, degradation of sample, or possible invalidation of results; listed here and at the critical steps in the procedure).

5. Procedure (identifying all pertinent steps, in order, and the materials needed to accomplish the procedure such as; Instrument or method calibration and standardization, Sample Collection, Sample handling and preservation, Sample preparation and analysis (such as extraction, digestion, analysis, identification, and counting procedures), troubleshooting, data acquisition, calculations and data entering requirements, data and records management, identifying any calculations to be performed, forms to be used, reports to be written and data and record storage information).

6. State the personnel qualifications/responsibilities (denoting the minimal experience the user should have to complete the task satisfactorily, and citing any applicable requirements (certification).

7. Health & Safety Warnings (indicating operations that could result in personal injury or loss of life and explaining what will happen if the procedure is not followed or is followed incorrectly; listed here and at the critical steps in the procedure). Safety considerations (Risk assessments and hazard identification (Control of Substances Hazardous to Health (COSHH) and Material Safety Data Sheet (MSDS) and manual handling-related risk) must be taken into consideration.

8. Result reporting, reference ranges, calculations, clinical interpretations and interferences (describing any component of the process that may interfere with the accuracy of the result or outcome).

9. Information on risk assessment associated with the procedure, identification of hazards associated and manual handling –related issues.

10. Describe next all appropriate QA and quality control (QC) activities for that procedure.

11. List any cited or significant references and a signature section

Equipment validation, calibration and new reagent testing. All newly procured equipment and instruments as well as new reagents being introduced and new reagent batches are subjected to a documented validation and testing (acceptance process) to demonstrate they perform as specified by the manufacturers and that they are suitable for intended use. It is important that a laboratory has a process to regularly monitor the performance of automated equipment and reagents. There should also be a process of how to manage equipment and reagent failure and what needs to be done before such reagents is put back in use.

Maintenance of all cold chain and mechanical equipments

All the cold chain equipment should be regularly inspected recorded of the performance including the alarms. Calibrate, if required and temperature to be recorded at periodic intervals. The important equipment is:

1. Blood Bank Refrigerators.
2. Deep Freezers. -40 & -80 deg C.
3. Refrigerated Centrifuge
4. Weighing Balance.
5. Electronic Sealers
6. Thawing Bath
7. Desk Centrifuges & Cell Washers.
8. Cell Separators.

Requirement and maintenance of records - record keeping. Keeping clear and accurate records is vital in transfusion. Remember the slogan in laboratory documentation is: If it is not documented then it was not done. The Following Registers should be maintained; ABO grouping and Rh typing register, blood collection register, preparation of stock of various components register, issue register for various components supplied, screening tests of blood donors for TTI'S register, compatibility register, stock register for all materials purchased, stocked and issued, transfusion requests received from clinicians, register for disposal of infected and contaminated materials, inspection record register for all Instruments, register for cold chain management of blood products and register for error detection and rectification. Clear and accurate records keeping will contribute to the success of diagnostic service delivery in the following ways:

1. Saves a lot of time and effort when in carrying out quality audit.
2. Keeps a good track of the costs of staff and their performance.
3. Allow for evidenced based decision when tendering for new equipment.

4. Highlights quickly areas where problems could arise and enable remedies to be put in place.

5. Fulfils statutory obligations and compliance.

6. Assists in effective investigation of incidents, adverse events and near misses.

7. Assists in providing information required by your bankers.

8. Helps in detecting non compliance to process.

9. Provides valuable information and details for the future decision of staffing levels.

10. May be required in case of litigation to prove a legal point.

Document Control. All blood transfusion records including compatibility slips, equipment monitoring records, quality control records and other associated are expected to be stored by law in a secured location un-tampered. In most developed countries these records are stored for up to 30 years. The aim is that if a ligation case arises as a result of the product transfused in the past, the records can be called for and analyzed to rule out liability. Blood transfusion service should develop and maintain documents that demonstrate the achievement of specified quality standards. Documentation provides' ability to trace prospectively and retrospectively all the steps in a procedure which are necessary for monitoring the techniques, component preparation and laboratory testing.

Quality Monitoring. A regular quality monitoring is essential to ensure that a full quality assurance system has been implemented and is effective. The purpose of a quality monitoring is to check the integrity of the QA programme. If during quality monitoring, problems are identified they must be resolved as soon as possible. A follow-up audit is required later to ensure that changes have actually been incorporated. A sequence of events can be followed from collection of a unit, passing through all the processes till it is issued, by checking all the necessary documentation. For example, during donor screening for HIV, data other than just the final screening results must be recorded:

1. Temperature monitoring record for the laboratory equipments (incubator, refrigerators used for storing kits, reagents, water baths and others).

2. Records of maintenance of equipment e.g. centrifuges, incubators, refrigerators, ELISA reader and others).

3. The results obtained should be reviewed in light of the test run validity and the control values.

4. Records of disposal of any positive donation.

Quality monitoring. The following quality monitoring should be carried out; monitoring of the results obtained, monitoring of the control values, monitoring of operation of the equipment, routine monitoring and calibrations of equipment (incubator, pipettes, centrifuges, platelet storage chamber, plasma thawer and others). Quality Control of Reagents. All reagents must be quality controlled before use in the analysis of a patient sample. The primary objective of a reagent quality control is to ensure that reagent is functioning as expected. The following principles apply to storage of reagents; The oldest reagents should be used first (first-in-first-out), there should be a system for indicating when supplies run low (effective stock control management), every new lot of reagents should be evaluated for potency and specificity. All the results should be recorded and a low potency, contaminated or defective reagent should never be used.

Reagent requirements

1. All reagents should be clearly labelled with batch number, expiry date and storage temp; instructions for use should be enclosed with each reagent packing.
2. All reagents and kit should be used according to the manufacturer's instructions.
3. Use of positive and negative controls should be done with each batch to show that reagents are potent and specific.
4. All reagents must be carefully stored at recommended temperature. Reagents to be kept at 4-8oC should never be frozen and are stored according to manufacturer's instructions only.
5. All reagents must be of high quality and have a shelf-life of at least one year.
6. Supply, storage and transportation of kits and reagents should be strictly standardized and manufacturer's instructions should be followed with ensured continuous power supply and periodic temperature monitoring.
7. All the reconstituted reagents should be stored and reused according to manufacturer's instructions.
8. If a reagent produces results outside the limits set by the manufacturer, the deficiency should be reported to the manufacturer.
9. Reagent records should include: The name of each reagent with lot number, batch number, expiry date and name of manufacturer and grade and strength of reactions.
10. Reagents that are out of date must never be used for patient testing.

Identification of Errors & Remedial Action. Each error must be analysed to assess the cause of error and should be properly documented. The major sources of errors are:

1. Clerical errors usually occur due to carelessness or during transcription of records.
2. Organizational errors may occur due to heavy workload or personal difficulties of staff members.
3. Technical errors may be caused due to human factors or by poorly standardized techniques, reagents or equipment.
4. Error can also occur if staff performing task has not been adequately trained.
5. Investigations would often reveal a breakdown in quality assurance system and remedial action should be taken for each error detected. Remedial action requires:
6. Investigation of the error
7. Reassessment of procedure, quality control, reagents and consumables and full documentation.
8. Conclusion and recommendation
9. Reporting and action to be taken

Role of Training and Personnel Proficiency Testing. Adequate and competent staffs are the backbone of a quality laboratory. Most of the failures in quality are caused by human error, carelessness or ignorance and not by defective technology. Usually the techniques are validated and well documented but staff validation is often ignored. As human factors are the most important variables in any procedure, training of staff and evaluation of training is of particular importance. Training must be well-planned, relevant and on-going. The training protocol should be constantly assessed and updated when required. All new staff members should be oriented to the workplace and adequately trained based on the SOP. All the staff members should be encouraged to enrol in a Continuous Professional Development (CPD) scheme and have regular in service update training and must be encouraged to attend formal courses, seminars, conferences to update their knowledge. All the personnel carrying out the test should follow the standard operating procedures. Periodic checking and review of results is another important step in a well-implemented quality assurance programme. The technical staff should be trained to carry out the test with prescribed quality control measures. The accuracy and precision of the work done by each Biomedical Scientist should be validated periodically. The external quality assurance samples will also help in performance evaluation.

41. Incident Reporting Procedure in Transfusion

Reducing mishaps from medical management is central to efforts to improve quality and lower costs in health care. Effective feedback from incident reporting systems in healthcare is essential if organizations are to learn from failures in the delivery of care. Risk rating of transfusion incidents (Severity) can either be; None, Minor, Moderate, Major or Catastrophic. The likelihood of a transfusion incident occurring can either be; rarely, unlikely, possible, likely or almost certain. All transfusion incidents, near misses and complaints must be investigated. Clinical Pathology Accreditation (CPA) standards, Blood Quality and Safety Regulations (2005) both of the UK and the MLSCN of Nigeria requires that all incidents in transfusion be investigated and reported in a timely fashion to obtain accurate data, ensure optimum learning outcome and to avoid subsequent occurrence of the incident. The aim and objectives of incident reporting includes:

1. To ensure that all incidents relating to quality and safety of blood transfusion are recorded promptly and appropriately in accordance with statutory regulation, principles of Good Laboratory Practice (GLP) and Good Manufacturing Practice (GMP).
2. To instill the culture of corrective and preventive action to prevent the re-occurrence of incident.
3. It ensures that accurate recored of incident is available in case of audit and investigation.
4. To facilitate the reporting of incidents to statutory authority like the MLSCN.

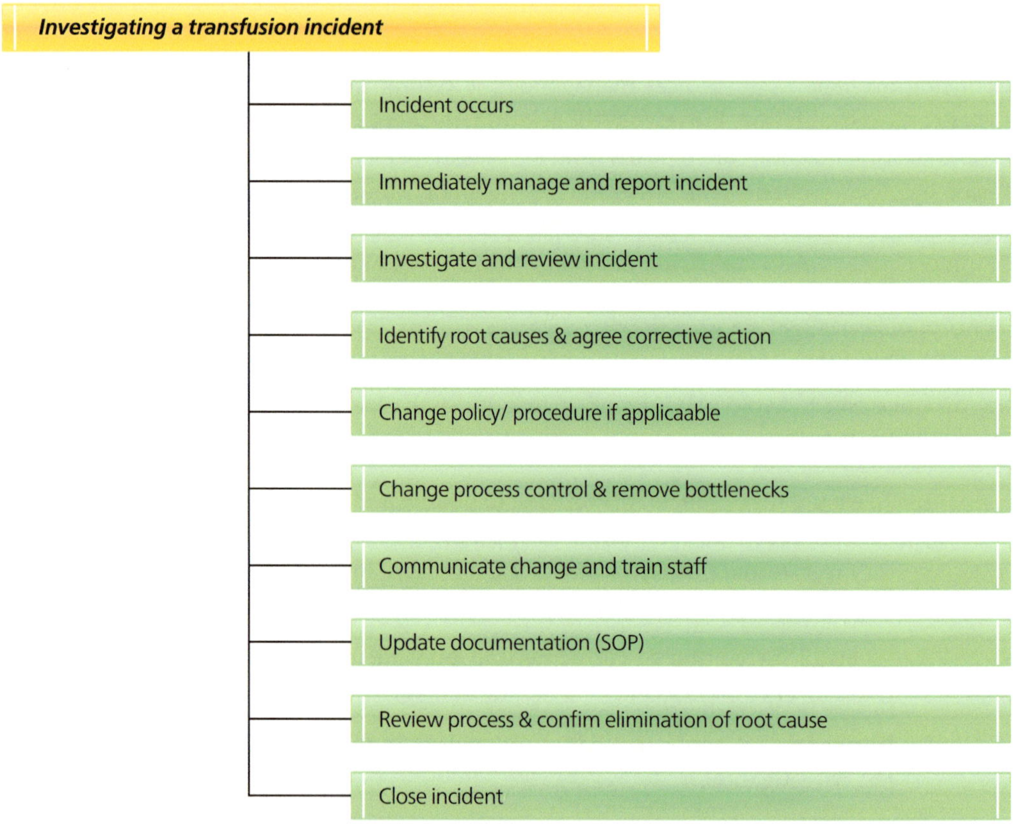

Method of investigating a transfusion incident

1. Gather all relevant document related to the incident. This may include documents like patient name, hospital number, date of birth, gender, request forms, compatibility slips, witness statements, root cause analysis information, telephone request documentation, computer records, transport records and temperature records of blood fridges.

2. Open an incident/non conformance file with relevant information of the date file opened, date of incident, nature of clinical incident (safety, quality or non conformance).

3. Collect information on immediate root cause analysis carried out after the incident, note the remedial action taken, the preventive active and corrective action taken to resolve the incident and prevent a re-occurrence of the incidents.

4. Investigate the incident based on information available determine the risk of incident to patient, likelihood of it re-occurring, non- conformances, root causes, the preventive and corrective action the laboratory

should put in place to prevent a re-occurrence of incident and a set a date to re-audit the process to ensure that the root causes has been dealt with.

Examples of Laboratory non-conformances

1. Equipment and calibration failure
2. Quality control failure
3. Manufacturers-associated reagent failure
4. Sub-optimal cold chain-related issues
5. Equipment downtime reated issues
6. Deviation from Standard Operating Procedure (SOP) with adverse outcome
7. Deviation from Standard Operating Procedure (SOP) with no adverse outcome
8. Customer complain about quality and safety of blood and blood products
9. External Quality Assessment failure or error
10. Any non-conformances identified in routine audits carried out in the laboratory.
11. Presence in the laboratory inventory of time expired reagents.

Examples of clinical incidents in Transfusion

1. Laboratory testing error.
2. Transfusion sample identification error.
3. Relevant blood transfusion documentation not signed.
4. Traceability –related issues related to non-returns of relevant transfusion documentation.
5. Inappriopriate transfusion or non-indicated transfusion.
6. Incorrect blood component transfused
7. Blood component wastage. Blood component (fresh frozen plasma, cryo-precipitate or platelet) ordered but not used and eventually wasted.
8. Blood component wastage due to negligent non observance of cold chain management requirement.

9. Blood transfusion reaction and other transfusion-related adverse events.

10. Blood administration errors

11. Issue of wrong component/specification (for example Kell positive unit given to woman of child bearing age, CMV positive unit transfused to HIV or immunocompromised patient and transfusion of non-irradiated blood and blood product for patient in whom it is indicated (patient on purine analogue chemotherapy and patient who are potential candidates for transplant).

12. Poor/inappriopriate component storage issues such as storage of platelet in the fridge and transfusion of units that has been out of cold storage for greater than 30 minutes.

13. Blood component quality problems such as bacterial contamination of blood products.

Example of an incident Investigation (Novo 7) to patient (X) **Incident: Issue of time expired product**

Investigator's name: Erhabor Osaro **Date of Incident: 3rd April 2010**

Give brief information of incident. On the 3rd day of April 2010 a time expired unit of batch product (NOVO 7) was mistakenly issued on a patient in HDU who had post partum haemorrhage and had continued to bleed even after the issue of several units of red cells, adult dose of fresh frozen plasma (FFP) and two units of platelet. The Novo 7 had been requested by the consultant to facilitate the immediate arrest of the life threatening haemorrhage. The discovery that the said batch product expired 4 months ago had been noted by the doctors and nursing staff during the pre- product administration checks by the patient bed side. The reconstitution fluid was however in date.

State the reasons for identifying this learning. I had identified this learning (incident) with the aim of carrying out a full investigation of the incident with the hope of determining the root causes, suggesting corrective and preventive measures to prevent the root causes, instigating policy and procedural changes and to enhance our drive as a department for continuous quality improvement.

Describe the root causes of this incident.

1. Poor inventory/stock control management of batch product (Novo 7).

2. Inadequate pre and post product allocation checks before issue of batch product.

3. Absence of SOP on inventory control management of batch products stipulating minimum, maximum and re-order level as well as lead time

between order and product availability for use. An SOP is a written document / instruction detailing all steps and activities of a process or procedure. These should be carried out without any deviation or modification to guarantee the expected outcome. Any modification or deviation from a given SOP should be thoroughly investigated and outcomes of the investigation documented according the internal deviation procedure. All quality impacting processes and procedures should be laid out in Standard Operating Procedures (SOPs). These SOPs should be the basis for the routine training program of each employee. SOPs should be available, followed strictly in laboratory analysis and regularly updated to assure compliance to CPA Standard F (Examination process) and sub standard F2 (Examination procedures) requirements. Changes of SOPs are in general triggered by process or procedural changes / adjustments.

Describe the immediate remedial action taken to prevent harm to patient:

1. Removed all remaining time expired Novo 7 out from stock to prevent re-occurrence of incident.
2. Rang the transfusion manager on call for advice.
3. Conveyed advice of consultant Haematologist to consultant managing the said patient in the high dependency unit.
4. On advise of the consultant Haematologist, requested an in date unit of the batch product from the nearest sister Hospital.

Non-compliances identified:

1. Issue of time expired batch product. This observation constitutes a non-compliance to CPA Standard D (Equipment, information system and materials) and sub standard D3 (Management of reagents, calibration and quality control).
2. Absence of SOP on inventory control management of batch products. This observation constitutes a non- compliance to CPA Standard F (Examination process) and sub standard F2 (Examination procedures).
3. Inadequate pre and post product allocation checks before issue of batch product. This observation constitutes a non- compliance to CPA Standard F (Examination process) and sub standard F2 (Examination procedure).

Describe the corrective and preventive action that could be taken to eliminate root cause.

1. Devise a more effective inventory /stock control system for batch products.

2. Draw up a standard operating procedure inventory /stock control system for batch products.

3. Train all employees carrying out the specific activity on the SOP and get them to sign the SOP as an attestation that they are aware of the presence of a standard procedure for the task and that they will continue to carry out the task based on the Standard operating procedure.

4. Re-iterate in the continuous improvement meetings held every morning the need to do a pre and post batch product allocation checks before despatching products to the wards or satellite fridges.

5. State the steps that should be taken to implement the corrective actions arising from this investigation and how lessons learnt from this incident enhanced the department quest for continuous improvement?

6. Amend SOP on issue of batch products (Novo 7) to reflect suggested change with regards to separating the batch product (Novo 7) from the diluents.

7. Communicate change to all staff performing task by way of training on new SOP.

8. Devise a more effective inventory control measure for batch products (Novo 7).

9. Draw up an SOP on inventory control management of batch products.

10. Review process in the next 3 months to ensure that the root causes has been eliminated.

42. Laboratory techniques and transfusion sample requirements

Blood banking reagents. The techniques used in blood bank involve mixing/reacting antigens, usually on red blood cells with antibodies. The environment where this reaction occurs can range in temperature from 4°C to 37°C. With the most common being room temperature for ABO and the initial Rh(D) testing and 37°C when screening and identifying other clinically significant antigen-antibody reactions. Situations for testing in the blood bank range from determination of antigens on the red cell (A or B antigens to determine a patient's ABO type and to determine the Rhesus group) to looking for particular antibodies that may cause transfusion reactions or hemolytic disease of the newborn. Depending on whether we are looking for a particular antigen or antibody will determine what reagents we are going to use. If we are looking for an antigen on a patient's red cells, we will use known antibody containing the group specific antibody that will cause agglutination of the antigens on the red cells.

If our aim is to detect the presence of antibody in the plasma or serum, we react the plasma/ serum against red cell panel containing known antigen to facillitae the identification of the corresponding antibody in the plasma. This reaction is based on the principle that antigen and antibody reaction are specific.

Sources of Antigen Testing. In almost all blood bank techniques we have red cells with antigens present. These red cells may either be reagent red cells with known antigens, patient red cells, or donor red cells. The reagent red cells are commercially prepared and have all the red cell antigens identified. When we use red cells where the antigens have already been determined, we can identify the possible antibodies present. A1 and B cells for confirmation of the ABO type in all patients and donors other than newborn babies. Antibody screening cells are O cells that have been studied to determine the presence of a number of antigens for specific antibodies that are known to cause transfusion reactions and hemolytic disease of the newborn. The antibody screening technique is part of all compatibility tests done before blood is transfused. Some of the more common antibodies detected are anti-D, anti-E and anti-K. Antibody identification cell panel are again O cells with the specific antigens known. Usually there are between 8 and 12 different cells in a cell panel. The pattern of positive and negative reactions helps identify the antibody.

Sources of Antibody for Testing. Antibody is found in serum. If it is the patient's serum that is being tested, we do not know what antibody may be present so we are using one of the 3 types of reagent cells listed above. If the serum is commercial reagent, the specific antibody present is already known. The commercial serum reagent is referred to as antisera. Therefore, we use Anti-A antisera to determine if a patient or donor has antigen A on his red cells. If we are trying to determine if the patient is Rh + or Rh -, we will use anti-Rho (D) antisera. Table 1 is a summary of known and unknown sources of both antigens and antibodies.

Source of antigen or antibody	Source with known component	Source with unknown component
Antigen	Reagent Red Blood Cells	Patient or Donor red blood cells
Antibody	Commercial Antisera	Patient or donors plasma/serum

Table: Sources of known and unknown antigen red cells and antibody plasma/ serum reagents

Testing procedures routinely done in blood banking. In a transfusion service there are a number of procedures routinely done. They include; ABO/Rh(D) typing, antigen typing from other blood group systems such as Rh antigens other than D, Kell, Kidd, and Duffy, allontibody screening for antibodies formed to blood group antigens other than A and B, alloantibody identification to determine the specificity of the antibodies detected in the antibody screening to allow for the selection of antigen negative red cells for transfusion, crossmatch, or compatibility testing, which determines whether donor blood can probably be safely transfused to the recipient. Other procedures include determination of Direct and indirect antihuman globulin test, dtermination of feto maternal haemorrhage (FMH), issue of prophylactic anti-D to pregnant rhesus negative women or following potentially sensitising event in pregnancy.

Procedure	Purpose	Source of antigen	Source of antibody
ABO/Rh typing	Detects A, B, and D	Patient's RBC's	Commercial anti-A, anti-B, and anti-D
Antigen typing	Detects antigens of other blood group systems (examples: K, E, C, Fya, Jka)	Patient's RBC's or Donor RBC's	Commercial antisera to the specific antigens (examples: anti-K, anti-E, anti-C, anti-Fya and anti-Jka).
Antibody screening	Detects antibodies with specificity of RBC antigens	Commercial Screening Cells	Patient's serum
Antibody identification	Identifies the specificity of RBC antibodies	Commercial panel cells	Patient's serum
Compatibility testing or Crossmatch	Determines serologic compatibility between donor and patient before transfusion	Donor RBC's	Patient's serum

Summary the sources of both the antigen and antibody

Grading agglutination reactions in the blood transfusion laboratory

Grading agglutination reactions gives an indication of the relative amount of antigen or antibody present. All tubes tests should be graded. The technique used in the resuspension of the cells will affect the grading of the reaction. The correct procedure for resuspending and grading reactions includes;

1. Use lighted agglutination viewer
2. Read only one tube at a time
3. Hold tube upright
4. Position cell button so it is facing you in the mirror
5. Very gently shake the tube and observe how the cells come off the cell button

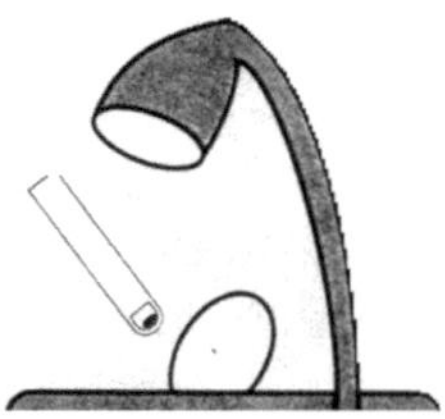

Figure : Example of lighted agglutination viewer

Grading Agglutination Reactions. Swirling off. A fine suspension indicates a negative reaction. Agglutination in chunks indicates a positive reaction. Continue shaking till all cells resuspended. Tilt tube, read and grade reaction. Solid agglutination clump is graded as 4+, several large clumps as 3+, small to medium sized clumps on a clear background as 2+, small clumps with cloudy background as 1+ and tiny aggregates with cloudy background as 0.5+. Sometimes agglutination can be observed microscopically and can either be positive upon microscopic examination or negative. Observation of small clumps amidst many unagglutinated cells is called mixed field reaction (MF). Haemolyzed reaction is indicative of a positive reaction. If no agglutination, the test is said to be negative. It is not advisable to use (-) to represent a negative reaction as it may be mis-understood. Rather it is more appriopriate to use either **Neg or 0.**

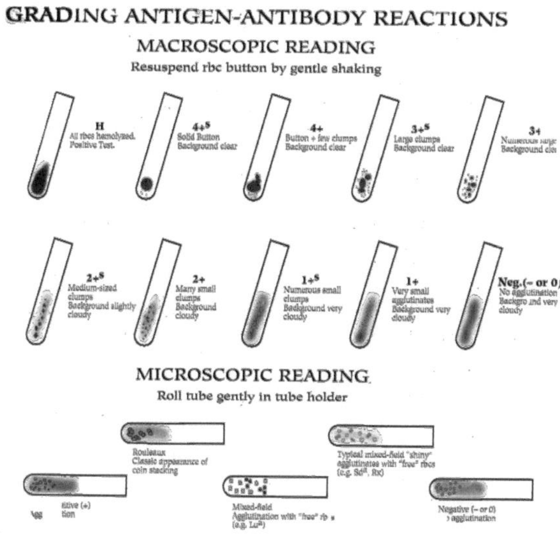

Preparation of red cells suspension. Between 2-5% cell suspension provides optimum antigen concentration for the tube method for red blood cells typing. To make sure your suspension is within this range use reagent red cells for comparison.

Washing red blood cells prior to preparing the 3% suspension. The purpose of washing the red blood cells is to remove plasma, which contains substance that may interfere with antigen-antibody reaction. The following may be in the plasma and may interfere with testing. Such substances include; soluble antigens such as A and B may be present and neutralize your reagent, interfering proteins such as Wharton's jelly that is seen in newborn cord blood, cold-acting autoimmune antibodies and increased levels of immunoglobulins that may cause either agglutination or rouleaux, haemolyzed red blood cells due to a difficult draw will interfere in your grading interpretation and fibrinogen can result in fibrin strands forming that makes grading reactions difficult.

Good technique in preparation of a 3% cell suspension involves the following

1. Place 1 to 3 drops of blood in the tube

2. Aim the tip of the saline bottle towards the center of the tube and forcibly squirt saline into the tube.

3. Fill the tube 3/4 full of saline (there will be less splattering in the centrifuge)

4. Centrifuge long enough spin to pull most of cells into a button in the bottom of the tube.

5. Decant the saline completely.

6. Shake the tube to resuspend cell button before washing the cells again. It will depend on the procedure being done as to how many types of washing are going to be done.

Sample Requirement in Blood Transfusion. Most samples for blood banking are drawn into an Ethylene Diamine Tetra Acetic Acid (red top tube). A few tests require an EDTA sample if complement is not to be activated. Serum must be tested while fresh to ensure good complement activity. Antigens on cells are stable longer (months) in a clot tube.

Patient Identification. The patient MUST be positively identified and preferably wrist banded. Some institutions use specific blood bank arm bands. Ask patient to state his/her name and date of birth. Responsible party should identify patient if he/she cannot. Verify information by comparing it to ID wrist band and ensuring that it matches what is on the request form. Resolve any differences before proceeding with the blood draw.

Labeling of Sample. The information on sample must match information on ID band, which would also need to be consistent with the order. Information on samples must be hand written (addressograph label is not allowed on a transfusion sample) must include the following; sample drawn should be 7.5 ml EDTA sample, name (last, first, middle initial) and no nicknames, unique identification number such as hospital number or medical record number or possibly social security number, ward, date and time sample drawn along with the signature or unique identifier of phlebotomist (on sample and on orders), gender and birthdate desirable but not mandatory. The date of birth provides another unique identifier along with the medical record number and full name of the patient. All unknown or unconscious patients admitted into Accident and Emergency (A&E) must be given a unique A&E identification number and an estimated date of birth until patient can be properly identified, sample labelling must be done at the patient bed side as one continuous uninterrupted process, mislabeled samples must not be accepted and all samples must be properly labeled. The following are what would warrant an improperly labeled specimen; missing information (Date of birth, hospital number, name), incorrect information (incorrectly spelt name, incorrect date of birth and incorrect hospital number), information on sample not matching information on orders, sample not signed by requesting clinician, unlabelled/ improperly labeled samples must be discarded if the problem cannot be resolved. In the case of an emergency blood drawn on a patient who is unidentified at that time can be tested but must have a unique identifier (A&E

number, estimated date of birth and name (for example Unknown Male) and blood specimen must also be discarded when both name and medical record number have changed (example: Erhabor Osaro and Hospital number 1365200 becomes Adias Teddy Charles 1423562).

Double bedside Check Procedure before transfusion. All patients to be transfused must have a wrist band. Details on the unit intended for transfusion must be checked by 2 nursing staff against the prescription and the patient medical notes. The following must be checked; surname, first name, hospital number, date of birth, blood group on the unit and patients blood group, donor number and expiry and suitability date. Finally check the wrist band to ensure that the unit is being transfused to the intended patient.

Administration of Blood component. Registered doctors, midwives, nurses and ODP's can administer blood. All transfusion must be prescribed on a transfusion record transcription. Drugs and other fluids **must not** be added to blood component or infused through the same cannula simultaneously. A blood giving set with a filter must be used to transfuse blood component. A drip giving set **must never** be used to transfuse blood component. The right sized cannula appriopriate for the size of the vein and the rate of transfusion must be used. The cannula must be flushed with 2-5ml of 0.9% saline pre and post transfusion. Red cell can be warmed prior to ensure that it attain ambient temperature to prevent hypotherma. Patient should be kept warm during the transfusion. Vital signs (temperature, blood pressure and pulse must be recorded before commencing transfusion and after the first 15 minutes of commencing transfusion, following any adverse events during transfusion and after each unit is transfused. There is no need to prime with saline before connecting the blood and there is no need to flush with saline after the residual volume is minimal. The blood giving set must be replaced after every 12 hours (after every 2-3 red cells, after a dose of FFP is given (4 units) and after 1-2 units of platelets) and when a different blood component type or fluid is being commenced. A unit of red cell must be transfused over 2-3 hours. Unit must be discarded after 4 hours. A unit of FFP or platelet is transfused over 30 minutes. If transfusion reaction is observed (mild febrile reaction with temperature < 38°C) review and give paracetamol and recommence transfusion but at a slow rate and observe. If symptom resolve, there is no need to report to transfusion laboratory. However one must be cautious if patient is neutropenic. If symptom do not resolve, stop the transfusion, report to transfusion laboratory for investigation of transfusion reaction. If urticaria, itching, wheals confirmed to the skin is observed, review patient and give piriton or hydrocortisone, slow down the transfusion and observe more frequently. If symptom do not resolve, stop the transfusion, report to transfusion laboratory for investigation of transfusion reaction. If there is severe transfusin reaction; fever >38°C with other symptoms such as rigors, flushing, restlessness, dyspnoea, headache, pain at infusion site, respiratory distress, loin and back pain, hypotension, tachycardia, haemoglobinuria, unexpected bleeding (DIC), anaphylaxis/haemolytic incompatible wrong blood incident, bacteremic shock and TRALI, the blood must be stopped, check the patient and unit ID, infuse normal saline to maintain systolic blood pressure, inform the transfusion laboratory and send reminant of unit and giving set, samples for blood culture on the patient and from sample taken from the blood bag, post transfusion blood and urine sample to enable the investigation of the transfusion reaction.

Pre-transfusion investigation of a patient's blood sample

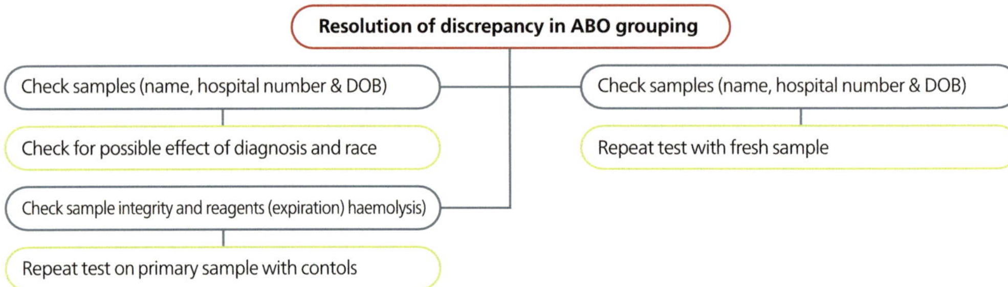

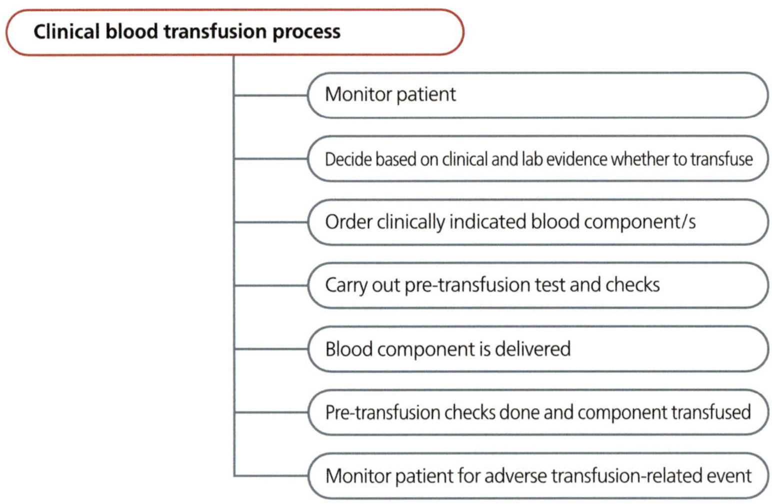

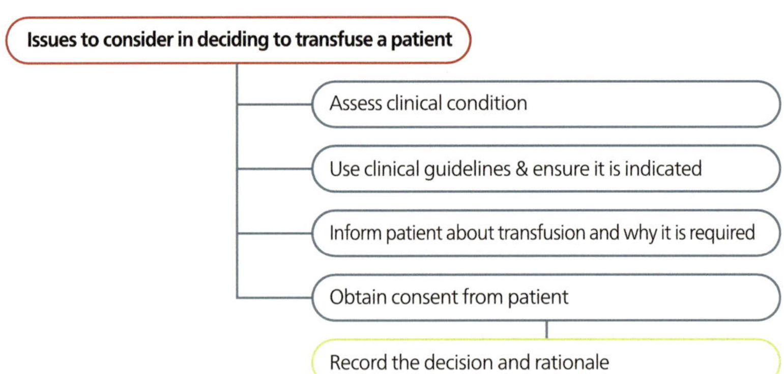

Cirical issues to remember when ordering blood component

- Identify the patient correctly
- Take blood sample and correctly label at patient bed side
- Complete the request/electronic order form correctly
- Take note of special transfusion requirements
- Send the sample and request form to the Blood Bank
- Communicate with Blood Bank if blood is required urgently

Process to consider during pretransfusion testing

- Determine patient's ABO and RhD type
- Carry out antibody screen on patient sample
- Detect clinically significant red cell antibodies
- Select and crossmatch appriopriate red cell units
- Apply compatibility label

Things to consider delivering blood component ward

- Check labelling & ensure it match patient identifiers
- Record removal of unit from storage location
- Deliver to appropriate person in clinical area
- Maintain correct storage conditions until transfusion

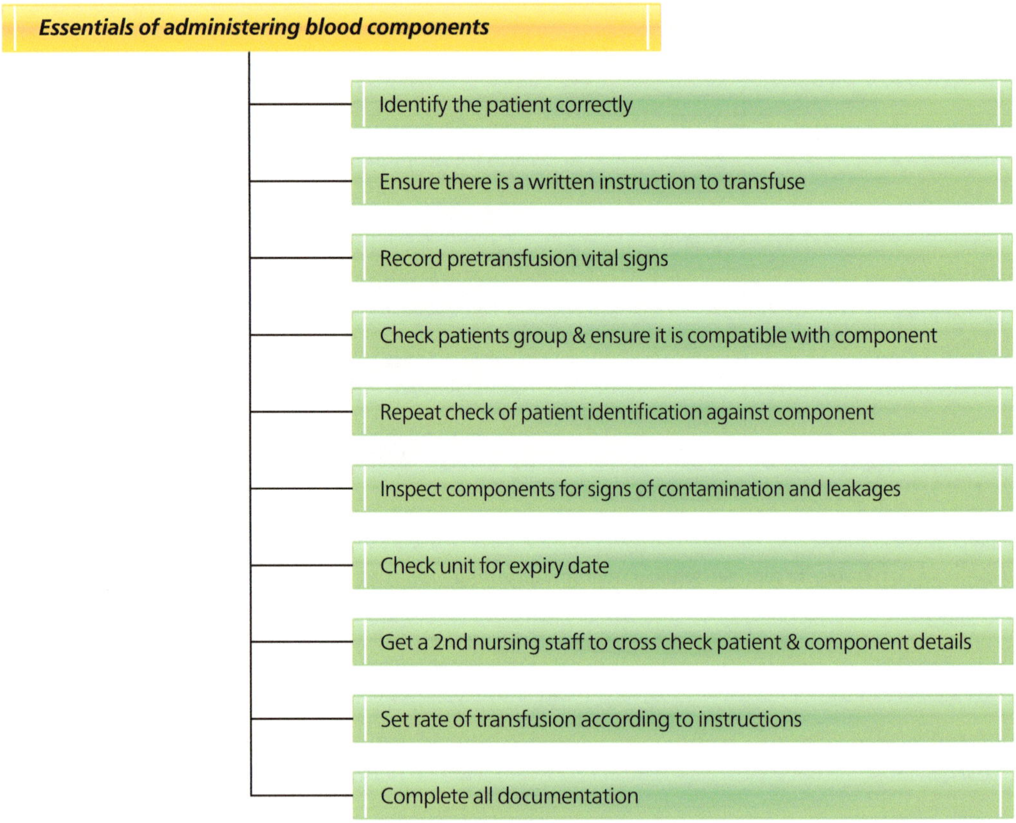

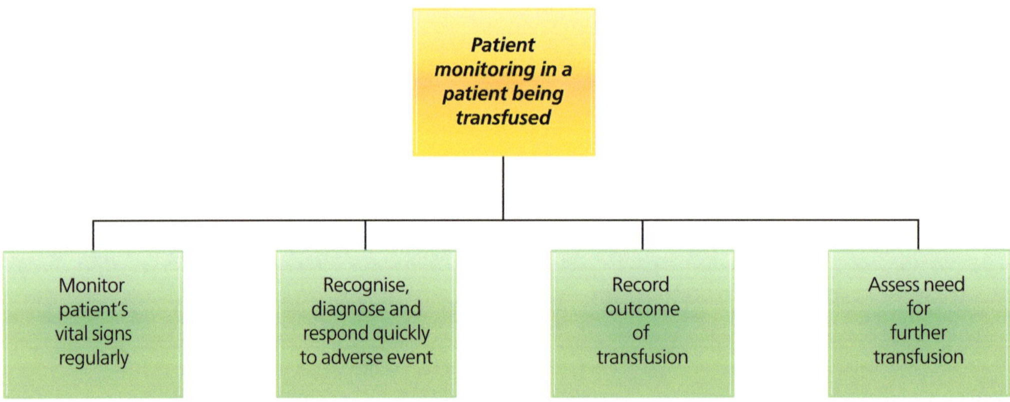

Essentials of patient monitoring transfused patient

Steps in the process	What can go wrong	Consequences to patient	Reasons why things goes wrong	Prevention and precautions
Assess clinical condition	Wrong clinical decision	Transfusion associated circulatory overload	Lack of transfusion knowledge or failure to follow guidelines	Ensure that clinical guidelines are available.
Decide if transfusion is indicated, which component and how many units to give	Unnecessary transfusion	Avoidable exposure to infection or immunological risk	Inadequate clinical Assessment	Ensure that guidiance are strictly complied with and that they are regularly audited.
Discuss with patient	Failure to give a necessary transfusion	Risk of myocardial ischemia	Unaware of importance of information and consent	Ensure that the prescriber has a thorough knowledge of the indications for blood components and the knowledge to answer Patient's questions.
Obtain consent	Patient case record lost	Patient makes complaint	No patient information Available	Written patient information is provided, at right time and is legible and understandable.
Record indication for transfusion and the discussion with patient	Wrong component given	No record available to defend medicolegal challenge	Information given at wrong time	Consent must be recorded.
	Wrong dose given		Patient couldn't read or understand information	Compliance with procedures is audited
	Patient not informed			Errors, events and reactions are investigated
	Decision not recorded			Ensures that procedures improved by lessons learned from root cause analysis of errors and near misses.

Clinical Decision toTransfuse

Steps in the process	**What can possibly go wrong**	**Consequences to the patient**	**Why things go wrong**	**Prevention/ precautionary measures**
Correctly identify the patient	Pretransfusion sample taken from the wrong patient.	Immunosuppressed patient put at risk of GVHD	Inadequate information on form.	Patient identification policy must be in place and being complied with.
Decide which component is needed and the quantity.	Failure to communicate special transfusion requirements for example CMV negative or irradiated component	Delayed haemolytic blood transfusion reaction.	Request form completed incorrectly.	Manimum data set for patient ID must be in place and being followed.
Complete blood request form.	Incorrect blood group in the patient record.	Young Rhesus negative female of child bearing age sensitized to produce immune anti-D by transfusing Rh positive unit.	Incorrect details on sample.	Prescriber must be trained on pre-transfusion sample requirement and request form.
Take pre-transfusion sample and label at patient bedside. Addressograph label is not acceptable.	Inappriopriate dose or volume requested.	Elderly patient transfused with wrong component (cryoprecipitate instead of FFP) or quantity (TACO).	Correct patient but sample tube wrongly labelled.	Prescriber must be aware of indication for particular components (CMV negative, irradiated, Kell negative units) and order component correctly.
Send blood sample and request to blood bank	Patient receives unit meant for another patient.	Fatal ABO incompatibility reaction	Sample taken from wrong patient.	Laboratory staff and transport staff 9porters) must be trained on major haemorrhage procedure.

Steps in the process	**What can possibly go wrong**	**Consequences to the patient**	**Why things go wrong**	**Prevention/ precautionary measures**
If a major haemorrhage, initiate a major haemorrhage procedure (MHP).	Failure to recongnise major haemorrhage.	Death or serious complication due to delayed transfusion.	Sample transport inappriopriate for crossmatch.	Major haemorrhage procedure must be practised periodically (drill).
	Failure to activate major haemorrhage procedure.		Ignorance of major haemorrhage procedure (MHP) and no MHP available.	Procedures must be audited regularly to ensure compliance to statutory requirement.
				All error, events, near misses and reactions must be investigated and corrective actions put in place.
				Procedures must be improved from lesion learnt from error, events, near misses and reactions.

Table: Analysis and prevention of errors in ordering blood components (Patient Sample and Request for Blood)

Steps in process	**What can go wrong**	**Consequences on patient**	**Why things go wrong**	**Prevetion/ precautions**
Note urgency of request. If in doubt confirm from requesting clinician.	Urgency misunderstood	Delayed transfusion-related risk of exsanguination.	Failure of communication	Major haemorrhage procedure should specify how urgent request are communicated.
Select appriopriate procedure for level of urgency.	Inappriopriate procedure selected.	Risk of incompatible transfusion due to mistaken identification.	Reluctance of transfusion lab to issue uncrossmatched red cells.	Blood bank must insist on correct identification and a fresh sample if necessary.
Check that patient ID on sample match what is on form and that both contains the minmum data set.	Patient sample and request form not checked. For consistency and completeness	Delayed transfusion.	Reluctance of clinical unit to transfuse uncrossmatched red cells.	Staff performing task must be trained and competency tested.

Steps in process	**What can go wrong**	**Consequences on patient**	**Why things go wrong**	**Prevetion/ precautions**
Note any specific requirement (CMV negative, irradiated units).	Requesting clinician does not specify special requirement.	Delayed haemolytic transfusion reaction due to missed alloantibody.	Staff failure to comply with SOP.	Blood bank must carry out internal qualiy control and participate in EQA programme.
Determine patient ABO, Rh group as well as antibody screen to detect presence of alloantibodies to enable the selection of antigen negative units.	Blood bank staff does not register the requirement.	Risk of GVHD.	Poor training of staff	Install effective computerised record system and train staff. There should be in place a paper back-up should the computer system fail.
Confirm that result of ABO and Rh group matches previous laboratory records.	Error in testing and recording of results		No SOP, failure by reqesting clinical staff, use of defective reagents and equipment.	Maintain apprioprate stock levels of blood component, reagents and consumables.
Select apprioprate unit and carry out compatibility testing.	Failure to check previous report or record. Failure to select apprioprate component and despatch of unit to wrong destination or using inappriopriate transport method		Inadequate records system in blood bank and suitable units not available.	
Label, record and dispatch selected units.			No SOP, failure by reqesting clinical staff, use of defective reagents and equipment.	
			Inadequate records system in blood bank and suitable units not available.	

Table: Analysis and prevention of errors in pretransfusion testing

Steps in the process	**What can go wrong**	**Consequences for the patient**	**Why things go wrong**	**Prevention/ precaution**
Pick up blood component from storage site.	Wrong unit selected	Fatal and serious haemolytic transfusion reaction.	Patient details not used to select blood unit from storage.	Staff collecting unit from fridge must go with patient ID.
Deliver blood component promptly to clinical area.	One or more patient receives an incorrect blood component.	Delayed haemolytic transfusion.	Delivery of blood to wrong location.	Staff collecting blood from fridge must be trained and competency tested.

Steps in the process	What can go wrong	Consequences for the patient	Why things go wrong	Prevention/ precaution
Blood component received in clinical araea	Delay in supplying blood	Uncorrected severe anaemia.	Clinical staff not aware that units have been delivered.	All procedures (SOP) must be documented
Blood component stored correctly until transfused.	Blood delivered to the wrong location.	Increased risk of transfusion of blood to wrong patient.	Component discarded due to inappriopriate storage.	Compliance to procedures must be audited regularly.
	Blood discarded due to incorrect storage condition.	Blood unit wasted		Errors, events, near misses must be investigated. Lessons learnt must be used as a learning process to improve procedures
	Wrong storage for example red cell placed in fridge or left in platelet storage area.	Transfusion reaction due to contaminated or thermally damaged blood		

Analysis and prevention of errors in delivering blood to the clinical area

Steps in the process	What can go wrong	Consequences for the patient	Why things go wrong	Prevention/ precaution
Check patient identity details.	Delay of transfusion	Transfusion-related sepsis	Pack not inspected.	Patient identification policy must be in place and bedside check must be observed.
Check written prescription	Contaminated pack not detected	Death due to contamination of contaminated unit.	Decolouration or change in colour of component not noticed.	Minumum data set for patient ID must be in place and observed.
Ensure IV line is in order.	Outdated pack not detected	Morbidity due to transfusion of haemolysed and outdated component.	Expired pack not identified.	Staff responsible for administering blood must be trained and competency tested.
Take baseline observation.	Patient receives incorrect component.	Death due to ABO incompatibility.	Check of patient and unit details not checked.	All Standard operating procedures must be documented and followed strictly.
Inspect contidion of unit	Component transfused too quickly.	Transfusion associated cardiac overload (TACO).	Instruction on rate of transfusion not clear and not followed.	Compliance to standard procedure must be audited regularly for compliance.

Steps in the process	**What can go wrong**	**Consequences for the patient**	**Why things go wrong**	**Prevention/ precaution**
Check expiry date.	Transfusion details not documented.	Unit not tracable.	Failure to adhere to SOP.	Errors, events, near misses must be investigated. Outcome of investigation must be used as a learning process to improve procedures.
Check and ensure that patient ID details on blood match that on the wrist band.				Computerized support system must be available.
Check and ensure that ABO and Rh D group on patient ID and component label match.				
Start transfusion at flow rate instructed.				

Table: Analysis and prevention of errors in administering blood

Steps in process	**What can go wrong**	**Consequences on patient**	**Why things go wrong**	**Prevention/precau-tions**
Observe patients vital signs and general condition	Adverse reaction not detected	Avoidable harm to patient.	Patient not monitored	Doctors and nurses responsible for trans-fusion must be trained on blood adminstra-tion and management of associated adverse events and compe-tency tested
Recongnise and re-spond appriopriately to adverse event.	Adverse reaction not managed correctly.	Delayed response to transfusion reaction.	Adverse reaction not recongnised.	Clinical guidelines must be available and being observed for the management of transfusion-related adverse events.
Record outcome of transfusion.	Delay in obtaining medical assistance.	Major morbidity or death due to transfu-sion event.	Adverse reaction not responded to apprio-priately and urgently.	Adverse reactions are investigated.

Steps in process	What can go wrong	Consequences on patient	Why things go wrong	Prevention/precautions
Assess need for further transfusion.	Delayed in assessing continued transfusion requirement.	Incomplete follow up of investigation.	Clinical help not called for.	Procedures must be improved by lessons learnt from the investigation of transfusion events.
		Incomplete transfusion records and non-compliance to legal and statutory requirement.	Clinician called fails to respond.	
			Clinician does not treat patient's reaction correctly.	

Analysis and prevention of errors in monitoring the transfused patient

43. Principle of informed consent in transfusion medicine

This topic will help transfusion practitioners understand the principles of patient confidentiality and the need for informed consent, understand the policies regarding informed consent for service users, know how to follow standard operational procedures to take and obtain informed consent, understand that it is part of their duty of care as health professional and that they are accountable for the release of information on a client or patient, understand that if patients or client's record need to be used to help student gain the knowledge and skills which they require or for research purposes, the same principle of informed consent applies. Transfusion practitioners must be able to:

1. Practice within local policy and procedures regarding patient confidentiality and informed consent.
2. Practice within national and local policies regarding informed consent.
3. Demonstrate the policies as they apply to diagnostic service users.
4. Carry out your professional duties and responsibilities appreciating the need to obtain explicit consent from a patient or client before disclosing specific information as well as understand that the client or patient can make an informed consent as to whether the information should be disclosed.
5. Carry out your professional duties and responsibilities appreciating the fact that it is the right and responsibility of every competent individual to advance his or her own welfare. This right and responsibility is exercised by freely and voluntarily consenting or refusing consent to recommended medical procedures, based on a sufficient knowledge of the benefits, burdens, and risks involved.
6. Treat with discretion the confidential information about patient or client and ensure that they are used for the purposes for which it was intended

and will not be released to unauthorised persons without their permission (consent).

7. Appreciate the fact that informed consent has legal, ethical, and clinical dimensions.

What is informed consent? A process of obtaining a patient's permission before disclosing specific information on the patient. A process of obtaining a patient's permission for a procedure after the patient and doctor have discussed the risks, benefits, and alternatives of the procedure and the patient understands them. A process by which a patient/client confirms his or her willingness to participate in a particular trial, after having been informed of all aspects of the trial that are relevant to the subject's decision to participate voluntarily in an experiment after understanding the risks involved.

What are the principles of informed consent? To trust another person with private and personal information about oneself is a significant matter. The patient or client has a right to believe that this information given in confidence will only be used for the purposes for which it was intended and will not be released to others without their permission (consent). It is impractical to obtain the consent of a patient every time you need to share information with other health professionals or staff involved in the health care of the patient or client. What is important is that the patient understands that some information may be made available to others involved in the delivery of their care. We need to obtain the explicit consent of a patient or client before we disclose specific information and it is important that the client or patient can make an informed consent as to whether the information should be disclosed.

How can disclosure of patient information occur?

1. With the consent (written or verbal) of a client or patient.

2. Without the consent of the patient or client when disclosure is required by the law or by the order of a court.

3. Without the consent of the patient when the disclosure is in the interest of public interest.

4. The public interest means the interest of an individual, or groups of individuals or of society as a whole and would cover issues such as; serious crime, child abuse, drug trafficking or other activities which places others at serious risk.

5. It is our responsibility as health professional (part of our duty of care) and we are accountable for the release of information on a client or patient. The deliberate release of patient information without their consent even in the interest of the public must be justified.

6. The organization that employs the health professions who make records are the legal owners of the records, but this does not give anyone in the organization the legal right to access or release this information to a third party without the consent of the client.

7. If patients or clients record need to be used to help student gain the knowledge and skills which they require, the same principle of informed consent applies. The person providing the training will be responsible for making sure the student understand the need for confidentiality and informed consent and the need to follow local procedures for handling and storing of records.

8. Informed consent includes being informed and giving consent. These two are closely related elements. Being informed requires offering information to potential human subjects. In any research on human beings, each potential subject must be adequately informed of the aims, methods, sources of funding, any possible conflicts of interest, institutional affiliations of the researcher, the anticipated benefits and potential risks of the study and the discomfort it may entail. Information provided by researcher should be simple and clear enough for the potential subject to understand and it is the duty of researcher to answer their questions. The subject should also be informed of the right to abstain from participation in the study or withdraw consent to participate at any time without reprisal. The principle of informed consent, aimed at the lawfulness of health assistance, tends to reflect the concept of autonomy and of decisional auto determination of the person requiring and requesting medical and/or surgical interventions. It is the right and responsibility of every competent individual to advance his or her own welfare. This right and responsibility is exercised by freely and voluntarily consenting or refusing consent to recommended medical procedures, based on a sufficient knowledge of the benefits, burdens, and risks involved. The ability to give informed consent depends on;adequate disclosure of information, patient freedom of choice, patient comprehension of information given and patient capacity for decision-making.

9. Three necessary conditions that must be satisfied in obtaining informed consent are;that the individual's decision is voluntary, that this decision is made with an appropriate understanding of the circumstances, that the patient's choice is deliberate insofar as the patient has carefully considered all of the expected benefits, burdens, risk and reasonable alternatives, legally, adequate disclosure includes information concerning the following;diagnosis, nature and purpose of treatment, risks of treatment and treatment alternatives.

Questions and answers on the principle of informed consent

Question 1: Mrs Ford came to the laboratory to have her blood taken for HIV screening. Later that morning her husband Mr Ford who is on warfarin also attends the clinic to have his blood taken for INR investigation. He enquires about whether his wife had attended clinic that morning and what the report of her HIV test was. How will you Handel this situation?

Answer 1: We need to obtain the explicit consent from a patient or client before we disclose specific information and it is important that the client or patient can make an informed consent as to whether the information should be disclosed.

Question 2: A staff nurse in Eye clinic that has no duty of care for a patient refereed from STD clinic has called the laboratory to enquire about the urine microscopy, culture and sensitivity result of her ex –partner who is suspected to have a sexually transmitted infection. How will you handle this enquiry?

Answer 2: The organization that employs the health professions who make records are the legal owners of the records, but this does not give anyone in the organization the legal right to access or release this information to a third party without the consent of the client particularly when the information accessed is not for the purpose of patient care.

Question 3: Mrs James goes to her family GP in Bolton to submit her early morning urine for pregnancy test. Later that afternoon a GP based in Wigan who has no duty of care to the patient but who introduces himself as a GP and partner of Mrs A rings to enquire about her pregnancy test result. How will you deal with such situation?

Answer 3: It is against the principles of patient confidentiality and informed consent to give confidential information on a patient to a relative clinician or healthcare worker who has no duty of care whatsoever to the patient and does not require the information for the management of the patient.

Question 4: Your brother's partner has just returned from holidays in the Caribbean. She presented to her GP with an episode of vomiting and abdominal pain. Her GP promptly referred her to the laboratory for pregnancy test. Your brother knowing you work in the laboratory in Port Harcourt Teaching Hospital rings you to enquire about his partner's laboratory results. How will you deal with this situation?

Answer 4: As healthcare workers, we are ethical bound not to disclose confidential information on patients or clients to third parties without their consent.

Question 5: A man has just been told that his son's blood group is O positive by his GP. The man however knows that his own blood group is AB positive and that his wife's blood group is O positive. He has read from the internet that a blood group AB parent cannot give birth to an O child. He rings you in the Laboratory to confirm the wife's blood group and enquire about the possibility of the child being his. How will you deal with this issue?

Answer 5: It is against the principles of patient confidentiality and informed consent to give confidential information on a patient or client to a third party without the consent of the patient. By giving such information without the consent of the wife, the husband will know that he is most likely not the putative father of the child.

Example of an informed consent form

Participant Consent Form

Study Title:

Name...

Address...

I give consent for myself / child to be a participant in this study. I have been fully informed what participation will involve and had all my questions answered. I understand that I can withdraw from this study at any time without giving reason and without penalty.

I also give consent for recordings to be made relating to my participation.

I also give consent for my personal data to be used by the research workers in any way they wish and passed to anyone they wish.

Date......................

Signed......................................

Participant

This study is approved by the hospital Research Ethics Committee

44. Stem cell transplantation

Hematopoietic stem cell transplantation (HSCT) is the transplantation of multipotent hematopoietic stem cell or blood, usually derived from either the bone marrow (BMT) or peripheral blood stem cells. In the case of a bone marrow transplant, the HSC are removed from a large bone of the donor, typically the pelvis, through a large needle that reaches the center of the bone, the technique is referred to as a bone marrow harvest and is performed under general anesthesia and Stored heparinized and the mononuclear cell count of 2-4 x 106 nucleated cells/kg is indicated). In peripheral blood stem cells transplant, the stem cells are collected using cell separator equipment. Mononuclear cells are collected (aphaeresis) after centrifugation before returning the red cells back into the patient. Stem cell content of PBSC is low and collection may be insufficient for transplantation. Prior chemotherapy (cyclophosphamide) and collection during the recovery phase. The peripheral stem cell yield is boosted a 100 times with daily subcutaneous injections of Granulocyte-colony stimulating factor, as well as treatment growth factor (at a dose of 10μg/kg/day for 4-6 days). GCFU help to mobilize stem cells from the donor's bone marrow into the peripheral circulation. Optimum yield with CD34+ cells of >2.5 X 106/kg and granulocyte-macrophage colony forming unit (CFU-GM) of 1-5 x 105/kg is considered optimal for transplantation. Other sources of stem cells include amniotic fluid and umblical cord blood. It is also possible to extract hematopoietic stem cells from amniotic fluid for both autologous and heterogonous use at the time of childbirth. Umbilical cord blood is obtained when a mother donates her infant's umbilical cord and placenta after birth. Cord blood has a higher concentration of HSC than is normally found in adult blood. However, the small quantity of blood obtained from an umbilical cord (typically about 50 mL) makes it more suitable for transplantation into small children than into adults.

History of stem cell transplant

Georges Mathé, a French oncologist, performed the first bone marrow transplant in 1959 on five Yugoslavian nuclear workers whose own marrow had been damaged by irradiation caused by a Criticality accident at the Vinča Nuclear Institute, but all of these transplants were rejected. Mathé later pioneered the use of bone marrow transplants in the treatment of leukemia. Stem cell transplantation was pioneered using bone-marrow-derived stem cells by a team at the Fred Hutchinson Cancer Research Center from the 1950s through the 1970s led by Donnall Thomas. Thomas' work showed that bone marrow cells infused intravenously could repopulate the bone marrow and produce new blood cells. The first physician to perform a successful human bone marrow transplant on a disease other than cancer was Robert A. Good at the University of Minnesota in 1968. Hematopoietic stem cell transplantation remains a risky procedure with many possible complications. It has traditionally been reserved for patients with life-threatening diseases. While it remains a procedure involving a high degree of risk, one must keep in mind that many disorders (mainly acute leukemias and neoplastic lymphoproliferative disorders) treated by this procedure. Stem cell transplantation is a medical procedure in the fields of hematology and oncology, most often performed for people with diseases of the blood, bone marrow, or certain cancers. It involves; elimination of a patient immune system using chemotherapy and or radiotherapy and replacement with patient stem cells previously harvested prior to chemotherapy or radiotherapy (autologous) or stem cells from another donor (allogeneic) or from an HLA -matched identical twin (syngeneic). Haemopoietic stem cells are indiated in the following disease conditions.

1. Non malignant disorders such as myelodysplastic syndrome, multiple myeloma and lymphoma.

2. Pediatric cases where the patient has an inborn defect such as severe combined immunodeficiency or congenital neutropenia with defective stem cells.

3. Leukemia (ALL, AML, CML and CLL) patients who would not benefit from prolonged treatment with or are already resistant to chemotherapy.

4. Children or adults with aplastic anemia who have lost their stem cells after birth including Fanconi's anaemia.

5. Inherited disorders such as sickle-cell disease, thalassaemia, immune deficiencies, inborn errors of metabolism.

6. Severe autoimmune disorders.

7. Neuroblastoma (Neuroblastoma is the most common extracranial solid cancer in childhood and the most common cancer in infancy. It is a neuroendocrine tumor, arising from any neural crest element of the sympathetic nervous system or SNS. It most frequently originates in one of the adrenal glands, but can also develop in nerve tissues in the neck, chest, abdomen, or pelvis).

8. Ewing's Sarcoma (A malignant round-cell tumour. It is a rare disease in which cancer cells are found in the bone or in soft tissue. The most common areas in which it occurs are the pelvis, the femur, the humerus, the ribs and clavicle.

9. Amyloidosis (A conditions in which amyloid proteins are abnormally deposited in organs and/or tissues. There are numerous symptoms that are associated with this disease. The most common ones have to do with the heart, such as heart failure, arrhythmia, and an irregular heartbeat. Also the respiratory tract can be affected and cause hemoptysis. Usually the spleen enlarges and sometimes ruptures. The gastrointestinal tract is usually affected and causes vomiting, hemorrhaging and diarrhea. The amyloidosis can also affect the motor functions and cause polyneuropathy. When the amyloid fibrils and oligomers get to the skin they can cause skin lesions and petechiae. One of the most famous symptoms is macroglossia.

10. Acquired severe marrow diseases (paroxysmal nocturnal haemoglobinuria, red cell aplasia and myelofibrosis).

11. Desmoplastic small round cell tumor.

12. Chronic granulomatous disease.

13. Hodgkin's disease.

Graft types

Autologous. In autologous HSCT patient is given a high dose of chemotherapy with or without radiotherapy with the intention of eradicating the patient's malignant cell population at the cost of partial or complete bone marrow ablation (destruction of patient's bone marrow function to grow new blood cells). Stem cells are extracted (aphaeresis) from the patient and stored frozen. The patient's own stored stem cells are then returned to his/her body, where they replace destroyed tissue and resume the patient's normal blood cell production. Autologous transplants have several advantages over alogenic transplant; lower risk of infection during the immune-compromised portion of the treatment, the recovery of immune function is rapid, the incidence of patients experiencing rejection (graft-versus-host disease) is very rare due to the donor and recipient being the same individual, graft versus host disease (GVHD) is not a challenge and the procedure-related mortality is low (<5%). These advantages have established autologous HSCT as one of the standard second-line treatments for such diseases as lymphoma. A limitation of this procedure is the risk of tumour cells contaminating the stem cell harvest.

Allogeneic. Allogeneic HSCT involves two people: the (healthy) donor and the (patient) recipient. Allogeneic HSC donors must have a tissue (HLA) type that matches the recipient. Matching is performed on the basis of variability at three or more loci of the HLA gene, and a perfect match at these loci is preferred. Even if there is a good match at these critical alleles, the recipient will require immunosuppressive medications to mitigate graft-versus-host disease. About 25 to 30 percent of allogeneic HSCT recipients have an HLA-identical sibling. Even so-called "perfect matches" may have mismatched minor alleles that contribute to graft-versus-host disease. Allogeneic transplant donors may be related (usually a closely HLA matched sibling), syngeneic (a monozygotic or 'identical' twin of the patient - necessarily extremely rare since few patients have an identical twin. Unrelated donors may be found through a registry of bone marrow donors such as the National Marrow Donor Program. Allogeneic transplants are also performed using umbilical cord blood as the source of stem cells. Transplanting healthy stem cells to the recipient's immune system, allogeneic HSCTs appear to improve chances for cure or long-term remission once the immediate transplant-related complications are resolved. The short arm of chromosome 6 contains a cluster of genes known as the Major Histocompatibility Complex (MHC) or the HLA region. These genes encode the HLA antigens and molecules like complement components, tumuor necrosis factor (TNF) and antigens related to antigen processing. A compatible donor is found by doing additional HLA-testing from the blood of potential donors. The HLA genes fall in two categories (type I and type II). In general, mismatches of the type-I genes (i.e. HLA-A, HLA-B, or HLA-C) increase the risk of graft rejection and are present in CD8+ cells. HLA-type 11 is present in CD4+ T-cells. A mismatch of an HLA type II gene (i.e. HLA-DR, or HLA-DQB1) increases the risk of graft-versus-host disease. In addition a genetic mismatch as small as a single DNA base pair is significant so perfect matches require knowledge of the exact DNA sequence of these genes for both donor and recipient. Leading transplant centers currently perform testing for all five of these HLA genes before declaring that a donor and recipient are HLA-identical. HLA typing is carried out either by serological technique using antibodies that are specific for individual HLA alleles or by molecular testing using PCR sequence-specific primers. The advantage of this procedure is associated graft versus leukemia (GVL). Mortality from allogeneic stem cell transplantation is higher for the following reasons; immunological incompatibility between donors and recipients despite HLA matching and immunological incompatibility - related immunodeficiency, GVHD and graft failure.

Allogeneic or syngeneic	Autologous
Acute lymphoblastic and myeloid leukaemia	Amyloidosis
Chronic myeloid leukaemia	Severe autoimmune disorders
Severe aplastic anaemia including Fanconi, s anaemia	Acute and chronic leukaemia
Haemoglobinopathies (thalasaemia and sickle cell disease)	Multiple myeloma
Inborn errors of metabolism in the haemopoietic and mesenchymal system such as osteopetrosis.	Hodgkins and non-Hodgkins lymphoma
Acquired marrow syndrome (aplastic anaemia, myelofibrosis, paroxysmal nocturnal haemoglobinuria)	
Malignant disorders (myelodysplasia, multiple myeloma, chronic lymphocytic leukaemia and lymphoma)	

Stem cell transplant indications

Storage of HSC. HSC because the cells must be harvested from the recipient months in advance of the transplant treatment. Bone marrow cells can be frozen (cryopreserved) for prolonged periods, without damaging too many cells. In the case of allogeneic transplants, fresh HSC are preferred, in order to avoid cell loss that might occur during the freezing and thawing process. Allogeneic cord blood is stored frozen at a cord blood bank because it is only obtainable at the time of childbirth. To cryopreserve HSC, a preservative called Dimethyl sulfoxide (DMSO) (DMSO has been used as a cryoprotectant and is still an important constituent of cryoprotectant vitrification mixtures used to preserve organs, tissues, and cell suspensions. Without it, up to 90% of frozen cells will become inactive. In a controlled-rate freezer DMSO prevent osmotic cellular injury during ice crystal formation. HSC may be stored for years in a cryofreezer, which typically utilizes liquid nitrogen.

Stem cell processing. After harvesting of HSC, it is processed (red cells are removed, the mononuclear cells are concentrated, autologous collections are purged by chemotherapy or antibody treatment to remove residual malignant cells and T-cells to reduce incidence of GVHD).

Conditioning. Prior to infusing stem cells into a patient, conditioning (chemotherapy and total body irradiation (TBI) is carried out. The aim of this is to; eradicate patient's haemopoietic and immune system, eradicate residual malignancy and to suppresses in case of allogeneic stem cell transplant the host immune system to prevent rejection of transplanted foreign stem cells.

Myeloablative transplants and non-myeloablative transplants. The chemotherapy or irradiation given immediately prior to a transplant is called the conditioning or preparative regimen, the purpose of which is to help eradicate the patient's disease prior to the infusion of

HSC and to suppress immune reactions. In recent years there has been a shift from the use of myeloablative to non-myeloablative conditioning regimens. Unlike myeloablative regimens, non –myeloablative agents do not completely ablate (destroy) the patient's bone marrow. TBI is used in patient with malignant disease. Drugs used include; cyclophoaphamide, bulsulphan, cytosine, arabinoside and etoposide or nitrosoureas. Stem cells are not transplanted immediately after TBI. It is preferable to allow for a period of 36hours post TBI to allow for the removal of residual chemotherapeutic agent from the patients circulation.

Myeloablative transplants. The bone marrow can be ablated with dose-levels that cause minimal injury to other tissues. In allogeneic transplants a combination of myeloablative options are available include cyclophosphamide with busulfan and total body irradiation is commonly employed. This treatment also has an immunosuppressive effect which prevents rejection of the HSC by the recipient's immune system. The post-transplant prognosis often includes acute and chronic graft-versus-host disease which may be life-threatening; however in certain leukemias this can coincide with protection against cancer relapse owing to the graft versus tumor effect.

Non-myeloablative allogeneic transplants. This is a newer treatment approach using lower doses of chemotherapy and radiation which are too low to eradicate all of the bone marrow cells of a recipient. Instead, non-myeloablative transplants run lower risks of serious infections and transplant-related mortality while relying upon the graft versus tumor effect to resist the inherent increased risk of cancer relapse. Also it requires high doses of immunosuppressive agents in the early stages of treatment; these doses are less than for conventional transplants. This leads to a state of mixed chimerism early after transplant where both recipient and donor HSC coexist in the bone marrow space. Decreasing doses of immunosuppressive therapy then allows donor T-cells to eradicate the remaining recipient HSC and to induce the graft versus tumor effect. This effect is often accompanied by mild graft-versus-host disease. Because of their gentler conditioning regimens, these transplants are associated with a lower risk of transplant-related mortality and morbidity and therefore allow patients who are considered too high-risk for conventional allogeneic HSCT to undergo potentially curative therapy for their disease. Examples of non-myeloablative regimens include; fludarabine, low dose irradiation, anti-lymphocyte globulin, low dose Busulfan and cyclophosphamide.

Engraftment. Engraftment is usually quicker with PBSC compared to BMT. Cytopenia typically occur within the first 1-3 weeks post transplant. First signs of successful engraftment include; increase in the monocyte and neutrophils followed by platelet coun, there is reticulosis, appearance of natural killer cells (NK) which are the earliest donor-derived lymphocytes to appear. G-CSF can be used to reduce the period of neutropenia, marrow cellularity gradually returns to normal but bone marrow reserve remains impaired for 1-2 years. Profound immunodeficiency persists for 3-12 months and is usually associated with low CD4 helper cells, high CD8 count and high CD8:CD4 for 6 months, after several weeks of growth in the bone marrow, expansion of HSC and their progeny is sufficient to normalize the blood cell counts and reinitiate the immune system, the offspring of donor-derived hematopoietic stem cells then populate many different organs of the recipient, including the heart, liver, and muscle and help in regenerating injured tissue in these organs and patient blood group changes to that of the donor and the antigen specific immunity becomes that of the donor in about 60 days.

Complications. HSCT is associated with a high treatment-related mortality and morbidity in the recipient (10% or higher), which limits its use to conditions that are themselves life-threatening. Major complications are: graft-versus-host disease, infection, veno-occlusive disease, mucositis, infections (sepsis), graft failureand the development of new malignancies.

Graft-versus-host disease. Graft-versus-host disease (GVHD) is an inflammatory disease caused by donor –derived immune cells (T lymphocytes) that react against recipient cells. It is an attack of the "new" bone marrow's immune cells against the recipient's tissues. Incidence is higher with increasing age of donor and recipient and in cases where there is HLA mismatch between donor and recipient. This can occur even if the donor and recipient are HLA-identical because the immune system can still recognize other differences between their tissues. Prophylaxis against GVHD usually involves use of ciclosporin (oral or intravenous) and methotrexate given to remove T cells from donor stem cell infusion. There are two types of GVHD (Acute and chronic).

Acute graft-versus-host disease. Typically occurs in the first 3 months after transplantation and may involve the skin, intestine, or the liver, and is often fatal. Skin rash typically affects the face, palms, soles, ears and sometimes the whole body. Diagnosis is usually by skin biopsy (cell necrosis in the basal layer of epidermis and lymphocyte infiltration). Diarrhoea and associated electrolyte depletion and imbalance may occur. Bilirubin and alkaline phosphatase are elevated although other hepatic enzymes may be normal. Treatment is usually by the use of high-dose corticosteroids such as prednisone. This immuno-suppressive treatment often leads to deadly infections.

Chronic graft-versus-host disease. Chronic graft-versus-host disease may also develop after 100 days following allogeneic transplant and it is the major source of late treatment-related complications. Chronic graft-versus-host disease may involve the joints, oral mucose, lacrimal glands and other serosal surfaces and often lead to the development of fibrosis, or scar tissue, similar to scleroderma. Sjogen's syndrome andlichen planus may develop. The immune system is impaired resulting in hyposlenism. Malabsorption and pulmonary abnormalities are common. Management often include use of drugs such as ciclosporin, azathioprine, mycophenolate, mofetil, thalidomide and corticosteriods.

Infection. Bone marrow transplantation usually requires that the recipient's own bone marrow be destroyed (myeloablation). Prior to engraftment patients may go for several weeks without appreciable numbers of white blood cells to help fight infection (Bacterial and fungal infection are frequent). This puts a patient at high risk of infections, sepsis and septic shock, despite prophylactic antibiotics. However, antiviral medications, such as acyclovir and valacyclovir, are quite effective in prevention of HSCT-related outbreak of herpetic infection in sero-positive patients. Use of oral antibiotics and sometimes intravenous broad-spectrum antibiotics may be commenced after blood cultures and other microbiological samples have been collected to prevent bacterial infection. Oral penicillin can be given prophylactically to reduce effects of gram negative encapsulated organisms affecting the respiratory tract. Antifungal agents such as amphotericin B and caspofungin or voriconazole, fluconazole and itraconazole may be used to prevent fungal infections such as Candida and Aspergillus species. The immunosuppressive agents employed in allogeneic transplants for the prevention or treatment of graft-versus-host disease further increase the risk of viral infections particularly herpes simplex, cytomegalovirus (CMV), varicella zoster virus (VZV). CMV is a major threat and is usually associated with potentially fatal pneumonitis, hepatitis, falling blood counts. Recipients who are CMV negative or whose CMV status is unknown must receive CMV negative donor stem cells and blood products. Immunosuppressive drugs are given for a minimum of 6-months after transplantation, or much longer if required for the treatment of graft-versus-host disease. Transplant patients lose their acquired immunity, for example immunity to childhood diseases such as measles or polio. For this reason transplant patients must be re-vaccinated with childhood vaccines once they are off immunosuppressive medications. Pneumocystis carinii pneumonitis may occur and can be prevented by prophylactic co-trimoxazole. Aciclovir may be a useful prophylaxis for varicella zoster virus infection. Epstein-Barr virus (EBV) and associated lympho-proliferative disease are rare. Haemorrhagic cystitis caused by the cyclophosphamide metabolite acrolein or adenovirus or polyomavirus can cause this complication. Mensa can help prevent this complication.

Veno-occlusive disease. Severe liver injury can result from hepatic veno-occlusive disease (VOD). Elevated levels of bilirubin (jaundice), hepatomegaly and fluid retention (ascites), weight gain and cardiac failures are clinical hallmarks of this condition. There is now a greater appreciation of the generalized cellular injury and obstruction in hepatic vein sinuses, and hepatic VOD has lately been referred to as sinusoidal obstruction syndrome (SOS). Severe cases of SOS are associated with a high mortality rate. Anticoagulants or defibrotide may be effective in reducing the severity of VOD but may also increase bleeding complications. Ursodiol has been shown to help prevent VOD, presumably by facilitating the flow of bile.

Graft failure. The risk of graft failure can occur in the following circumstances; patients with aplastic anaemia and in patients in whom T-cell depleted donor stem cells is used for transplant or as a GVHD prophylaxis. T –cell depletion of donor stem cells prevent donor T-cells form overcoming resistance from host.

Mucositis. The injury of the mucosal lining of the mouth and throat and is a common regimen-related toxicity following ablative HSCT regimens. It is usually not life-threatening but is very painful, and prevents eating and drinking. Treatment is usually with pain medications plus intravenous infusions to prevent dehydration and malnutrition.

Graft-versus-tumor effect. Graft-versus-tumor effect (GVT) or "graft versus leukemia" effect is the beneficial aspect of the Graft-versus-Host phenomenon. HSCT patients with either acute or in particular chronic graft-versus-host disease after an allogeneic transplant tend to have a lower risk of cancer relapse. This is due to a therapeutic immune reaction of the grafted donor T lymphocytes against the diseased bone marrow of the recipient. This lower rate of relapse accounts for the increased success rate of allogeneic transplants compared to transplants from identical twins, and indicates that allogeneic HSCT is a form of immunotherapy. GVT is the major benefit of transplants which do not employ the highest immuno-suppressive regimens.

Other complications

1. Oral carcinoma. Patients after HSCT are at a higher risk for oral carcinoma. Post-HSCT oral cancer may have more aggressive behavior with poorer prognosis, when compared to oral cancer in non-HSCT patients.
2. Haemolysis and microangiopathic haemolytic anaemia because of ABO blood group incompatibility between donors and recipients.
3. Relapse of original or residual disease for example acute and chronic leukaemia.
4. Delayed pulmonary complications including restrictive pneomonitis, bronchiolitis obliterans.
5. Endocrine complications including hypothyroidism particularly associated with TBI and eye problems (cataracts).
6. Autoimmune disorders including myasthenia, rheumatoid arthritis, anemia and thrombocytopenia.
7. Secondary malignancies such non-Hodgkin's lymphoma as well as CNS complications (neuropathies).
8. Growth failure associated with low growth hormone levels in children.
9. Impaired sexual development and infertility.

Blood products support following SCT. Severe pan-cytopenia is often associated with SCT in the first 1-3 weeks. Blood product support may be required in these critical moments. Red cells concentrates are given to treat anemia, platelet concentrate are given to maintain the platelet count above 10 x 10^9/L. All blood product giving post transplant **must be** irradiated (to kill any lymphocytes) and prevent GVHD.

Prognosis of SCT. Prognosis in HSCT varies widely dependent upon a number of factors; disease type, stage, stems cell source, HLA-matched status (for allogeneic HCST), and conditioning regimen. A transplant offers a chance for cure or long-term remission if; the inherent complications of graft versus host disease does not manifest, an Immuno-suppressive treatment does not produce a negative life threatening effect and if the recipient survives the spectrum of opportunistic infections. In recent years, survival rates have been gradually improving across almost all populations and sub-populations receiving transplants. Mortality for allogeneic stem cell transplantation can be estimated using the prediction model created by Sorror and colleagues using the Hematopoietic Cell Transplantation-Specific Co-morbidity Index (HCT-CI). The Hematopoietic Cell Transplantation-Specific Co-morbidity Index (HCT-CI) was developed to identify relevant comorbidities in the allogeneic stem cell transplantation population and to enable risk assessment before allogeneic transplant. Use this calculator to identify comorbidities in the allogeneic stem cell transplantation population and to enable risk assessment before allogeneic transplant using the Hematopoietic Cell Transplantation-Specific Co-morbidity Index (HCT-CI). The following co-morbidities can to a larger extent determine the success of a transplant.

Hepatic disease

- None
- Mild (chronic hepatitis, bilirubin > Upper Limit of Normal (ULN) to 1.5 x ULN, or AST/ALT > ULN to 2.5 x ULN).
- Moderate or severe (cirrhosis, bilirubin > 1.5 x ULN, or AST/ALT > 2.5 x ULN).

Pulmonary disease

- None or mild disease
- Moderate pulmonary (DLCO and/or FEV1 66% to 80% or dyspnea on slight activity).
- Severe pulmonary (DLCO and/or FEV1 = 65% or dyspnea at rest or requiring oxygen).

Other factors

- Arrhythmia (Atrial fibrillation or flutter, sick sinus syndrome, or ventricular arrhythmias).
- Inflammatory bowel disease (Crohn's or ulcerative colitis)
- Cardiac (CAD, CHD, myocardial infarction or ejection fraction = 50%).
- Inflammatory bowel disease (Crohn's or ulcerative colitis).
- Inflammatory bowel disease (Crohn's or ulcerative colitis).
- Diabetes (requiring insulin or oral hypoglycemic)
- Psychiatric disturbance (depression or anxiety requiring psychiatric consult or treatment).
- Obesity (body mass index > 35 kg/^{m2})
- Infection (requiring continuation of antimicrobial treatment after day 0.
- Cerebrovascular disease (TIA or cerebrovascular accident).
- Rheumatologic (SLE, RA, polymyositis, polymyalgia rheumatica).
- Peptic ulcer (requiring treatment)
- Moderate or severe renal failure (serum Cr > 2 mg/dL or 177 μmol/L, dialysis, or prior renal transplant).

- Prior solid tumor (excluding non-melanoma skin cancer).
- Valvular Heart Disease (except mitral valve prolapse).

45. Alkaline denaturation test

The alkaline denaturation test is a test used for differentiating between foetal and adult blood. It is sometimes necessary to establish the origin of a blood sample (foetal, maternal or adult). The principle of the test is based on the resistance of foetal red cells containing haemoglobin F to alkaline denaturation. Examples of cases where it may be necessary to determine the origin of a blood sample include:

- In cases of PV bleed in a pregnant mother (particularly Rhesus negative mother)
- Inadequate or mis-labelling of samples (cord and maternal samples)
- In cases of a blood tap from amniocentesis
- In cases of forensic investigation to determine if blood spot on a crime scene is foetal or adult blood.

Sample requirement. Sample must contain macroscopic unaltered blood free from contamination by faeces and vomit. The sample must be less than 3 days old. Each test is controlled using a cord sample as positive control and an adult sample as a negative control.

Instrumentation /reagents required

1. 2 Plastic coombs tube (75 x 12mm) per test and control

- Tube rack
- Pasteur pipettes
- Centrifuge
- 0.12N NaOH
- Water

Method

1. Prepare 0.12N NaOH by diluting 0.3N NaOH by adding 200mls of 0.12N NaOH to 500mls of distilled water.
2. Label the 75x12mm tubes appriopriately and prepare a haemolysate of the test and control samples by adding 2 drops of blood into a tube and

filling it with distilled water. Test haemolysate can be prepared from blood samples, blood stained sheets and sanitary pads.

3. Place the tubes with the haemolysate in a centrifuge for 60 seconds to remove the stroma

4. Transfer 8 volumes of the haemolysate into a second tube and add 2 volumes of 0.12N NaOH, mix and observe immediately. Compare the colour against the original haemolysate. Include positive 9 known foetal sample) and negative controls (known adult maternal sample).

Result. Foetal red cells containing haemoglobin F remains pink (resist denaturation) while adult maternal sample containg adult haemoglobin turns brown.

INDEX

A

B

C

D

E

F

G

H

I

M

P

Q

R